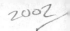

SAY GOOD-BYE TO ILLNESS

by

Devi S. Nambudripad
M.D., D.C., L.Ac., Ph.D.

Author of
Living Pain Free With Acupressure,
The NAET Guide Book
and
Say Good-Bye To...Series

THIS BOOK HAS ALREADY REVOLUTIONIZED
THE PRACTICE OF MEDICINE!

The doctor of the future will give no medicine,
but will interest his patients in the care of
the human frame, in diet,
and in the cause and prevention of disease.

– Thomas A. Edison

Published by
Delta Publishing Company
6714 Beach Blvd.
Buena Park, CA 90621

(888) 890-0670 • (714) 523-8900 • Fax (714) 523-3068
www.naet.com

DEDICATION

This book is dedicated to
my loving parents,
my husband, Kris Nambudripad
and
my son, Roy

Love can make you survive! My life is living proof of that. I received unconditional love and support from my parents while I was growing up. Later, the same love from my husband encouraged me to push forward, one more day, looking for the thread of a miracle to survive, just to please my loved ones. When my son, Roy, came along, I had a need to remain alive, by all possible means, with or without pain, to take care of him and to nurture him. If it were not for these knots of love, which I was bound with from childhood, I doubt if I would be alive today to write this. *We all need love for survival. Love is so powerful, it conquers all!*

First edition, 1993
Second edition, 1999
Third edition, 2002
Copyright © 2002 by Devi S. Nambudripad
M.D., D.C., L.Ac., Ph.D. (Acu)
Buena Park, California
All rights reserved.

Library of Congress Control No: 2001119632
ISBN: 0-9704344-8-0
Printed in U.S.A.

The medical information and procedures contained in this book are not intended as a substitute for consulting your physician. Any attempt to diagnose and treat an illness using the information in this book should come under the direction of an NAET physician who is familiar with this technique. Because there is always some risk involved in any medical treatment or procedure, the publisher and author are not responsible for any adverse effects or consequences resulting from the use of any of the suggestions or procedures in this book. Please do not use this book if you are unwilling to assume the risks. All matters regarding your health should be supervised by a qualified medical professional.

TABLE OF CONTENTS

ACKNOWLEDGMENTS

I am deeply grateful to my husband, Dr. Kris K. Nambudripad, for his inspiration, encouragement and assistance in my schooling and later, in the formulation of this project. Without his cooperation in researching reference work, revision of manuscripts, word processing and proofreading, it is doubtful whether this book would ever have been completed. My sincere thanks also go to the many clients who have entrusted their care to me, for without them I would have had no case studies, no technique and certainly no extensive source of personal research upon which to base this book.

I am also deeply grateful to Mary Karaba, Karen Watts, Meg Brazil, Shirley Reason, Ileen Garcia, Joyce Baisden, Helene Singer, Lettie Vipond, Toby Weiss, Amy Clute, Michael Magrutsch, Karen Tuckerman, Rosemary Depauw, Margaret Davies, Dikran Ayarian, to name a few among many of my devoted patients, for believing in me from the very beginning of this research until the present, and by supporting my theory and helping me to conduct the ongoing detective work. I also have to express my thanks to my son, Roy, who assisted me in many ways in the writing of this book. Roy was one year old and very sick when I practiced my technique on him at the beginning of my search for an allergy cure. Now, he is a 21-year-old, healthy, levelheaded, responsible young man who is pursuing his goal to become a medical doctor.

Additionally, I wish to thank Robert Prince, M.D., Chi Yu, Fong Tien and many of my friends who wish to remain anonymous for proofreading and assisting me with this work, and Mr. Sri at Delta Publishing for his printing expertise. I am deeply grateful for my professional training and the knowledge and skills acquired in classes and seminars on chiropractic and kinesiology at the Los Angeles College of Chiropractic in Whittier, California; the California Acupuncture College in Los Angeles; SAMRA University of Oriental Medicine, Los Angeles; University of Health Sciences, School of Medicine, Antigua; and the clinical experience obtained at the clinics attached to these colleges.

My special thanks also go to Mala Moosad, N.D., R.N., L.Ac., Mohan Moosad, M.S., L.Ac, who supported and stood by me. They helped me immensely by taking over my work load at the clinic so that I could complete the revision of this book. I also would like to acknowledge my thanks to my dear mother for nourishing me emotionally and nutritionally while working on this book forever. My heartfelt thanks also go to Barbara Cesmat, an NAET trained practitioner, who has dedicated her time to help desperate allergy sufferers by assisting me in many ways to promote my mission of making NAET available to every needy person in the universe. She spends many hours daily answering the hundreds of e-mails I receive from all over the world. I would also like to acknowledge my everlasting thanks to my office manager, Janna Gossen, who worked with me from the first day of my practice, and all the other staff members for their support.

I would like to remember the late Dr. Richard F. Farquhar at Farquhar Chiropractic Clinic in Bellflower, California. Under Dr. Farquhar, I accumulated many hours of special instruction and hands-on practice in kinesiology. I am grateful to Dr. Victor Frank for developing "Total Body Modification" seminars, where I first learned about the activator, a pressure device I now use in my NAET practice. Before I learned to use the activator, I was applying NAET with acupuncture needles, sometimes having to use needles as long as 6-7 inches. It was not a very pleasant experience for the patient to have 6-7 inch long needles threaded along the spine. Certainly, the procedure was not pleasant for me either. Discovery of the activator technique in Dr. Frank's class changed my acupuncture practice to acupressure, and I was able to teach NAET to medical practitioners who were not licensed to apply acupuncture to their patients. I later attended a few classes with Dr. Arlan Furr in activator methods, which gave me a thorough knowledge in using activator techniques; and, of course, this made my life and my patients' lives easier.

I am grateful to Dr. Scott Walker for developing Neuro-Emotional Techniques (NET). Before I took his class, I was afraid to use emotional treatments on my practice. I thought my observations about food and environmental allergies in connection with emotional blockages were purely unconfirmed assumptions. I limited the use of emotional treatments solely to my family and a few patients who were very close to me. I was apprehensive about treating others for emotions, believing that they might not find me credible. When I attended Dr. Scott's seminar, I was relieved to learn I was not the only one finding an emotional component involved in patients' treatments. Even though the emotional blockage elimination method in NAET is totally different than that used in NET, I felt confident in using the approach more freely after I attended Dr. Scott's class.

I do not have enough words to express my heartfelt thanks and appreciation to the California Acupuncture State Board for supporting NAET from the beginning, permitting me to teach other licensed acupuncturists by making me a CEU provider instantly. Perhaps the California Acupuncture State Board will never know how much they have helped humanity by validating my new technique and allowing me to share the treatment method with other practitioners and, through them, to the thousands of patients like me who now live a normal life. I am forever indebted to acupuncture and Oriental medicine. Without this knowledge, I would still be living in pain. Thank you for allowing me to share my experience with the world!

I extend my sincere thanks to these great teachers. They have helped me to grow immensely at all levels. My mentors are also indirectly responsible for the improvement of my personal health as well as that of my family, patients, and the health of other NAET practitioners and their countless patients.

Many of my professors, doctors of western and Oriental medicine, allopathy, chiropractic, osteopathy, kinesiology, as well as nutritionists, were willing to give of themselves by teaching and committing personal time, through interviews, to help me complete this book. I will always be eternally grateful to them. They demonstrated the highest ideals of the medical profession.

Devi S. Nambudripad, M.D., D.C., L.Ac., Ph.D.

Dr. "Devi" has developed an amazingly effective treatment technique which continues to bring relief to thousands of patients. Based on our preliminary clinical research results, as well as the numerous case studies presented from around the world, NAET works on many levels to improve the lives of those it touches. I foresee widespread acceptance of NAET as we continue to obtain excellent results in our clinical research studies.

Robert Cohen, M.D.
Research Director
NARF (Nambudripad's Allergy Research Foundation)
Buena Park, CA
April, 2002

"Allergy ELIMINATION?!? Is it possible?" I asked, when I first heard about Dr. Devi and NAET. "Absolutely!" is the answer to that question, I later discovered, after meeting Devi and learning her amazingly simple, most effective technique. Bar none, no other allergy treatment in my practice has been as effective as NAET. Dr. Devi is truly a medical pioneer, and she has my deepest respect, both personally and professionally. TELL EVERYONE YOU KNOW about the best-kept secret in the world of allergy diagnosis and therapy: NAET.

Ann McCombs, D.O.
Medical Director
Center For Optimum Health
Seattle, Washington
April, 2002

CHARLES G. GABLEMAN, M.D.
Diplomate, American Board Of
Allergy And Immunology
5105 River Bluff Drive
Fort Worth, Texas 76132

I have been acquainted with Andrew Pallos, D.D.S, for about twenty years as a patient and a friend. I have been a friend and a patient of George Weinand, N.D., for about a year. I regard my friendship with these gentlemen as a very valuable asset in both their roles as practitioners and friends.

Dr. Pallos is very well trained and uses his professional knowledge with outstanding expertise. The benefits of his dental work have been most satisfactory and gratifying to me. However, unlike the majority of dental professionals, he has not been content to be confined to the conventional focus on teeth. He has not hesitated to become involved in other segments of the healing spectrum.

He is board certified in acupuncture for dentists and has familiarized himself with the use of acupuncture and its electronic variants to general healing. This application has proven particularly productive and effective in treating all types of allergies via the Nambudripad's Allergy Elimination Techniques (NAET). The theoretical physiologic basis of this method has now been verified by its successful employment in medical offices and clinics all over the country.

Speaking as a board certified allergist, retired after ten years of practice in internal medicine and thirty years in allergy and immunology, as well as a patient over these many years, I am in a position well qualified to evaluate the Nambudripad's Allergy Elimination Techniques. It exceeds, by far, any other presently extant. Not only is it speedy, specific and immediately productive, but also the recent refinements appear to be yielding an actual cure of the problem. Heretofore, only temporary suppression of the allergy symptom was possible, necessitating continual repetition of the therapeutic doses for many years.

This fact severely limits the benefit of conventional allergy care. Furthermore, except for its modifications promulgated by Drs. Hansel,

Rinkel and Lee, it is inherently relatively nonproductive and potentially dangerous, even fatal, at times. Conventional allergy treatments may spawn the appearance of new allergies, e.g., to the chemical media in which they are injected.

No such hazard exists in the NAET approach. It is non-invasive, eliminating the danger of induced infection, tissue necrosis or embolism. This alone would render its value high above any others. The fact that immediately after the treatment the allergic reaction to the offending substance is eliminated further enhances the worth of NAET.

As a patient I can state unequivocally that my allergies are under much better control than ever before. This procedure is applicable not only to allergies, but also to chronic fatigue, immune dysfunction syndrome, asthma and other chronic conditions.

I can vouch for this allergy elimination technique with authority, and have just completed a course of desensitization to many of my allergies at Dr. Weinand's hand. Should the opportunity occur, I shall pursue this excellent therapy further (I am unable to do so now as I have recently relocated to another part of the country).

Without qualification, I recommend this amazing method as practiced by Dr. Weinand and Dr. Pallos (students of Dr. Nambudripad) to anyone seeking relief from any allergy-related diseases.

Charles G. Gableman, M.D.
Diplomate, American Board of
Allergy and Immunology

A FEW WORDS ABOUT NAET FROM NAET PRACTITIONERS!

Dear Devi:

We just had a fantastic change in a patient using NAET and wanted to let you know.

She is a 50 year old woman who is an RN and runs a medical office near us. She had had severe Diabetes for two years and has been on two oral hypoglycemics and very strict low carbohydrate diet. She got her basic ten and then we determined the combination treatment with sugar. After completing the combination treatment with sugar, insulin, pancreas, and stomach acid she woke up the next morning with a blood sugar of 80.
She has not had any diabetic medicine for over two weeks and her sugars have remained normal! She has even started eating bread and potatoes and the sugar level remains within normal range.

Just thought you would like to know this wonderful news!

David Minkoff, M.D.
Clearwater, FL

Dear Devi:

I thought you might rejoice sharing this boy's happiness. Kevin was unable to eat eggs. When he ate any products with eggs in them, his mouth turned into fire, his throat swelled, and he had to be rushed to the hospital ER or given an epipen injection. He was unable to enjoy birthday cakes and other delights made with eggs for four of his seven years. After his first NAET clearing for eggs, he was able to have a small egg product. After clearing many combinations associated with eggs, including mayonnaise, cake frosting, stomach acid, grains and finally soybean oil and lecithin, Kevin is now able to eat any egg products — as much as he wants — without any reaction whatsoever. He's one very happy child, thanks to NAET!"

Gary Erkfritz, D.C.
Thousand Oaks, CA

NTT (Nambudripad's Testing Technique) gave me the best tool to evaluate my patients' health disorders, and NAET taught me the greatest healing technique to eliminate the problems, almost instantly and painlessly. NAET has truly revolutionized the practice of medicine! I applaud Dr. Devi for developing this unique technique and sharing it with the world. I have no doubt — this is going to be the "Medicine of the Future."

Robert Prince, M.D.
North Carolina

Devi Nambudripad has pioneered the greatest leap in the field of energy medicine technology on the doorstep to the 21st century, a time when there is greater suffering from allergies than ever before. The extension of NAET into the holistic veterinary community revolutionizes the medical care that we are able to provide to animals. NAET makes it possible to impact the lives of animals and their owners — and does so without the use of drugs. This book offers a glimpse into the miracles that NAET can bring to the lives of all creatures on the planet.

Rahmie Valentine, L.Ac., O.M.D.
Santa Monica, CA

Practicing NAET for the past five years has greatly enhanced both my professional and personal life. I have witnessed the dramatic elimination of life-threatening allergies, the routine reversal of bothersome allergies, and the gradual rebuilding of vitality and wellness from debilitating allergies. NAET is excellent.

Andrew Pallos, D.D.S.
Laguna Niguel, CA

Dr. Devi's technique represents a profound understanding of the body's reset mechanism which allows the allergic patient to return to normal function. This is an easily tolerated, systematic approach which shows excellent results in clinical practice.

Randol Christman, L.Ac., O.M.D.
Kihei, Maui

After 13 years of practice as a chiropractor, I had the opportunity of a rebirth as a holistic practitioner when I first learned NAET. NAET gives me the opportunity of integrating mechanical, biochemical, and neuro-electrical concepts to create a conceptual model that gives practical effective results. NAET has enhanced my personal health and understanding of the human body and, therefore, the human condition. Bravo, Dr. Devi!

Helen Thomas, D.C.
Santa Rosa, CA

NAET offers an opportunity for me to evaluate the current status and chief complaint of the patient and administer the treatment effectively. It is accepted because the patients are involved in the procedure and they experience the results in a short time. They know instantly if it worked or not.

George W. Edwards, D.M.D.

This simple, yet powerful, technique saved my life. I now enjoy LIVING! My family, friends and patients experience a wellness that they had not known, some of them for years. The energy of the body and mind flowing freely is the true expression of LIFE... God Bless You, Dr. Devi!

Barbara Cesmat, DCH, Ph.D.
Woodland Hills, CA

Woman 21 years old had eczema. She got eczema when she was 1 year old over her whole body. After 20 treatments, there was no eczema anymore.

Ray Rosekrans
Acupuncturist, Holland
31(0) 228 510182

Dr. Devi's allergy elimination technique is the most incredible practice tool I have seen in health care in my 40 years of practice.

John H. Kasler, D.C.
Charlotte, NC

NAET has given me great satisfaction in treating my patients of all ages. My patients and I love the results with NAET...no doubt, NAET brings the PRACTICE OF MEDICINE into the 21st century.

David Minkoff, M.D.
Clearwater, FL

I have treated patients from age two months to 70 years old and find enormous pleasure in watching how their lives change from such simple acupuncture techniques. One says, "I felt as if I was let out of jail!" Another describes it as, "escape from allergy hell." My patients' improvement in health, mood and behavior are, in some cases, incredibly profound and the credit goes to NAET. Thank you, Devi, for a technique that so quickly transforms so many lives.

Carolyn Reuben, L.Ac.
Sacramento, CA

NAET has changed my life and practice. NAET is a profound and fascinating technique of correcting allergies, which is an underlying cause of most health problems and diseases.

Sue Anderson, D.C.
Ann Arbor, MI

In February 2002, a patient at our center was being seen for vomiting which was occurring daily since 9/11. She worked downtown and saw the second plane hit. She had already been seen by a gastroenterologist who found no cause for her vomiting. I was called by the practitioner seeing her to treat her for the emotional allergy to what she witnessed. Following the treatment, the vomiting stopped.

Geri Brewster RD, MPH, CDN
The Atkins Center for Complimentary Medicine
New York, NY

NAET has added a new dimension to my practice. My patients are thrilled to have a return of their regular and favorite activities since their symptoms have been relieved.

Mary Schultz, DC, RCRD / WI

Pollen allergies (Kafun Shou) and environmental allergies can be successfully treated with NAET.

Teruaki Nozawa
2-4 Mitojima-honcho
Fuji-city, Shizuoka
Japan 416-0924

It is certainly a "Good-bye To Illness" technique. The results that my patients and I receive from Nambudripad's Allergy Elimination Treatments are incredible.

Carol Cooper, L.Ac., LCSW
Chandler, AZ

First, I was a patient. Now I am a practitioner. My patients have regained their health after decades of chronic illness. NAET is a remarkable treatment that forces everyone to rethink how the body works.

Dr. Karen F. Bates D.C., L.M.T.
Colorado Springs, CO
(714) 649-4091

After treating a variety of health ailments with outstanding success, for the past four years using NAET, I can't help but wonder if NAET is the link we were missing in the health industry.

Eric Roth, M.D., D.O.
New York

Dr. Devi's method has brought the understanding and approach to healing to a deeper level. It still puzzles me everyday how easily and thoroughly my patients are relieved of symptoms, layer after layer, and can enjoy a healthy life again — or, in some cases, experience it for the first time. There is no turning back now. Medicine can only progress from here.

Frederique Nault, ND
Bali, Indonesia

I have always been on the lookout for a technique which could deliver better results for my patients. With Dr. Devi and NAET, this has become a possibility. I believe a technique is only as good as the long-term results it produces. Even after a year of using NAET everyday, I am still astounded by the results it is producing. For the first time in my chiropractic career, I now feel that by incorporating NAET into my practice, I can offer my patients totally holistic "WELLNESS" Care.

Dr. Phil Barham, D.C.
Brisbane, Australia

NAET has given me even greater thrills in healing than chiropractic alone. Many patients are suffering a life of hell when they begin their therapy. Each allergy elimination brings them better health, and certainly more comfort. Never do you promote the therapy; it sells itself so naturally. Beautiful, holistic healing.

Kate Willesee B.Sc., D.C.
Mosman, NSW, Australia

NAET is truly the medicine of the future. It is exciting to be using it in the present. The results and satisfaction are mind boggling. I can hardly believe it, even though I see the results over and over again, each and every day. The scope of the many health problems that NAET routinely helps continues to astound me, and amazes my patients. The only problem is there are not enough hours now to treat the many patients wanting treatment with this wonderful technique.

Terry Power BSc., Grad DC, MChiroSc, DAc.
Port Macquarie, NSW, Australia

Since I have started treating patients with NAET the results have been phenomenal, greater than my wildest expectations. Children who had life threatening allergies (asthma) are now symptom-free. Young adults who were unable to go to university, school, or even walk down the street because they were hypersensitive to the environment, can now go nightclubbing without ill effect. My practice has expanded by at least 200% since treating patients with NAET. Thank you, Devi, for coming to Australia and imparting this wonderful technique which has enabled me to bring health to my patients.

Maria Colosimo N.D.
Melbourne, Australia

I have practiced chiropractic and holistic health for 34 years. I've studied with many different teachers in many different disciplines, but I have to say that studying NAET has helped me get more people better than most — if not all — of the other techniques I've studied. NAET truly is a blessing to living beings on planet Earth. When people have an inkling of the extent that NAET enables people to become healthy once again, they will give the Nobel Prize to Dr. Devi for her discoveries. All my thanks, Dr. Devi!

Gary E. Erkfritz, D.C.
Thousand Oaks, CA

I am a pharmacist, practicing NAET since 1994, in the Philippines with excellent results. I have found NAET truly an amazing natural treatment. Many of my patients have solved their chronic health problems through NAET and, years after treatment, they still remain free of their previous health problems.

Dr. Mila Ting
Manila, Philippines

Based on my experience and the results of thousands of NAET treatments in my clinic, Dr. Nambudripad has elevated integrative medicine to a new whole level.

Gary Trott, O.M.D., L. Ac., TX

NAET is like a blessing from the Heavens! It never stops amazing me. I suffered from a lung infection since four months, with the result that I became asthmatic with frequent coughs, fatigue, and no interest in life. Antibiotics and other treatments didn't offer any relief. Then I contacted Dr. Devi. Her NAET testing revealed that I was reacting to a special brand of olive oil I was using since four months. To my amazement, 20 minutes after the NAET treatment for this oil, I became free of my symptoms!

Jean-Michel Belin
Annecy, France

My patient had constantly re-occurring bladder infections for the past 5 years due to a prolapsed bladder. Acupuncture helped, but with NAET the infections have stopped!

Pam Mills
4310 N.Troy
Chicago, IL 60618
(773) 588-2912

Julie, a 34 year old woman, suffered from migraine headaches since the 4th grade. She knew that eggs always triggered her migraines. After one NAET treatment for egg mix, Julie happily eats eggs with absolutely no headaches.

Dr. Ron Arconati, D.C.
St. Louis, MO 63129
(314) 846-2100

When I brought NAET to Czech republic two years ago and started to use it, I felt like Don Quichote fighting the windmills. Nobody believed in it. I convinced couple of clients and treated them for free. After their first pollen season they did not believe it again. But now to the positive results ... their friends and families fill up my office. With little exaggeration and humor I can say Allergic people from Czech Republic thanks Dr. Nambudripad from the bottom of their hearts for this wonderful treatment - NAET that is changing their lives!

Ivana Rusnak M.
Czech Republic

FOREWORD

"Sandra, you need to see Dr. Devi," I was told while waiting to be seen by another doctor. "Why?" I asked in a frustrated tone. By that time, I was pretty fed up with doctors even though I was one myself. I had suffered from chronic fatigue syndrome for the past year and a half. To add proverbial insult to injury, I had been hospitalized with my first attack of asthma and was placed on very high doses of steroids, antibiotics and four different broncho-dilators (the very substances I was accustomed to helping my patients successfully discontinue). No one seemed to know the cause of my medical condition.

After "escaping" from the hospital, I contacted an acupuncturist who was able to get me off the medications. However, I was at a standstill, unable to work because of the asthma and chronic fatigue. The acupuncturist (not my internist nor pulmonary specialist) had given me a "peak flow meter" to monitor my progress. For more than three months, the meter seemed stuck on 300 (normal for me is 500). Within 15 to 30 minutes after eating certain foods, the meter repeatedly dropped to 250. This was my first clue to my identifying many of the foods and environments that were adversely affecting me. Finally, I traveled to Los Angeles for help.

"Yes, you must see Dr. Devi. She takes away "allergies," said my friend. "Takes away allergies?" I raised my eyebrows in disbelief. "That's impossible! I'm a clinical ecologist, and I've treated allergies for years. You can't take them away. You can make people better by giving them shots or drops under the tongue, but you don't take an allergy away. You just make the patient less sensitive or reactive." I was so sick and desperate, however, that I followed the suggestion.

Dr. Nambudripad's waiting room was filled with people, each man and woman recounting incredible stories of the results of "Allergy Elimination

Treatment." Although skeptical, I began to have hope. As Dr. Devi began testing me using clinical kinesiology, I was shocked to find that I was reacting to many vitamins and minerals, including vitamin C, B complex, zinc, iron, vitamin A, table salt and other essential nutrients of my every day diet. Most foods were actually causing me problems. One by one, she began eliminating them, using her special treatment technique. To my amazement, in just nine days my peak flow meter rose 140 points and remained there. Then vitamins and other nutrients, instead of causing problems, now assimilated and began repairing damaged cells. Foods that had been a problem before did not even budge the peak flow meter. More importantly, I was able to return to work within a few days. I have continued to heal.

An allergic reaction is simply an improper response of the immune system to an otherwise harmless substance, such as foods, vitamins, medications, pollens, flowers, weeds, grasses, trees, dust, formaldehydes, plastics, metals, etc. The body reacts by releasing powerful chemicals that cause classic symptoms such as runny nose, watery eyes, rashes, depression, anger, asthma, fatigue, headaches, insomnia and various pains which can present in almost any part of the body. She pointed out to me that many health problems in people all over the world are undiagnosed allergic reactions or are due to the lowering of the immune system by multiple allergic reactions that allow diseases to attack the weakened host.

A few months later, I was privileged to attend a seminar taught by Dr. Nambudripad and learned how to implement the Nambudripad's Testing Techniques (NTT) and Nambudripad's Allergy Elimination Techniques (NAET) in my office. The practice of medicine hasn't been the same ever since. What a thrill to treat a patient for an allergy to B complex and see her hip pain of 40 years duration disappear instantly!

Obtaining a patient's medical history takes on a different meaning as Dr. Nambudripad teaches the art of detective sleuthing. Rarely do I recommend a supplement or vitamin without first testing to check for allergy or effectiveness. Eliminating allergies to medications allows the medicines to be more effective while you are tracking down and eliminating the cause of the problems. Once the cause has been found and eliminated, the same amount of medication no longer may be necessary.

Certain patterns have been observed by practitioners of NAET and provide useful protocols for helping our own patients. For example, those suffering from arthritis should be checked for allergy to table salt, corn products, dried beans, and pepper, nutmeg and other spices. People with clinical depression, without any help from known antidepressants, should be checked for allergy to B complex vitamins, sugar and trace minerals. Those plagued with addictions to alcohol, drugs, chocolate, caffeine or cigarettes are shown to be helped more effectively if allergy to vitamin B complex and sugars are eliminated prior to treating the allergy to the addicting substance.

Many symptoms and diseases are very often tied in one way or another to allergies to seemingly harmless substances in our environment. Eliminating an allergy to her lipstick relieved one person's chronic cough. One woman had suffered hypertension for many years and yet was on a good diet, exercised daily and had a positive attitude. Extensive searching finally revealed the culprit: an allergy to nylon. She has remained normotensive for several months now after eliminating the nylon allergy...good-bye hypertension! Since that case, I have discovered and successfully treated three people with hypertension related to allergy to nylon. A telephone operator's eczema disappeared when NAET was done on the plastics found in her keyboard.

Anyone who has tried to wrestle with an elimination or rotation diet knows how frustrating that can be, not only for the dieter, but also especially for students. How wonderful it is to know that one doesn't have to give up allergic items such as wheat, corn, chocolate, home furnishings, pets, favorite clothes, the job that one loves, perfumes, make-up items or a computer, etc., with such an easy, painless treatment!

Thank you, Dr. Nambudripad, for persevering in the development and documentation of this fantastic allergy elimination technique. I also applaud you for the countless hours you spend in teaching patients to test themselves and determine hidden allergies that might be causing trouble. Giving the patients that information helps them to take responsibility for their own health and puts them in charge instead of leaving them to play victim. Once she's in charge, the patient and doctor can work together to achieve a mutual goal: to *Say Good-bye To Illness!*

ADDENDUM TO FOREWORD TO SAY GOOD-BYE TO ILLNESS...

Several years have gone by since I was privileged to write the foreword to Dr. Devi's book. I continue to be amazed at the repeated cases whose lives have been changed by this technique. In my office, NTT is used to determine the appropriate nutritional supplementation or medication and the correct dosage for each patient. No more guesswork or merely copying a protocol out of a book. The therapy can be tailored to the individual. Even the contents of intravenous solutions are verified by NTT and cleared by NAET if an allergy to one or more of the ingredients is found. Doing this enhances the therapy and causes us to witness the desired results more quickly.

Emotional problems that have, in some cases, required years of professional treatment cleared within one or two emotional NAET's. What a blessing to these people! Many family conflicts turned out to be merely allergy between those involved and resolved once properly treated by NAET.

What a difference this technique has made in my own health and in my practice. Even more exciting, we are still learning new ways to utilize this wonderful therapy. Once again, Thank you, Dr. Nambudripad, for your contribution toward helping us regain and keep our health!

Sandra C. Denton, M.D.
Alaska Alternative Medicine Clinic
3333 Denali St., #100
Anchorage, Alaska 99503
(907) 563 6200

February, 2002

PREFACE

Since childhood I suffered from a multitude of health problems. Because of this prolonged and first-hand knowledge of ill health, it is no wonder that I became focused on health-related problems, particularly those related to allergies; and this, in turn, undoubtedly resulted in my natural inclination to pursue medicine as a profession. Eventually, I became a *registered nurse, a chiropractor, a kinesiologist, an acupuncturist and a doctor of allopathic medicine.* I began specializing in the treatment of the allergic patient, using methods I learned through an intensive study of Oriental medicine, combined with the more traditional western methods learned from my training as a nurse.

During my studies and early practice as an allergist, using eclectic methods of allergy treatments, I discovered a technique that eliminated most of my health problems. *Integrating the relevant techniques from the various fields I studied, combined with my own discoveries, has become the focus of my practice.* There is no known successful method of treatment for food allergies using western medicine except avoidance, which means deprivation and frustration. Each of the disciplines I studied provided bits of knowledge which I used in developing a new treatment to eliminate allergies permanently called *Nambudripad's Allergy Elimination Techniques,* or *NAET* for short.

As an infant, I had severe infantile eczema, which lasted until I was seven or eight years old. I was given western medicine and ayurvedic herbal medicine without a break. Ayurveda is the traditional Indian system of medicine based largely on herbs and naturopathy. Western medicine did not help me at all. While I was taking the herbal medicines, my symptoms were under control. Whenever I went off the herbs, my eczema recurred. When I was eight years old, one of the herbal doctors told my parents to feed me white rice cooked with a special herb formula. (The ingredients in this special blend were coriander leaves, dry coriander seeds, lemon leaves, lemon rind, black pepper, ginger root, brown sugar, dandelion leaves, coconut oil, turmeric, cumin seeds, rock salt, garlic, dried pomegranate skin and clarified butter. The action of each of these herbs, according to Chinese medicine, is explained in more detail in the footnote to follow.)

This special diet helped me a great deal. The herbalist seemed to know what he was doing. This simple herbal diet was selected from a regular kitchen shelf, yet it was a powerful cleanser for the body. Through this special diet, my body was able to eliminate the toxins I produced daily. The only drawback was that I had to be on this diet constantly. As I was growing up, I began cheating every so often by going on and off this special diet. If I missed one day, I suffered consequences; so my parents made sure that I stayed on it faithfully. In a few months my eczema cleared up, but my good health did not last. I began to experience symptoms of arthritis. On certain days, all of my joints ached. The pain became so severe I stayed in bed for days at a time. Whenever I ate the white rice cooked with herbs, I felt better. I started liking white rice more and more. It became a staple diet for me. In 1976, I relocated to Los Angeles. I became more health-conscious and tried to change my eating habits by adding more fruits, vegetables, whole grain products and complex carbohydrates. All of a sudden, I became very ill. I suffered from bronchitis, pneumonia and my arthritis returned. My symptoms multiplied. I suffered from insomnia, clinical depression, constant sinusitis and frequent migraine headaches. I felt extremely tired all the time, but remained wide awake when I went to bed. I tried many different antibiotics and medicines, changed doctors and consulted nutritionists. All the medication, vitamins and herbs that I took made me sicker, and the consumption of good nutrition made me worse. I was nauseated all the time. Every inch of my body ached. I lived on aspirin, taking almost 30 a day to keep me going.

During this time, I had three miscarriages, which affected me emotionally. In order to keep my sanity, I decided to go back to school, coughing and puffing my way through. I might as well have been a lifelong smoker! Following my mother's advice, I turned to God and began to observe all of my family's traditional religious holidays. I fasted, with only water intake on all the Hindu religious holy days. The day after the fast I felt better, had more energy and my mind was clearer. I became very religious. I know now that staying away from foods that I was allergic to was the reason for my feeling of well being the next day. Of course, I know that God played a great role, too.

According to the Hindu bible, "Gita," God, will only help you if you take the initiative to help yourself first. If you try and reach half-way, He will meet you there and travel with you the rest of the way. So, fasting, avoiding the allergenic foods, discovering the allergy elimination techniques, eliminating my allergies and related illnesses, were part of the half-way deal. At last, I had reached the half-way point on the journey to my destination.

In 1981, I started my medical school training at the Los Angeles College of Chiropractic. By then, I had been fighting a two-year attack of chronic bronchitis. My nutrition teacher at the college advised me to go on a juice diet. In two days, I had severe laryngitis, my bronchitis got worse, and I had a fever of 104 degrees. She said I was going through a healing crisis. In the southern part of India where I come from, when a person gets sick with a common cold or fever, cooked soft rice was the prescribed food. So, I stayed home for three days, eating cooked soft white rice and appeared to partially recover from that episode.

When I returned to college, we had a guest speaker who was an acupuncturist. I was sitting in a corner of the classroom, coughing frequently. He watched me for a while and commented that I was suffering from *an attack of wind/heat* (common cold in Chinese medicine). At the time, I did not understand what he meant. He explained a few things about acupuncture and gave me a quick treatment using acupressure on acupuncture points. His treatments made me feel very good and, to my surprise, I stopped coughing. Up until that moment, I had only heard about acupuncture; now I had a personal first-hand experience with the procedure. I felt very happy to learn about this new branch of medicine and was very impressed with it because it gave me some relief from my nagging symptoms.

My mind was thinking only about acupuncture. After the class was over, I went up to the guest speaker, got the address of an acupuncture college, called the school the same day and signed up for classes. The very first class was in acupressure, entitled *Touch for Health.* My instructor decided to teach *muscle response testing, to detect food allergies,* that first day. By then, my cough had returned. He noticed my chronic, raspy cough, and suspected that I was suffering from food allergies. He tested me for various allergies to food items through muscle response testing. I reacted to almost everything he tested, except for white rice and broccoli. He suggested that I might do better if I ate only white rice and broccoli exclusively for a few days. (I suddenly had flash backs to age eight when I was put on a white rice diet by another doctor.)

By that time, I had been examined and treated by many doctors, including neurologists, cardiologists, psychologists, nutritionists and herbalists. Nobody suspected food allergies as a cause of my chronic ill health. I was excited by this possibility. I was willing to try anything to get better. I followed my teacher's advice and ate white rice and broccoli exclusively. Within one week's time, my bronchitis cleared up, my headaches became infrequent and less intense, my joint pains eased and my back ceased hurting. My thinking and concentration became clearer. My depression of two years disappeared. I did not have insomnia anymore. My general body aches cleared. For the first time in my life, I experienced pain-free days. Until then, I was under the impression that everybody was supposed to experience a certain amount of body aches and pains all the time, because I had never known otherwise. It was a delight for me to go to bed without pain and wake up in the morning without pain.

After a week's restricted diet, I tried eating some other foods but my symptoms returned. I began eating only white rice and broccoli again. I could not eat salads, fruits or vegetables, because I was very allergic to vitamin C; whole grain products because they contained B complex; fruits, honey or any products made from sugars because I was very allergic to sugar; drink milk or eat milk products because I was very allergic to calcium; fish groups because I was allergic to vitamin A; egg products because they caused skin problems. I was allergic to all types of dried beans, including soybeans, which gave me severe joint pains and backaches. Spices gave me arthritis and migraines. Almost all the fabrics, except silk, gave me itching, joint pain and caused extreme tiredness. My teacher at the acupuncture college confirmed my doubts: I was simply allergic to everything under the sun, including the sun by radiation.

While I was growing up in India, I complained to one of my doctors about the constant body aches and electric shock-like sensations in my body that I experienced frequently. He diagnosed me as suffering from hysteria and psychosomatic disorders. I was saddened by this diagnosis, because I knew that I did not have hysteria nor psychosomatic disorders, but pure pain. I hoped and prayed that someday, somehow, I would find relief from pain. Now I know all about "hysteria;" it is simply a scapegoat diagnosis by frustrated doctors who have not learned to properly diagnose their patients.

It seemed that I was allergic to everything except white rice, broccoli, silk and aspirin. What a combination! At least I was lucky to have a few items I was not allergic to. In my practice, I see many less fortunate patients with allergies to everything you could imagine. Most of them were living lives equivalent to living in a bubble before they were treated with NAET. *When you are chemically and environmentally allergic to almost everything around you, it usually takes two to three years of continuous treatments with NAET* (two to three sessions a week), before you can come out of the bubble and into the real world filled with its assorted pollutants, fumes, chemicals, formaldehydes, pesticides and smog.

I was happy to live with a few limited non-allergenic items. I lived on white rice and broccoli for three and a half years. Then, one day around noon, I came home from school. I didn't have anymore cooked rice. I put some rice for cooking and ate a few pieces of carrot while I was waiting for the rice to cook. In just a few minutes, I felt tired and lethargic. I felt like I was going to pass out. The rest is history. Please read the rest of the story of discovery of NAET in Chapter 9. When I awoke I felt strangely different. I was not sick or tired anymore. Instead, I felt a renewed, pleasant energy.

Suddenly, I wondered whether there could be any connection between my sense of well-being and the contact between the carrot and my skin. During that semester I was attending a class in *electromagnetic field and acupuncture* at the acupuncture college. This helped me understand the connection between the electromagnetic force of my body and the carrot. In class, we were taught that every object on earth, whether living or non-living, possesses a surrounding electromagnetic energy field. Earth has its own energy field. Every object is attracted to Earth. Every object is also attracted to one another. All these different energies can attract or repel, depending upon their energy differences.

I tested the carrot for allergy and determined I was not allergic to it. I sensed that during the treatment, something strange had happened. I ate one whole carrot stick and did not have any reaction. I tried some other foods I was known to be allergic to and reacted as before, so I knew my assumption was correct. *My allergy to carrot was gone* because of my contact with the carrot while undergoing acupuncture. My energy and the carrot's energy were repelling prior to the acupuncture treatment. After the treatment, their energies became similar — no more repulsion!.

The repulsive energy between my body and the carrot was presented as an allergy in me. During the acupuncture treatment, my body probably became a powerful charger and was strong enough to change the adverse charge of the carrot to match with my body's charge. This resulted in removing my allergy to the carrot. I continued to treat for other items that I previously could not eat. I tested and treated my husband and my son for many of their respective allergies. In a few weeks, we were no longer allergic to many foods that previously made us ill. We could eat and enjoy a variety of foods without getting sick. Later, I extended this to my patients who suffered from a multitude of symptoms that arose from allergies.

My amazing recovery and return to health has now been duplicated over and over in thousands of my patients. I am convinced that I have discovered something truly wonderful about the treatment of allergies that does not include strict diets, stringent potions of any kind or isolation to avoid the allergy-producing environmental elements. It is this knowledge, as well as the urgent prompting of thousands of my patients who no longer suffer from symptoms of their allergies, that convinced me to write this book.

The more extensively I studied the subject of allergies, the more I found it to be a truly fascinating, yet highly complex field. Although food allergies as causes for multiple physiological problems have been gaining acceptance as a separate area of medical study in the last few years, it certainly has not been given the recognition it deserves. In fact, knowledge of the field is still quite limited, not only among the general public but also among those who treat allergies, because of the limited volume of research conducted.

After learning about the prevalence of allergies and gathering a great deal of clinical hands-on experience with patients, I felt motivated to write a book on allergies that might be of use to students and professionals within the health care field. However, as I thought about the book, I came to understand that good health care really depends on the patient. It is just as imperative to inform the general public about allergies as it is to educate the health-care professional. Therefore, this book is written not only for the health-care professional, but also for lay persons wishing to acquire an understanding of the allergy process within the body.

The framework of this book is drawn from a formal dissertation I submitted as a basis for my doctorate degree to SAMRA University of Oriental medicine, Los Angeles, in June of 1986. It only differs slightly from the doctoral dissertation in content and focus. The principal difference is the fact that a dissertation is typically a scholarly treatise. Accordingly, my dissertation was a comparison of the Oriental with the modern western medical approaches to the treatment of patients suffering from allergic reactions. Technical terminology was used throughout.

This book, on the other hand, has been condensed and is written with a different thrust. It is designed to provide up-to-date information about the current state-of-the-allergy-treatment methodologies; to create a book that can be of value to people suffering from allergic symptoms regardless of their level of exposure to medical terminology, and to enhance the reader's knowledge and understanding of allergic reactions and possible alternative treatment methods.

I am aware that technical terminology or jargon is a part of any highly specialized field. After all, technical terminology is necessary for the professional because it reduces the need for unnecessary words and clarifies instructions. It is also clear that use of technical jargon severely reduces the ability of the uninitiated to understand important facts. Thus, the technical jargon developed around any highly technical field actually creates a significant communication barrier between the professional and the lay person.

In this book, I do use some specialized terminology, that may give some lay readers a harder time and diminish their reading pleasure and understanding. But rest assured, technical terms are kept to a minimum.

Caution has also been exercised in determining the depth of the subject matter. For instance, the way allergies and the nervous system are inextricably interrelated is just now being understood. But since the human nervous system is one of the most complex areas of human anatomy and remains largely uncharted, I decided to deal with it in a sweeping fashion, drawing the reader's attention only to the close link between the nervous system and allergic reactions.

I would feel gratified, indeed, if the up-to-date material compiled in this book were to contribute to all of my readers achieving, maintaining and enjoying good health; and if, through these readers, an even larger number of people received benefits through methods available today. *The companion book to Say Good-bye to Illness (The NAET Guide Book) and Living Pain Free with Acupressure* (a self-help book to manage your pain) should also provide you with some help when you are desperate. To enhance your understanding of the subject matter, you should check out some of the other relevant books and articles quoted as a part of this book. You will find them under the section marked "BIBLIOGRAPHY" at the conclusion of this book.

Since the main focus of this presentation is acupuncture, an understanding of that medical system and an introduction to the basis of Traditional Chinese Medicine (TCM) is mandatory. You should keep in mind, however, that an in-depth introduction to Oriental medicine was neither intended nor considered appropriate within the scope of this publication. Therefore, I urge you to refer to appropriate books for more information on this topic. Some of the references are listed in the bibliography.

Stay Allergy-Free and Enjoy Better HEALTH!

Dr. Devi S. Nambudripad,
M.D., D.C., L.Ac., Ph.D.
Los Angeles, California

May, 2002

Footnotes:

Coriander leaves clear the neurotoxins from the brain and nervous system and thus strengthens the nervous system. Coriander seeds cleanse the sinuses and glandular system. Lemon rind and rice cleanse and strengthen the lung meridian. Pepper strengthens the heart and circulatory system. Ginger root strengthens the stomach meridian.

Brown sugar strengthens the spleen meridian. Dandelion leaves strengthen the liver meridian. Coconut oil strengthens the gall bladder meridian. Turmeric and cumin seed have antibacterial properties and can help to clean and strengthen the small intestine meridian. Rock salt rejuvenates the kidney meridian; lemon leaves strengthen the bladder meridian; pomegranate strengthens the large intestine meridian and garlic is a natural antibacterial, antiparasitic and antioxidant that helps to clean the toxins from the whole system.

INTRODUCTION

Say Good-bye To Illness Through NAET

You Deserve Perfect Health!

I t is your *HUMAN RIGHT* to: eat whatever you want, live in whatever environment you want to live in, wear whatever clothes or cosmetics you want to wear, live or associate with whomever you want to, and be happy. If you are able to do all these things, you can say that you are healthy, physically, physiologically and psychologically; if you are not able to do these things, you have an illness. This book, "Say Good-bye to Illness," will help you to understand about your illness and assist you in finding the right help you need to achieve better health.

This book will show you how a harmless, commonly used product can cause the most complicated, familiar health problems. The central nervous system reacts to foods or other substances as if they are toxic when they are really neutral or beneficial. You can now reprogram your brain to perfect health.

You'll learn how genetically passed allergies and allergy-related illnesses can now be controlled with ease.

WHAT IS NAET?

Nambudripad's Allergy Elimination Techniques, also known as NAET, is a non-invasive, drug free, natural solution to eliminate allergies of all types and intensities (mild sensitivity, to severe hypersensitivity reactions, to severe anaphylactic reactions (successfully treated peanuts, penicillin, aspirins, mushroom, shellfish, etc., and the patients can use them in their everyday life now without any adverse reactions) and allergy-related disorders (some of the examples: common colds to severe infections; learning disabilities to autism and ADHD; anger and clinical depression to schizophrenias and various other mental disorders; mild joint pains, arthritis of different types and intensities, small cysts and skin eruptions to tumors and growths, angina pains, high blood pressure to strokes, all arising from allergies to food, environmental toxins, chemical toxins, and emotional stressors) and often with lasting results. NAET uses a blend of selective testing and treatment procedures from acupuncture/acupressure, allopathy, chiropractic, nutritional, and kinesiological disciplines of medicine to balance the body bioenergetically with various unsuitable electromagnetic energies found in one's living environment. Using NAET methods, one can also learn to balance the body from most adverse reactions that happened in the body from the interactions between certain unsuitable energies and the body itself; for example: depression or crying spells after eating certain food, hyperactivity or mental fog after exposure to pesticides, insomnia after applying a certain body lotion, sudden lower backache after wearing a shirt that was dry cleaned a week ago, sudden migraine after drinking one's favorite chocolate milk shake, etc. The unsuitable energies include: food, chemicals, pathogens, natural environmental resources like grass, wood, rocks, radiation, etc., physical sensitivities like heat, cold, humidity, dampness, wind, dryness, vibrations of various kinds, etc. NAET was discovered by Dr. Devi S. Nambudripad in November of 1983.

NAET is a completely natural, non-invasive and drug-free holistic treatment. Over six thousands licensed medical practitioners have been trained in NAET procedures and are practicing all over the world. Please look up the NAET website: www.naet.com for more information on NAET and a NAET practitioner near you.

WHAT IS AN ALLERGY?

A condition of unusual sensitivity of one individual to one or more substances (may be inhaled, swallowed or came in contact with the skin), which may be harmless or even beneficial to the majority of other individuals.

In sensitive individuals, contact with these substances (allergens) can produce a variety of symptoms in varying degrees ranging from slight itching to swelling of the tissues and organs, mild runny nose to severe asthmatic attacks, general tiredness or fatigue to severe anaphylaxis. The ingested, inhaled or contacted allergen is capable of alerting the immune system of the body. The frightened and confused immune system then commands the white blood cells to produce immunoglobulins type E (IgE) to stimulate the release of the chemical defense forces, like histamines, from the mast cells. These chemical mediators are released as part of the body's immune response to the foreign substances; and these chemicals produce abnormal physical, physiological and psychological symptoms in the sensitive person.

WHAT CAUSES ALLERGIES?

Energy blockages and imbalances caused in the body's energy circulation by various factors:

a. Heredity (inherited from parents, grandparents, uncles, aunts, etc.).

b. Toxins from various sources:

Toxins are produced from the interaction between the person and the unsuitable energies of foods, drinks, chemicals, pesticides, environmental factors, bacteria, fungus, virus, mercury, MSG, etc.

c. Lowering the immune system due to extra stress put on the person's body, causing the body to become weak and over-reactive towards other energies. The commonly seen stressors are: physical injuries, accidents, surgery, serious illness, and emotional injuries.

d. Deficiency and malabsorption disorders, producing abnormal enzymes leading to abnormal functions in the body (poor digestion, causing anaphlaxis, hormonal disorders, abnormal thyroid functions, etc.)

e. Overexposure to toxic substances (chemicals, attic insulation material, pesticides, allergic foods and drinks, food additives, food colorings, extreme cold, heat, etc.,) over a period of time.

f. Emotional factors and traumas creating sudden stops in the energy functions leading to chronic blockages in the energy circulation (sudden sadness, joy, trauma, etc., or painful memories of various incidents from past and present, causing the unusual immune response).

g. Toxins caused from physical exertion like vigorous exercise, running, playing sports, etc. Toxins (produced in the body from: bacterial or viral infections; molds, yeast, fungus or parasitic infestation; constant contacts with certain irritants like mercury, lead, copper, chemicals, etc.).

h. Radiation (excessive exposure of television, sun, radioactive materials, etc.).

WHAT ARE SOME COMMON ALLERGENS?

- Inhalants: pollens, flowers, perfume, dust, paint, formaldehyde, etc.
- Ingestants: food, drinks, vitamins, drugs, food additives, etc.
- Contactants: fabrics, chemicals, cosmetics, furniture, utensils, etc.
- Injectants: insect bites, stings, injectable drugs, immunization, etc.
- Infectants: viruses, bacteria, contact with infected persons, etc.
- Physical Agents: heat, cold, humidity, dampness, fog, wind, dryness, sunlight, sound, etc.
- Genetic Factors: inherited illnesses or tendency from parents, grandparents, etc.
- Molds and Fungi: molds, yeast, candida, parasites, etc.
- Emotional Factors: painful memories of various incidents from past and present.

HOW DO I KNOW I HAVE ALLERGIES?

If you experience any unusual physical, physiological or emotional symptoms in the presence of any of the above items, you can suspect an allergy.

WHO SHOULD USE THIS BOOK?

Anyone who is suffering from food and environmental allergies or anyone suffering from an allergy-related disease or condition should read this book. This drug-free, non-invasive technique is ideal to treat infants, children, grown-ups, old and debilitated people who suffer from mild to severe allergic reactions.

HOW IS THIS BOOK ORGANIZED?

- Chapter 1 explains the definition of allergy in various disciplines of medicine and also in laymen's terms.

- Chapter 2 describes the various categories of allergens and how they affect an allergic person.

- Chapter 3 is a step-by-step method of evaluating your allergic history.

- Chapter 4 explains Nambudripad's Testing Techniques and gives you information about various allergy testing techniques.

- Chapter 5 describes the normal function of the human nervous system and how it creates allergies by receiving wrong stimuli.

- Chapter 6 discusses kinesiology, acupuncture and how energy blockages can cause allergies and diseases in the human body.

- Chapter 7 explains Muscle Response Testing (MRT) to detect allergies, the main testing technique used in NTT (Nambudripad's Testing Techniques) and Nambudripad's Allergy Elimination Techniques (NAET).

- Chapter 8 discusses various causes of diseases.

- Chapter 9 is about this revolutionary treatment technique and how it was discovered.

- Chapter 10 explains the major acupuncture meridians, their normal and pathological functions.

- Chapter 11 describes and illustrates self-balancing and using acupressure techniques to give the reader more control over his/her health.

- Chapters 12 - 22 describe various health conditions, system by system, which can be affected by energy blockages that cause allergies and allergy-related illnesses. The colors in these chapters symbolize the *Five-Element Theory of Oriental Medicine*: yellow/earth; white/metal; blue/water; green/wood; and red/fire.

Case studies are given following the explanation of each allergic condition. Actual patients' testimonials are also included where appropriate to help the reader understand the severity of the symptoms and the process involved in undergoing treatment to eliminate the allergic reactions.

The glossary of terms will help you to understand the appropriate meaning of the medical terminology used in certain parts of the book.

The resource guide is provided to assist you in finding products and consultants to support you in dealing with your allergies..

A detailed index is included to help you locate your area of interest quickly and easily.

CHAPTER 1

WHAT IS AN ALLERGY?

Over a period of 10 years, Carolyn had been hospitalized a total of 12 times, her stays lasting from a few days to weeks, for seizure episodes, bronchitis, acute asthmatic attacks and frequent bouts of pneumonia. For several months following the hospitalization her health would improve. However, by the time she regained her strength, another episode of asthma or pneumonia would land her back in the hospital. A talented musician, she could not work or play an instrument even as a leisure activity. She was forced to go on disability.

Carolyn had tried everything she could think of to end her suffering. Several physicians in general medicine had long ago given up trying to help her. She had seen an internist, a neurologist, a vascular surgeon, a lung specialist and at least four doctors specializing in the treatment of allergies from a western perspective. She had undergone nearly every diagnostic procedure known to modern medicine. On the advice of one physician, she even underwent psychiatric evaluation. Still, the ongoing headaches persisted, as did the asthmatic symptoms, muscle and joint pains, epileptic-type seizures, persistent dry cough, postnasal drip, chronic diarrhea, bladder infections, yeast infections, frequent urination, dyslexia, disorientation and extreme mental and physical fatigue.

This is the story of a real person who, like so many others around us, suffers from the frustrating and agonizing symptoms of allergies; symptoms that not only confuse and frustrate patients and their doctors, but also place tremendous stress on their families and employers.

The facts of this actual case history are typical and quite common. The heavy doses of cortisone and antibiotics Carolyn received during her hospitalization produced temporary and sometimes permanent relief from the symptoms of allergies in a majority of allergic patients. However, the possibility of recurrence waits just around the corner. The side effects of cortisone and other antiallergenic medicines increase the risk of heart disease, obesity, joint disorders and moonface (a temporary deformity caused by allergic reactions to the cortisone prescribed to reduce the original allergic symptoms).

> An allergy is an adverse physical, physiological, and/or psychological response of an individual towards one or more substances also known as allergens.

DEFINITION OF AN ALLERGY

A condition of unusual sensitivity of one individual towards one or more substances from one's living environment which may be harmless or even beneficial to a majority of other individuals. In other words, an allergy is an energy imbalance between the electromagnetic energy of the person and the substance causing unpleasant physical, physiological and/or psychological reactions in the person's body.

According to Oriental medical principles, the Yin-Yang state represents the perfect balance of energies. Any imbalance in a Yin-Yang state causes an energy difference. Any imbalance in the Yin-Yang state causes disharmony. This disharmony is allergy.

An allergy is a hereditary condition: an allergic predisposition or tendency is inherited, but the allergy itself may not manifest until some later date. The age of onset of an allergic condition depends on the degree of inheritance. The stronger the genetic factor, the earlier in life is the probable onset. Studies have shown that when both parents were or are allergy-sensitive, 75 to 100 percent of their offspring react to those same allergens. When neither of the parents is (nor was) sensitive to allergens, the probability of producing allergic offspring drops dramatically to less than 10 percent. Most of us suffer from allergic manifestation in varying degrees because of our different levels of parental inheritance.

In some cases, even when parents had no allergies, their offspring still suffered from many allergies since birth. In these cases, various possibilities exist:

Parents may have suffered from a serious disease or condition. For example, parents had malaria before the child was born that caused alteration in the genetic codes. The pregnant mother may have been exposed to harmful substances: radiation (X-ray), chemicals (an expectant mother taking too much caffeine, alcohol, drugs or antibiotics), toxins as the result of a disease (streptococcal infection as in strep-throat, measles or chicken pox). Pregnant mother may have suffered severe emotional trauma(s). The parents may have suffered severe malnutrition (not getting enough food or not assimilating due to poor absorption or allergies), possibly causing the growing embryo to undergo cell mutation during its development in the womb. The altered cells do not carry over the original genetic codes or do not go through normal development. The organs and tissues that are supposed to develop from the affected cells have impaired function, may be due to emotional factors and stress-induced imbalances.

It is estimated that 50 percent of the population throughout the world suffers from allergies. But the estimate is just that, an estimate, due to the various definitions of allergies among researchers. There is no specific definition for allergy that has been universally agreed upon. If medical researchers were willing to broaden their views on allergies to include hypersensitivity, intolerances, IgE mediated and non-IgE mediated reactions, we would clearly recognize the overwhelming percentage of allergy sufferers going above 90%.

Many medical professionals and patients ask me the same question: "Are you treating true allergies or just treating sensitivities?" The symptoms, diagnosis and treatments of sensitivities, hypersensitivities and intolerances, (non-IgE mediated reactions) and allergies (IgE mediated reactions) often overlap. Both intolerances and allergies, in varying degrees, can be tested by Muscle Response Testing (MRT). In the case of an allergy, weakness of the test muscle is noted while doing muscle response testing, and a strong resistance is experienced by the test muscle while doing MRT when there is no allergy. The "Naeter," (developed by "Startechhealth.com"), a recently developed, a noninvasive computerized electrodermal testing device has been found very affective in detecting hypersensitivies, intolerances, IgE mediated allergies and non-IgE mediated allergies in allergy-sufferers, validating the efficacy of NAET Muscle Response Testing for allergies. All of these allergic reactions can successfully be treated and eliminated by NAET. MRT and NAET are explained in detail in Chapter 7.

The literal meaning of allergy comes from the Greek word *allos*, which translates *altered action*, or put another way, a reaction. The term *allergy* was first proposed in 1906 by an Austrian pediatrician, Clemens Von Pirquet (1874-1929), who worked a great deal with tubercular children, studying the immune system and what we now call allergic reactions. It was Pirquet who developed a scratch test for tuberculosis, a forerunner of the allergy scratch testing done in many clinics today. By combining the two Greek words *allos* (altered) and *ergion* (action or reactivity), Pirquet created the word *allergy*, literally meaning *altered reactivity*. This describes a biological hypersensitivity in certain individual to substances, which in similar amounts and circumstances, are harmless to most people.

Somewhere around mid 400 BC, nearly 2500 years ago, Hippocrates, the Greek physician considered the "Father of Medicine," noted that cheese caused severe reactions in some men, while others could eat and enjoy it with no unpleasant aftereffects. Three hundred years later, the Roman philosopher Lucretius said, "What is food for some may be fierce poison for others." From this we derive the expression, "One man's meat is another man's poison." This is a simple and concise definition of allergy, although the condition was not recognized as such until only very recently.

The activation of immunoglobulin type E (IgE) antibodies causes true allergies; however, millions of people experience various allergic symptoms every day in varying degrees without producing these antibodies. These types of reactions can be called either *intolerance* or *hypersensitivity*.

When the body is exposed to what it thinks is a foreign and dangerous substance, a normal immune system will immediately release chemical mediators that are appropriate to the condition to counteract the allergic reaction. The body will come to a settlement with the allergen in seconds without causing any obvious ill-health symptoms in the person. But when the immune system perceives what should be harmless substances as dangerous intruders and stimulates antibody production to defend the body, things do not settle down as pleasantly as in the person with a normal immune system. Here, the first contact with an allergen initiates the baby step of an allergic reaction inside the body. The body will alert its defense forces in response to the alarm received about the new invader and will immediately produce a few antibodies, storing them in reserve for future use.

In most people, a first contact or initial sensitization will usually not produce many symptoms. During the second exposure to the allergen, the body will alert the previously produced antibodies to action, producing more noticeable symptoms. If you have a strong immune system, the second exposure may not cause too many unpleasant symptoms either. But often, with the third exposure, the threatened immune system will begin serious action by producing massive amounts of antibodies to defend against the invader, causing what we call an allergic reaction.

There are various types of immunoglobulins produced in the body at various instances as a natural defense mechanism to protect the body. Some of the known ones include:

IgE - The antibody that is responsible for immediate hypersensitivity and reactions in the body when it comes in contact with an allergen.

IgA - This is produced when the reactions are associated with the mucous membranes.

IgD - This is found on the surface of the B-cells.

IgG - Also known as gammaglobulin, which produces a delayed reaction, with symptoms taking anywhere from a few hours to 3-4 days to appear. IgG is the major antibody in the blood that protects against bacteria and viruses.

IgM - This is the first antibody to appear during an immune response.

Some people could have just the IgE mediated allergies only, in which case IgE antibodies can be found in the blood sample. Some people can have more than one antibody in their blood, depending on how many allergens they have reacted to in the past.

An allergic reaction may be manifested in varying degrees as mild to severe itching, rashes, hives or swelling anywhere within the body. The most commonly affected areas are the skin, eyes, nose, throat, mouth, rectum and vaginal mucosa. An allergy can also affect the patient systemically, also known as anaphylactic shock. An anaphylactic shock can affect a few or all organs at the same time, giving rise to exaggerated systemic symptoms, manifesting in sharp pains in the head, abdomen and chest. It can also cause swelling of the tongue and throat, leading to constriction and breathing difficulties, or a partial shutdown of blood circulation, causing low blood pressure, fast heart rate and thready pulse or no pulse at all. Additional symptoms we've seen include: decrease in body temperature, leading to cold and clammy skin; sensation of chills; internal cold; pallor; rolling eyes; sensation of fear; fever; unresponsiveness; lightheadedness; nausea; diarrhea; panic attack, fainting and, at times, even death, due to a complete shut down of the system.

Many people, including some health professionals, upon hearing the word "allergy" think only of a runny nose, sneezing, hives and, perhaps, asthma or hay fever. In some instances, the reactions of allergy sufferers are predictable, but for others, the reactions are not at all what would be expected. These reactions vary radically and appear unexpectedly, making diagnosis elusive and pretreatments nearly impossible. Curiously, an increasing number of medical doctors and researchers are now considering that allergic factors may be involved in most illnesses and medical disorders.

According to the statistics released by the American College of Allergy, Asthma and Immunology (ACAAI) in January 1999, approximately 40-50 million Americans have some form of allergy, only one to two percent of all adults are allergic to foods or food additives. Eight percent of children under age six have adverse reaction to ingested foods; only two to five percent have confirmed food allergies.

Without question, there are many undiagnosed allergies hiding beneath the myriad of unresolved health problems inflicted on unsuspecting patients worldwide. The research and experience gathered from my allergy specialty practice confirms that only a fraction of allergies are regularly diagnosed by traditional medical diagnostic measures. My conclusion is based on 15 years' experience and thousands of case histories, not only from my practice, but also from the thousands of doctors I have trained in the NAET method. These reactions render the sufferers and their loved ones many anxiety-filled moments, days, and in some cases, months or longer. The practitioner may doubt his/her knowledge and ability to practice medicine or get frustrated about the situation and give a "scapegoat diagnosis" like *viral, incurable, genetic, strange, idiopathic* or *psychosomatic.* A scapegoat diagnosis gives the patient temporary satisfaction and some momentary peace of mind to the doctor; however, the result is not long-lasting to either party.

The shocking fact is that there are hardly any human diseases or conditions in which allergic factors are not involved directly or indirectly. Any substance under the sun, including sunlight itself, can cause an allergic reaction in any individual. In other words, potentially, you can be allergic to anything you come in contact with. If you begin to check people around you—even so called healthy people—you will find hidden allergies as a causative factor in almost all health disorders.

For those whose lives are merely disrupted by the discomfort of the reaction, simple antihistamine or topical remedies bring temporary relief until the particular allergy season passes. But for those whose lives are literally being threatened, either long-term immunotherapy or complete avoidance is the only hope the traditional medicine has been able to offer so far. Immunotherapy, of course, is very expensive and time consuming, and it often does not present a satisfactory outcome. Most people finally resort to a lifetime of depriving themselves of the many things in life that would otherwise bring them joy and fulfillment. Common complaints are, *"My allergies have taken control of my life,"* and *"The very things that I want to make me happy are the very things that I react to the most."*

Even with total isolation from potential allergens, there is no guarantee that allergy sufferers will be able to stay away from every situation and still remain reaction free. With the progress of science and technology, our modern life-styles have changed dramatically. New products, which are potential allergens for many people, are being developed every day. The quality of life has improved; but for some allergic patients, the scientific achievements have created more nightmares.

We cannot ignore the fact that we are moving into the twenty-first century where technology will be even more predominant than today. There is nothing wrong with the technology. In fact, modern technology has provided a better quality of life-style. But the allergic patient must find ways to overcome adverse reactions to chemicals and other allergens produced by the technology in order to enjoy the new world. Even though it requires a series of detailed treatments, NAET offers the prospect of relief to those who suffer from constant allergic reactions by reprogramming the brain to perfect health. Just like rebooting a computer, we can reboot our nervous system through NAET and overcome the adverse reactions of the brain and body.

In my opinion, it is certainly better than submitting to or seeking "mercy killing" to overcome the constant pain and struggle.

To comprehend NAET, some understanding of the brain and its functions is necessary. Many books on the subject of the brain are available in bookstores and libraries. A brief introduction to the brain function related to NAET is given here. For more information, please consult the references in the bibliography.

THE BRAIN AND THE NERVOUS SYSTEM

Study of the nervous system is a complex subject even to students of the neurological sciences. I do not expect every reader to comprehend all the material presented below on the nervous system and its functions. Let us also attempt to review the relationship between the nervous system and one of its functions—the immune response.

To understand the nervous system, one must know its organization, the mechanism of communication and the signaling pathways.

ORGANIZATION

The nervous system is comprised of the central nervous system and the peripheral nervous system. The spinal cord and brain are the two components of the central nervous system.

THE BRAIN CAN BE DIVIDED INTO SIX MAJOR PARTS:

1. Medulla

2. Pons
3. Cerebellum
4. Midbrain/Thalamus
5. Cerebral cortex and hemispheres

The brain is the master control center of the body and constantly receives information from the sensory nerve fibers about conditions both inside and outside the body. It rapidly analyzes this information and then sends out messages that control body functions and actions. It also stores all information from past experiences, which makes learning and remembering possible. In addition, the brain is the source of thoughts, moods and emotions.

EXPLORATION OF THE BRAIN THROUGH THE YEARS

Before the invention of the compound microscope, nervous tissue was thought to function like a gland. In the beginning of the first century, Greek physician Galen proposed that nerves circulate a special kind of fluid secreted by the brain and spinal cord to the body's periphery. In the eighteenth century, the microscope revealed the true structure of the cells of nervous tissue. Even so, nervous tissue did not become the subject of a special science until the late 1800's, when the first detailed descriptions of nerve cells were undertaken by Camillo Golgi and Santiago Ramon Y Cajal.

Golgi was able to view the neuron under the microscope. He was able to see that the neurons had cell bodies and two major projections, a branching dendrite at one end and a long cable-like axon at the other. Ramon Y Cajal was able to stain individual cells, thus showing that nervous tissue is not one continuous web, but a network of discrete cells. In the course of this work, Ramon Y Cajal developed some of the key concepts and much of the early evidence for the principle that individual neurone are the elementary signaling elements of the nervous system.

Physiological investigation of the nervous system began in the late 1700's when the Italian physician and physicist Luigi Galvani discovered that living, excitable muscle and nerve cells produced electricity. Modern electrophysiology grew out of work in the 19th century by three German physiologists—Emil Du Bois-Reymond, Johannes Muller, and Hermann

Von Helmholtz—who were able to show that the electrical activity of one nerve cell affects the activity of an adjacent cell in predictable ways.

At the end of the nineteenth century, pharmacology made its first impact on our knowledge of the nervous system and behavior when Claude Bernard in France, Paul Ehrlich in Germany, and John Langley in England demonstrated that drugs do not interact with cells arbitrarily, but rather bind to specific receptors typically located in the membrane on the cell's surface. This discovery became the basis of the all-important study of the chemical basis of communication between nerve cells.

The brain works like a computer. Brain cells produce electrical signals and send them from cell to cell along pathways called *circuits*. These electrical circuits receive, process, store, and retrieve information. The brain creates its electrical signals by chemical means. The proper functioning of the brain depends on many complicated chemical substances produced by the brain cells.

The spinal cord consists of 31 pairs of spinal nerves. Parasympathetic and sympathetic nerves emerge from the spinal cord and travel to various parts of the body, including body surfaces. There are special sensory receptors called *nociceptors* seen in certain areas in the peripheral tissue. Nociceptors are activated by perceived or actual tissue damage. Harmful stimuli to the skin, subcutaneous tissue or muscle activate several classes of nociceptor receptors, or the peripheral endings of the nociceptor fibers, whose cell bodies are located in the dorsal root ganglia. Nociceptive afferent nerve fibers terminate on neurons in the dorsal horn of the spinal cord. Nociceptive information is transmitted from the spinal cord to the thalamus and cerebral cortex along five ascending pathways.

Synaptic transmission between nociceptors and dorsal horn neurons is mediated by chemical neurotransmitters. Some of these neurotransmitters released by the sensory nerve endings are: neuropeptides, glutamate, serotonin, bradykinin, histamine, prostaglandins, leukotrienes, tryptophane, and substance P. Neurons in several regions of the cerebral cortex respond selectively to nociceptive input. Some of these neurons are located in the somatosensory cortex. Chemical mediators can sensitize and sometimes activate nociceptors. Insult to tissue releases bradykinin and prostaglandins, which activate nociceptors. Activation of nociceptors leads to the release of substance P. Substance P acts on mast cells near the sensory nerve endings, causing the release of histamines and other immune system mediators.

Sensory information in the central nervous system is processed in stages, in the sequential relay nuclei of the spinal cord, brain stem, thalamus, and cerebral cortex.

The cerebral hemispheres consist of cerebral cortex, basal ganglia, hippocampus and the amygdala. The basal ganglia helps in regulating motor and sensory activities; the hippocampus participates in storing the memory; and amygdala is involved in coordinating the autonomic and endocrine responses at various levels including emotional level. The cerebral cortex can be further divided into three areas according to their functions:

1. The *sensory cortex* receives messages from the sense organs (eyes, nose, ears, tongue, and fingertips by touching), as well as messages of pressure, pain, and temperature.

2. The *association cortex* analyzes, processes and stores information about all internal and external stimuli received from the sense organs. Due to this unique functional ability of the association cortex, man is able to display higher mental abilities, such as thinking, speaking, storing, retrieving, correcting and restoring information about everything that happened around him/her.

3. The *motor cortex* sends out responses to the peripheral nervous system through spinal nerves about the stimuli received from the sense organs. It also controls the movements of all skeletal muscles.

THE MECHANISM OF COMMUNICATION

The nervous system obtains sensory information from the environment, evaluates the significance of information, and generates appropriate responses. The peripheral nervous system relays information to the central nervous system through the afferent nerves; and when the responses are generated in the brain, the efferent nerves bring them back to the spinal cord and to the peripheral nervous system. The *axon* carries nerve impulses from the cell body to other neurons. The *dendrites* pick up impulses from the axon of other neurons and transmit them to the cell body. The point where any branch of one neuron transmits a nerve impulse to a branch of another neuron is called a *synapse*. Each neuron may form synapses with thousands of other nerve cells.

THE SIGNALING UNIT

Nerve cells are the main signaling units of the nervous system. A typical neuron has four morphologically defined regions: the cell body, dendrites, the axon, and presynaptic terminals. Each of these regions has a distinct role in the generation of signals and the communication of signals between nerve cells.

The nervous system obtains sensory information from the environment, evaluates the significance of the information, and generates appropriate responses. The peripheral nervous system relays information to the central nervous system through the spinal nerves and ganglia when the commands are generated in the brain; the same nerves bring them back to the spinal cord and to the peripheral nervous system.

When the sensory nerve endings (from nasal mucosa, lung, mouth, alimentary tract, skin, fingertips, etc.) gather information about an antigen close to its proximity (allergen), it transmits information via afferent nerve fibers to the brain (hypothalamus and to associated parts of the cerebral cortex). The hypothalamus and the parts of the cerebral cortex will relay the information about the allergen's proximity to the rest of the body via electrical signals and alert the entire body. Along with every nerve cell, the body's immune system will be alerted to call upon the defensive forces. With the result, the the immune response will begin immediately by stimulating lymphocytes to mature into plasma cells, and the plasma cells to produce antibodies (IgE and IgG, etc., suitable for the condition) as needed to handle the situation.

The allergens are small antigens that commonly provoke an IgE antibody response. Such antigens normally enter the body at very low doses by diffusion across mucosal surfaces and, therefore, trigger an immune response. The specific IgE produced in response to the allergen binds to the high-affinity receptor for IgE on mast cells, basophils, and activated eosinophils. IgE production can be amplified by these cells. The tendency to IgE overproduction is influenced by genetic and environmental factors. Once IgE is produced in response to an allergen, re-exposure to the allergen triggers an allergic response. The allergen triggers the activation of IgE-binding mast cells in the exposed tissue, leading to a series of responses that are characteristic of allergy.

We propose that NAET intercepts here and put a stop to the immune response, with the result that the anticipated allergic reaction no longer takes place. Not only that, by stimulating the specific afferent and efferent nerves and nociceptors in dorsal root ganglia while the person is in physical contact with the said allergen, the NAET treatment is able to change the characteristics of the previous stimulus into a new one with a different signal. These altered stimuli will carry new information about the antigen via synapses to the appropriate areas of the cerebral cortex. In return, the brain will relay its response about this new information to every cell in the body. The previously activated immune response will get deactivated or replaced by a newly relayed signal, thus effectively rendering the previously perceived harmful substance into one which the nervous system now recognizes as being relatively harmless. This process has been observed in numerous patients to give them an instant, non-allergic response when re-exposed to the previous noxious substance.

Our experience to date has shown that the IgE and IgG antibody levels take a period of months to drop to lower levels upon retesting for specific antigens. This is quite similar to the findings of traditional allergists that persons who lose reactivity to certain allergens which caused positive Double-Blind Placebo Controlled Food Challenges (DBPCFC's) during childhood will continue to have positive skin tests for these allergens for up to two years after DBPCFC has become negative.

NAET involves the whole brain and its network of nerves as it reprograms the brain by erasing the previous harmful memory regarding the allergen, and imprinting a new, useful memory in its place.

EMOTIONS

The psychological investigation of behavior dates back to the beginnings of western science, to classical Greek philosophy. Many issues central to the modern investigation behavior, particularly in the area of perception, were subsequently reformulated in the seventeenth century, first by Rene Descartes and then by John Locke. In the mid-nineteenth century, Charles Darwin set the stage for the study of animals as models of human actions and behavior by publishing his observations on the continuity of species in evolution. This new approach gave rise to ethology, the study of animal behavior in the natural environment, and later to experimental psychology, the study of human and animal behavior under controlled conditions.

In fact, by as early as the end of the eighteenth century, the first attempt had been made to bring together biological and psychological concepts in the study of behavior. Franz Joseph Gall, a German physician and neuroanatomist, proposed three radical new ideas. First, he advocated that all behavior emanated from the brain. Second, he argued that a particular region of the cerebral cortex controlled specific functions. Gall asserted that the cerebral cortex did not act as a single organ but was divided into at least 35 organs (others were added later), each corresponding to a specific mental faculty. Even the most abstract of human behaviors, such as generosity, secretiveness, and religiosity, were assigned their spots in the brain. Third, Gall proposed that the center for each mental function grew with use, much as muscle bulks up with exercise. As each center grew, it caused the overlying skull to bulge, creating a pattern of bumps and ridges on the skull that indicated which brain regions were most developed. Gall sought to establish an anatomical basis for describing character traits by correlating the personality of individuals with the bumps on their skulls. His psychology, based on the distribution of bumps on the outside of the head, became known as *phrenology.*

In the late 1820's, Gall's ideas were subjected to experimental analysis by the French physiologist Pierre Flourens. By systematically removing Gall's functional centers from the brains of experimental animals, Flourens attempted to isolate the contributions of each *cerebral organ* to behavior. From these experiments, he concluded that specific brain regions were not responsible for specific behaviors, but proposed that all brain regions, especially the cerebral hemisphere, were able to perform all the functions of the hemisphere. Injury to a specific area of the cerebral hemisphere would, therefore, affect all higher functions equally.

In 1823, Flourens wrote: "All perceptions, all volitions (willingness) occupy the same seat in this organ (Cerebrum); the faculty of perceiving, of conceiving, of willing merely constitutes therefore a faculty which is essentially one."

The emotions we experience involve many areas of the brain as well as other body organs. A part of the brain structure called the *limbic system* plays a central role in the production of emotions. This system consists of parts of the temporal lobe, hypothalamus and thalamus. An emotion may be provoked by a message from a sense organ or by a thought in the cerebral cortex. In either case, nerve impulses are produced and reach the limbic system. These impulses stimulate different areas of the system, depending on the kind of sensory message or thought. For example, the impulses might activate parts of the system that produce pleasant feelings involved in   emotions like joy and love. We can easily be inspired and energized by impulses that activate parts of the system that uplift our spirits and bring forth feelings of harmony and well being. These grand moments of reverie are in our power. On the other hand, the impulses that stimulate unpleasant feelings associated with anger and fear can produce negative results.

Scientists have only an elementary understanding of the extraordinarily complicated processes of thinking and remembering. Explanations for much of this area of thinking are still beyond our grasp.

THE BASIS OF NAET

A thorough treatise on biochemistry is not appropriate for the purpose of an introduction to this new method of treatment for people suffering from allergies. Instead, this discussion will concentrate on the basic constructs of this treatment method and give some insight into the lives of the people it has helped. This is not a new technology. It is actually a combination of knowledge and techniques that uses much of what is already known from allopathic (western medical knowledge), chiropractic, kinesiology, acupuncture (Oriental medical knowledge) and nutrition. Each of the disciplines I studied provided bits of knowledge which I used in developing this new allergy elimination treatment. There is no known successful method of treatment for food allergies using western medicine except avoidance, which means deprivation and frustration.

I developed this new technique of allergy elimination, to identify and treat the reactions to many substances, including food, chemicals, environmental allergens and emotional imbalances caused from allergies.

Through many long years of research, and after many trials and errors, I devised this combination of allergy elimination treatments to eliminate energy blockages (allergies) permanently and to restore the body to a healthy state. These energy blockage elimination techniques together are called *Nambudripad's Allergy Elimination Techniques,* or **NAET** for short.

ALLOPATHY AND WESTERN SCIENCE

Knowledge of the brain, cranial nerves, spinal nerves and autonomic nervous system from western medicine enlightens us about the body's efficient multilevel communication network. Through this network of nerves, vital energy circulates in the body carrying negative and positive messages from each and every cell to the brain and then back to the cells. Knowledge about the nervous system, its origin, travel route, organs and tissues that benefit from its nerve energy supply (target organs and tissues) and its destination, helps us to understand the energy distribution of the spinal nerves and the importance of ventral and dorsal root ganglia. If the energy supply reaches all the respective organs and tissues, through their miles-long nerve fibers, they all remain healthy and happy. If the energy distribution is reduced or stopped in one or more of the spinal nerves, the respective organs and tissues will have diminished function or partial or complete shut down. By evaluating the condition of its target organs and tissues, changes in energy distribution via any spinal nerve can be detected (Gray's Anatomy, and Principles of Neural Science, 4th ed.).

KINESIOLOGY

Kinesiology is the art and science of movement of the human body. Kinesiology is used in NAET to compare the strength and weakness of any muscle of the body in the presence or absence of any substance. This is also called Muscle Response Testing to detect allergies.

It is hypothesized that a measurable weakness in a particular muscle is produced by the generation of an energy disturbance in the particular spinal nerve route that supplies to the corresponding weakened muscle when a specific item is brought into its energy field. Any item that is capable of producing energy disturbance in any spinal nerve route is called an allergen. Through this simple kinesiological testing method, the allergens can be detected; disturbed spinal nerves and their nerve routes can be identified; and the target organs, tissues, and other body parts can be uncovered.

PILOT STUDY OF MRT

Muscle testing to detect allergies is supported by the pilot study done by WALTER H. SCHMITT, Jr. and GERRY LEISMAN, "Applied Neuroscience Laboratories," N.C., USA, and the College of Judea and Samaria, P.O. Box 3, Ariel, 44837, Israel, titled "Correlation Of Applied Kinesiology Muscle Testing Findings With Serum Immunoglobulin Levels For Food Allergy," August 1998.

This pilot study attempted to determine whether subjective muscle testing employed by applied kinesiology practitioners, prospectively determine those individuals with specific hyper-allergenic responses. Seventeen subjects were found positive on applied kinesiology muscle testing screening procedures indicating food hypersensitivity (allergy) reaction. Each subject showed muscle weakening (inhibition) reactions to oral provocative testing of one or two foods for a total of 21 positive food reactions. Tests for a hypersensitivity reaction of the serum were performed using both a radio-allergosorbent test (RAST) and immune complex test for IgE and IgG against all 21 of the foods that tested positive with Applied Kinesiological muscle screening procedures. The serum tests confirmed 19 of 21 food allergies (90.5 %) suspected based on the applied kinesiology screening procedures. This pilot study offers a basis to examine further a means by which to predict the clinical utility of a given substance for a given patient, based on the patterns of neuromuscular response elicited from the patient, representing a conceptual expansion of the standard neurological examination process.

CHIROPRACTIC

Chiropractic technique helps us to detect the nerve energy disturbance in a specific nerve energy pathway by finding and isolating the exact nerve root that is being pinched. The exact vertebral level in relation to the pinched spinal nerve root helps us to trace the travel route, the destination and the target organs of that particular energy pathway.

ACUPUNCTURE / ORIENTAL MEDICINE

Yin-Yang theory from Oriental medical principles also teaches the importance of maintaining homeostasis in the body. According to Oriental medical principles, *when the Yin-Yang is balanced in the body (a state of perfect balance between all energies and functions), no disease is possible.* Any disturbance in the homeostasis can cause disease.

NUTRITION

You are what you eat! The secret to good health is achieved through correct nutrition. What is correct nutrition? How do you get it? When you can eat nutritious food without discomfort and assimilate the nutrients from the food, that food is said to be the right food. When you get indigestion, bloating, and other digestive troubles upon or after eating a particular food, that food is not helping you to function normally. However natural, expensive or packed with high quality nutrition, if a food item causes one or more of these symptoms upon ingestion, it is not the right nutrition for you. This is due to an allergy to that food. Different people react differently to different foods, so it is very important to clear the allergy to the nutrients. Allergic people can tolerate foods low in nutrition better than nutritious foods. After clearing the allergy, you should try to eat more wholesome, nutritious foods. Above all, you should avoid refined, bleached food that is devoid of nutrients.

Many people who feel poorly due to undiagnosed food allergies may take vitamins or other supplements to increase their vitality. This can actually make them feel worse if they happen to be allergic to these nutrients as well. Only after clearing those allergies can their bodies properly assimilate them. So, nutritional assessment should be done periodically and, if needed, appropriate supplements should be taken to receive better results.

INCOMPATIBILITIES / IMBALANCES

Study of the functions of the nervous system is an ongoing study. Western scientists do not have all the answers yet to substantiate the multitudes of activities taking place in our brain-body-mind everyday. But thousands of years ago, Oriental medical pioneers explored the body system and its functions through meridian theory. Meridian theory explained the mechanisms of energy blockages in the energy meridians and how the energy blockages lead to functional imbalances and incompatibilities in a human body. Cumulative effect of imbalances and incompatibilities eventually produced diseases. They also demonstrated that, by removing the energy blockages from the energy pathways, diseases could be healed and health could be restored.

Meridian theories are not easy to describe using western terminology. Meridian concept is summarized in Chapter 10. If the reader wishes to learn more about Oriental medicine or meridian theorem, please read the appropriate books given in the bibliography.

There are energy imbalances in daily activities like eating, digesting, sleeping and exercising. There are energy imbalances in our relationships, such as disharmony between parents, siblings, spouses and friends. You experience energy imbalances in day-to-day activities, like spending, buying, saving, working without rest, studying without a break, traveling day and night, etc. Every one of these activities affects your Yin-Yang balance and can cause disharmony in your life. Therefore, unbalanced functions of all types, stemming from incompatible energies of food, material, people, thoughts, or behavior are addressed as *allergies* in this book.

SOME POSSIBILITIES FOR IMBALANCES IN HEALTH ARE:

■ **Overeating:** Indulgent eating of rich and fatty foods. We now know that an allergy to fats and sugar causes addiction to such foods.

■ **Indigestion:** May be arising as a result of a disharmony between the food and digestive juices.

■ **Sleeping:** A person may have the desire, for example, to sleep 18 hours a day. This may be due to an imbalance in the functions of the internal organs causing a number of energy pathways to slow down. When there is minimal available energy in the body, the brain wants to preserve the energy for more important functions in the body. Sleep requires minimum energy. While the person sleeps, the body can utilize the available energy for other functions, like digestion, etc. This disharmony of the internal organs may be due to poor absorption of the vital nutrients from the food due to an allergy to the nutrients that are supposed to regulate the functions of the internal organs.

■ **Exercising:** Some people continue their aerobic workout for many hours a day. Exercise can increase the blood and energy circulation. When the circulation of blood and energy improves, some of the energy blockages are pushed out of the energy pathways. When one has a lot of energy blockages, the brain demands him/her to do more exercise for hours, hoping to get the energy blockages out of the pathways.

■ **Energy imbalance in relationships:** Spouses, siblings or children, engaging in or being subject to verbal, mental or physical abuse.

■ **Imbalances in daily activities:** Spending the paycheck the very first day it is received, or spending only a small portion and depositing the rest in the bank while living in poverty the rest of the time.

These examples exhibit imbalances caused by disharmonies. Due to the alteration of the genetic codes caused from allergies, nerve receptors supplying energy to certain organs remain dormant and are unable to conduct messages from and to the spinal cord. In some instances, these dormant receptors become *hyposensitive (hidden allergies)* toward certain items, whereas in other people they become *hypersensitive (Active allergies)*. Neither type functions normally. Both types can be tested by MRT. Most other standard medical allergy tests available today are unable to detect hidden allergies successfully.

In 1983, I developed NAET to detect and successfully wake up such dormant sensory nerve fibers those were forced to remain dormant by numerous allergies from one's living arrangement, and restore their normal functions and of the target tissues and organs that depend on their integrity for their normal functions in the body.

In our highly technological age, the numbers of substances that are potentially allergenic are constantly being expanded as we learn what it truly means to *live better through chemistry.*

A substance capable of producing an allergic reaction is known as an allergen and may be different for every person. For instance, most people are allergic to poison oak or poison ivy. For the same reason, most people find roses to be nothing more than beautiful and fragrant flowers. No matter what the substance may be, for the person in whom a substance produces an allergic reaction, that is an allergen.

Further explanation is necessary to understand the changes that actually take place in the body when an allergic manifestation occurs. An allergy is an unusual or exaggerated response to certain substances. It is believed to be a normal response that has been abnormally exaggerated.

For instance, when an inflammation of the eye occurs, it is an effort on the part of the eye to throw off some irritating substance. When the nose begins to drip and the hay fever victim sneezes, this is an effort on the part of these organs to eliminate some of the irritants (such as pollen). When giant hives occur, watery fluid becomes present in the tissues, for the purpose of washing away whatever substance is causing the trouble. When asthma occurs, the bronchial tubes contract in an effort to prevent the irritant from penetrating deeper into the lungs.

These reactions are controlled by the autonomic nervous system, which is composed of the sympathetic and parasympathetic nerves. They control such organs as the lachrymal glands (which secrete tears), the salivary glands (which secrete saliva), the respiratory organs, the digestive system and the heart. These processes are controlled by the two systems of nerves that act antagonistically against each other. The sympathetic nerves cause relaxation in the muscles, and the parasympathetic nerves cause muscles to contract. When the two systems are functioning properly, we are not aware of these processes. When one system overreacts on the other, certain things occur in the body that make us aware of their existence.

For instance, when we are frightened or angry, the adrenal glands secrete additional adrenaline into the bloodstream, stimulating the activity of certain organs and tissues of the body. The heart works more rapidly, perspiration flows more freely and the body summons all its defense forces to ensure protection and save the body from any possible harm—preparing the body for "fight or flight."

According to Oriental medical principles, this is the state when the energy pathways displace "free flowing of energy." Free flowing energy ensures perfect balance of the body. When the body is in perfect balance, and the sympathetic nerves are in control, allergic reactions are not possible. In fact, people who have severe allergic symptoms, such as asthma, do not have these symptoms when they are very angry, frightened, or when sympathetic nervous system activity is heightened. It is a well-known fact that on a battlefield, even chronic asthmatics have no symptoms whatsoever. With this knowledge, the basis of our modern wisdom and use of adrenaline as a drug in treating allergic patients was formed.

The parasympathetic nerves act in the opposite manner. They contract rather than relax the muscles. They also can cause relaxation of vigilance on the part of certain organs, such as the blood vessels, which become more permeable when these nerves are in control. When asthma occurs, the bronchial tubes are contracted and the air is prevented from escaping, as it should, and does, in normal breathing. When giant hives occur, it is because proper control of the blood vessels has been relaxed and the blood vessels become more permeable, permitting fluid to escape into the tissues.

Illness is a warning given by the brain to the rest of the body of the organism regarding energy disturbances within the energy channels of the organism. Through illness, pain, inflammation, fever, heart attacks, strokes, abnormal growths, tumors and various discomforts, the brain signals the body concerning the possible dangers if the energy disturbances are allowed to continue within the channels. If the symptoms are minor, disturbances are minor. If the symptoms are major, the disturbances are major. Minor disturbances can be removed easily, whereas major disturbances take a long time to resolve.

The brain, through 31 pairs of spinal nerves, operates the best network of communication ever known. Energy disturbances take place in a person's body due to contact with adverse energy of other substances. When two adverse energies come closer, repulsion takes place. When two compatible energies get together, attraction takes place.

The repulsion of energies can take place between two living organisms; for example: between two humans (father and son, doctor and patient, etc.), two siblings, a husband and wife, two friends, a person and a group, an animal and human being, etc. Repulsion can occur between one living organism and one nonliving object, (a human being and fabrics or food); one living organism and energies of different substances (chemicals, work materials, various types of radiation from television, microwave, radio, sun, etc.). It can also occur in one living organism and its actions or reactions (a man and his disturbed emotions).

When a person's energy tries to fight other adverse energies from his/her surroundings at the same time, the person's energy becomes weaker against all other energies. The failure to overcome the attack of adverse energies causes the energy pathways of the weakened body to create blockages toward all the adverse energies around it. As a result, whenever an adverse energy comes near, the energy pathways contract and become blocked. When such a person is surrounded by numerous adverse energies all the time, his/her energy pathways remain blocked all the time. The continuous blockage of the energy pathways causes poor body function. The symptoms resulting from such blockage can be severe in intensity.

NAET can unblock the blockages in the energy pathways and restart normal energy circulation through the energy channels. This will, in turn, help the brain to work and coordinate with the rest of the body to operate the body functions appropriately. When the brain is not coordinating with the vital organs, physiological functions are impaired.

Poor functions of the organs due to lack of energy circulation will create toxic build-up in:

■ The network of the nervous system, causing poor memory, brain fog, brain fatigue, insomnia, hyperactivity, neuralgia, anger, etc.; the respiratory system, giving rise to shortness of breath, sore throat, sinus troubles, cough, asthma, bronchitis, pneumonia, etc.

■ The circulatory system, causing high blood pressure, irregular heartbeat, atherosclerosis, varicose veins, vascular abnormalities, chest pains, heart abnormalities, etc.

■ The gastrointestinal system, leading to lack of absorption of the nutrients, indigestion of all kinds, overweight, underweight, high cholesterol, high triglycerides, diabetes, hypoglycemia, abdominal bloating, abdominal pains, colitis, irritable bowel syndrome, ulcers, constipation, flatulence, fatigue, body aches, etc.

■ The urinary system, causing sluggish kidney function, urinary disturbances, frequent urination, water retention, etc.

■ The reproductive system, leading to poor sexual functions, male infertility, female infertility, prostate problems, endometriosis, premenstrual disorders, menopausal disorders, tumors, cysts, various other inflammatory conditions, etc.

■ The joints, muscles and ligaments, giving rise to various types of arthritis, scleroderma, fibromyalgia, muscle aches, spasms, pains, and joint problems; the skin, causing itching, rashes, hives, eczema, psoriasis, warts, moles, rough skin, etc.

■ The emotional area of each vital organ, causing disturbances in the associated vital organs:

  ◆ *Lung* - grief, sadness, intolerance, low self-esteem

  ◆ *Stomach* - disgust, bitterness, aggressive behaviors, attention deficit disorders, depression, nervousness, obsession

  ◆ *Spleen* - worry, over-thinking, anxiety, shyness, unable to make decisions, easily hurt

  ◆ *Heart* - joy, lack of joy, self-confidence, compassion, guilt, hostility, insecurity

  ◆ *Liver* - anger, rage, aggression, mood swings, depression

  ◆ *Kidney* - fear, confusion

When the circulation in the energy pathways is restored, the vital organs resume their routine work with adequate responsibility. The brain and body together will remove any toxic buildup through the body's natural excretory mechanisms.

When the energy channels are filled with vibrant energy, and the energy circulates through the channels freely, the body is said to be in perfect balance, or in *homeostasis*. When the body is in homeostasis, it can function normally, and allergies and diseases do not affect the body. In this state, the body can absorb all the necessary nutrients from foods consumed.

The energy channels need energy to function normally. This energy is produced from the nutrients consumed, such as vitamins, minerals, sugars, etc. The attraction or repulsion of the *electromagnetic energy field* is created in the body by the interaction of the various charged nutrients inside the body. Each cell is an electricity-generating unit loaded with positively charged potassium and some sodium. Most of the sodium is outside the cell. The sodium and potassium keep circulating in and out of the cell in the presence of water with the help of other nutrients, like proteins and sugars. These charged molecules inside the body make the whole body an electrical unit with an electrical field around it.

Whenever a body becomes imbalanced, allergic manifestations appear. Any number of things may cause an imbalance: a serious accident, a major operation, a childhood disease (whooping cough, chicken pox, etc.), an emotional shock: the loss of loved ones or loss of a job or property, childhood molestation, betrayal, battering, cult victimization, child abuse, etc. It may be that the patient has been repeatedly exposed to particular hypersensitive allergens over a short period and the body's defenses have become exhausted due to overwork.

These symptoms may be more acute at certain times of the year, particularly when pollens, which are more prevalent during specific seasons, cause the allergy. The symptoms may be worse in certain locations and under certain conditions, such as major holidays.

With this understanding, you can look at the relationship between hospitalized patients with acute health problems and the food they consumed before getting sick. Statistics of heart attack victims show that many heart attacks take place after or during elaborate meals such as Thanksgiving, Christmas, New Year's Day, weddings, etc. Until recently, blame for these incidents were placed on emotional triggers. Few individuals connected heart attacks with food allergies.

On emotional and sentimental occasions, an allergic person may go for "one more bite" of any of the available foods. With the first bite of an allergic food, the brain begins to block the energy channels, attempting to prevent the adverse energy of the food from entering deeper into the energy pathways. To accomplish this, the brain calls upon its defensive forces for protection. With the second bite, the rest of the defensive forces go to work to protect the body. The more the allergic food is ingested, the more the body's defense forces are weakened.

When the sympathetic and parasympathetic nerves are not coordinating well, the highly blocked area or the weakest parts of the body fail first. If the lungs are the highly blocked areas of the body, the patient can have an asthmatic attack. If the stomach is the weakest, the person may have acute abdominal pain, or a related migraine headache. Chronic effects of stomach blockages can also affect brain function. A person can demonstrate manic disorders, schizophrenia, depressive disorders, etc.

You can suffer from general body ache, nausea, extreme fatigue, fibromyalgia, etc., if the spleen is weak; and sugar intolerance or absorption problems (hypoglycemia or diabetes) if the pancreas is affected. If your liver is weak, you may suffer from chemical toxicity, fatigue, skin disorders, emotional imbalances, anger, mood swings, depression and premenstrual symptoms. If your kidneys are affected, you may have various types of arthritis, chronic backache, yeast type infections, frequent urination and become fearful all the time. You may suffer from eye infections if the bladder is affected, and latent asthma, knee pains, constipation, overweight problems and low-backache if the colon is affected.

If the heart is affected, you can experience cardiac symptoms. Follow the heart attack victim further. When he/she has a heart attack, the victim may stay alive until help arrives if only a small amount of the allergen has been consumed. When the paramedics arrive, if the victim is not sensitive to the emergency drugs they inject, the heart attack victim will continue to breathe and function. In the cardiac unit, the victim will be given complete rest from physical activities by being kept in bed. He/she will get rest from emotional activities by *sedation,* and rest from the ingestion of food allergens by abstinence from mouth feeding. In 48 to 72 hours, the allergic food will have had a chance to clear the body, the heart will begin to beat normally once again, and the patient will be labeled as stabilized.

On the other hand, if the victim was allergic to all or part of the drugs he/she received, the pain or symptoms may very well become progressively worse, and the heart will eventually stop functioning. In this case, the last report will say: "In spite of all revival attempts, the patient expired."

BENEFITS

Wouldn't it be wonderful if allergy sufferers could be taught a simple test, which could detect and predetermine the potentially harmful reactions between substances and people before the adverse electromagnetic energies create havoc in their systems, bringing on ill health and unhappiness?

You are now able to do just that. You can manipulate your brain and nervous systems as you desire and for your benefit using Oriental medical principles. You can reprogram your brain to accept incompatible energies as suitable ones and use them for your own benefit, rather than allow them to cause energy blockages and imbalances, and finally diseases. It is not necessary to stay away from certain food items that you like or throw away your favorite clothes because they make you sick. You do not have to hide indoors during the pollen season or spend the rest of your days in metropolitan areas instead of vacationing in the mountains because of your fear of poison oak and mosquitoes. You do not have to look pale, sick, and aged instead of using the latest cosmetic products that would make you look at least 20 years younger because of your fear of skin rashes and hives. You do not have to hide from sunny beaches for fear of skin problems and skin cancers. You do not have to end up in divorce court a month after your marriage that you thought would last forever. You could even avoid seeing your teenagers using drugs and alcohol, some even ultimately ending up in suicides, if you are able to uncover the problems in time, before they take over their lives.

Our psychiatric hospitals might be empty if the causes of the psychiatric patients' energy blockages could be found and removed. Our county jails would not be packed if inmates' emotional allergies were tested and treated. Heart attacks and other tragic deaths due to cancer and other incurable diseases might be prevented if everyone in the world could be taught to find their suitable electromagnetic fields, stick to them, and avoid unsuitable energies from a very early age. NAET could be used to change the unsuitable energies into suitable ones. If everyone learned and practiced these techniques from childhood on, it might be possible to stop many disease processes, perhaps even delay the aging process.

Now NAET treatments are available to the whole world. It is up to the health professionals to learn them and use them on their patients.

Doctors of allopathic, chiropractic, osteopathy, dentistry, naturopathy and acupuncture/Oriental medicine from all over the United States, Canada, Europe, Australia, Asia and other countries, have been trained to treat their patients with this new, revolutionary technique. Regular training sessions are conducted several times a year to prepare many more licensed medical professionals to meet the challenge. This book will teach you to test yourself and locate the cause of your problem. Steps of treatments are not given here, because that is beyond the scope of this book. NAET training is limited to actively licensed medical practitioners only. The information about the training seminars is available from the following sources:

NAET Seminars

6714 Beach Blvd.
Buena Park, CA 90621
Tel: 1-714-523-0800/Fax: 1-714-523-3068

E-mail: naet@earthlink.net
website: naet.com

CHAPTER 2

CATEGORIES OF ALLERGENS

Y ou can be allergic to anything: foods, drinks, prescription drugs, over-the-counter drugs, illicit drugs, herbs, vitamins, tap water, purified water, rain water, clothing, jewelry, ice, cold, heat, wind, work materials, your own body secretions, body organs, chemicals, formaldehyde, building materials (sick building syndrome), paints, pressed wood, naturally seen plant enzymes (terpenes or phenolics, aldehydes, acetaldehydes, synthetically made additives), silica, silicone, latex, plastics, synthetic fibers and products, pollens, grasses, trees, wood and wood work, etc. Undiagnosed allergies can produce symptoms, illnesses, and even chronic diseases. You may suffer from: asthma, emphysema, chronic lung disorders, addictions (to alcohol, caffeine, drugs, tobacco, sugars, carbohydrates, fats), arthritis, candida, yeast problems, parasitic infestation, chronic fatigue, immune disorders, tumors, cancer, premenstrual disorders (PMS), menopausal disorders, hormonal imbalances, infertility, eye disorders, ear troubles, upper respiratory complications, sinus troubles, chronic infections, inflammatory conditions, fibromyalgia, other unexplained pain disorders, prostate troubles, migraines, headaches, pediatric problems, ear infections, attention deficit disorders, autism, hyperactivity, mental disorders, anxiety, depression, digestive disorders, circulatory disorders, sleep irregularity, chemical sensitivity, nutritional disorders, restless leg syndrome, skin ailments, genito-urinary disorders, and various emotional imbalances, etc.

By learning the simple Nambudripad's Testing Technique (NTT), anyone, professional or public, can easily learn to recognize various allergens and the health conditions they cause. This will help the sufferer begin to seek the appropriate diagnostic studies and pursue proper health care as needed. When the patient's diagnosis is correct, results are less frightening than an uncertain explanation.

Science and technology have altered the life-style of mankind enormously. The reactions and diseases arising from responses to these changes are also very different. Our quality of life has improved from these scientific achievements; yet, these same scientific accomplishments have become everlasting nightmares for some allergic patients.

Technology is becoming more pervasive over time. It will always be with us. But allergic patients must find ways to overcome adverse reactions to new chemicals and other allergens created by the new technology they are exposed to. Even though it requires a series of detailed treatments, NAET offers the prospect of relief to people who suffer from constant allergic reactions and "incurable" diseases.

Various allergic reactions can be grouped according to the clinical manifestations of the person with allergies.

1.   **People suffering from food allergies:**
      They have no seasonal symptoms, but suffer from varying numbers of unusual or unpleasant physical, physiological or emotional symptoms whenever they eat a food item to which they are sensitive (for example, eggs, milk, fruits, wheat, sugar, raisins, fish, oils, fats, spices, nuts, etc.).

2.   **People suffering from chemical allergies through external sources:**
      They have no unusual symptoms if they do not come in contact with any chemicals. They can be happy and healthy when they live in a natural environment surrounded by natural life, eating organically grown, unprocessed food. But, whenever they come near or in contact with any chemicals they are sensitive to, they suffer from a varying number of unusual or unpleasant physical, physiological, or emotional symptoms.

Chemicals from city water, synthetic fabrics, fabric softeners, detergents, hair products, pesticides, fungicides, herbicides, food grown with artificial fertilizers, prescription drugs (antibiotics, pain relieving medication), vitamins, herbal supplements, massage oils, insect bites, cleansing agents, formaldehyde, cosmetic products, personal protective equipment (latex gloves, masks), hospital supplies (oxygen tubes, rubber or plastic catheters, surgical instruments, surgical sutures, hospital cleaning agents, disinfectants, anesthetics, drugs), dental materials and equipment, food additives, artificial food coloring, newspaper inks, paper products, hydrocarbons, perfumes, gasoline, exhausts, tobacco smoke, plastic products, light and radiation from different sources, etc., can cause allergic reactions.

3.   **People suffering from chemical allergies from internal sources:**
This group of people react to their own body secretions (sweat, urine, feces, mucous, semen, tears and saliva), body parts (hair and nails), different organs (stomach, spleen, lungs, kidney, liver, heart, brain, etc.). The body's defense mechanism is derailed, and the body makes antibodies against its own tissues and/or fluids. The immune system attacks the body that it inhabits, which eventually causes damage or alteration to its own cells, tissues, organs and functions. Such damage results in cancer, abnormal tissue growths and tumors, kidney failure, organ failure, hearing loss, poor vision, heart attacks, liver failure, cataract, adrenal depletion, diabetes, thyroid malfunctions, etc.

4.   **People suffering from pollen and natural environmental allergies:**
These people have frequent tearing from the eyes, sneeze, wheeze, have asthma and other upper respiratory disturbances, suffer from fatigue, irritability and hay-fever symptoms during pollen season (pollens from weeds, trees, flowers and grasses), allergic to cotton, natural materials, but feel reasonably well for the rest of the year if they avoid natur and products made from natural substances.

5.   **People suffering from only environmental allergies:**
This group suffers from allergies to all the chemical factors, pesticides, and environmental substances like pollens, grasses, weeds, wood, tree,

flowers, sand, precious stones, dirt, dust and insects, etc. They do not react to nutrients or to food without chemicals. They can eat organic foods without any chemical involvement. But if the food is prepared in plastic containers, or if any food coloring or additive containing unnatural items is present, they have allergic reactions. As long as they wear or use 100% cotton, silk or any natural fabrics, they function well. If they use any synthetic materials like polyester, acrylic or other such materials, they become nonfunctional.

6. **People suffering from allergies to animals and other humans:**
    These people have no allergies to food, drinks or the materials around them. They react to the electromagnetic energy of other living beings, which makes them allergic to other human beings, like their mother, father, spouse, brother, sister, children, partners, employee and employer. They can also have allergies to pets, cats, dogs, insects, bees, ants, etc.

7. **People with emotional allergies:**
    The people in this group have allergies to actions and interactions of everyday life: thoughts or feelings (fear, anger, self-esteem, creativity, power, self-worth, inferiority, superiority, etc.); concepts: ("I can never get healthy," "I can never lose weight," or "I can never make enough money," etc.); a memory of a certain incidence: (nightmares, fear or anxiety while driving due to a memory of a highway auto accident that happened 10 years ago); emotions, like hating jobs or obsessions with careers (teaching, acting, cooking, gardening, writing, etc.), and interactions (fighting with co-workers, classmates, boss or teachers). Some people enjoy going against rules and regulations, acting against the norm in situations or disobeying authorities (running red lights when the police are not watching, etc.).

8. **People with combination allergies:**
    This group of people reacts to what seems to be an infinite number of combinations of food, pollens, chemicals, other humans, animals, thoughts, memories and concepts.

9. **People who are universal reactors:**

This group has multiple chemical sensitivities and suffers from severe reactions to all of the above allergens. These people suffer from severe allergies, sensitivities, and many other health problems. They are grouped as ecologically and environmentally ill. Ecological illness is the result of adverse reactions to substances in the air, water, food, living environment, work environments, and chemicals. They do not feel safe anywhere. They can suffer from varied, chronic symptoms of any and every organ or system of the body. These are the people who would be better off living in a protective "bubble."

CATEGORIES OF ALLERGENS

Common allergens are generally classified into nine basic categories, based primarily on the method in which they are contacted, rather than the symptoms they produce.

1. Inhalants
2. Ingestants
3. Contactants
4. Injectants
5. Infectants
6. Physical agents
7. Genetic factors
8. Molds and fungi
9. Emotional stressors

INHALANTS

Inhalants are those allergens that are contacted through the nose, throat and bronchial tubes. Examples of inhalants are microscopic spores of certain grasses, flowers, pollens, powders, smoke, cosmetics, perfumes, different aromas from spices, coffee, popcorn, food-cooking smells, different herbs, oils, chemical fumes, paint, varnish, pesticides, insecticides, fertilizers, flour from grains, etc.

It is difficult to say that there is a typical or predictable allergic reaction in response to a given allergen. However, if there is a predictable response, it is in this general category of inhalants that it comes closest to being found.

Most of us have suffered discomfort from accidentally breathing a toxic substance. For example, when we smell chlorine gas from a bottle of common household bleach, our immediate reaction makes our eyes water, noses run, and breathing can become difficult as our bronchial tubes go into spasm. This experiment can be duplicated repeatedly if we wanted proof that bleach is directly responsible for the given set of reactions. Of course, most of us learn very quickly that it is the bleach that caused our discomfort, and learn not to breathe deeply when near it.

The cause of the discomfort was very closely associated with the reactions to the bleach, the burning eyes, runny nose, and restricted breathing. In this case, a simple scientific deduction can be drawn from this cause-and-effect relationship. A correct diagnosis based on a similar cause-and-effect relationship is not always this easy. For example, it was more difficult to diagnose one of my patients as being allergic to olive pollen because the reaction had a delayed effect. The time lapse makes the causal link less obvious.

Consider how much more difficult it is to make a proper diagnosis when the patient's physical responses to a given allergen differ radically from those that would normally be anticipated. For instance, there was the case of a man in his early 60's who came to my office, nearly incapacitated by lapses of memory and seizures that resembled some form of epilepsy, Alzheimer's disease or perhaps a mild stroke. He often wandered off in total confusion or complete amnesia, sometimes losing track of significant blocks of time.

Neurological examination and a CAT scan showed his brain-wave pattern to be completely normal. After considerable detective work, the cause in this case turned out to be the airborne spores of a fern tree he had recently planted in his backyard. His atypical reaction to the inhalant was totally illogical physiologically. In his case, diagnosis and treatment was delayed for several months because of the lack of respiratory distress seen in other patients who suffer sensitivities to inhalants. This added frustration and potential danger for the patient.

This clearly points out that there are no typical responses to allergens in the real world. If you are depending on allergies to produce a uniform set of responses for all people, you may misdiagnose and provide the wrong treatment. You cannot duplicate and package a standard medication as an antidote for any specific allergy—each individual case is different. Treatment of patients must not be oversimplified. Not everyone exhibits typical allergic symptoms (whatever you perceive "typical" to be). Should you do so, you risk missing a myriad of potential reactions that may be produced in some people in response to their contact with substances that are, for them, allergens.

INGESTANTS

Ingestants are allergens which are contacted through the mouth and thus find their way into the gastrointestinal tract. These include foods, condiments, drugs, beverages, chewing gum, vitamin supplements, etc. We must not ignore the potential reactions to things that are touched, then inadvertently transmitted into the mouth through our hands.

The area of ingested allergens is one of the most difficult to diagnose because the allergic responses are often delayed from several minutes to several days. This makes the direct association between cause and effect very difficult. Some people can react violently in seconds after they consume an allergen. In extreme cases, one has only to touch or come near the allergen to forewarn the central nervous system that it is about to be poisoned, resulting in the premature allergic reaction. Usually more violent reactions are observed in ingested allergens than in any other forms.

Such was the case of Steve, a young man in his early teens, who came to my office for a sports-related injury. He also had a history of asthma. On one occasion his mother brought attention to the fact that her son had continuous itching in an area four finger widths below the knee, on the outer side of the anterior tibial crest. The itching was on the stomach meridian, which meant that the cause of the allergic rash was related to something he was eating. After further questioning, it was found that he broke out in a rash whenever he ate his favorite breakfast cereal.

We set up a simple experiment to confirm it. One by one, Steve was given all his regular breakfast items: juice, toast and rice cereal. Then he was given time to chew. All went well until he placed one, and only one, rice cereal flake in his mouth. He immediately complained of feeling hot and began to redden in an allergic rash; and in a few more seconds, he had almost slipped into an anaphylactic shock. After several tense minutes and continuous treatment by NAET, his symptoms subsided.

Literally, any substance you eat can be an allergen for someone. For instance, people have been known to faint every time they eat an orange without exhibiting any other food allergies. By avoiding the allergen, they can prevent the occurrence of unnecessary allergic reaction. However, one should keep in mind that in minor allergy cases, untreated patients tend to manifest allergic symptoms to other similar allergens. For example, a patient who faints when she eats an orange might develop asthma or migraine headaches when she eats a banana at a later date.

Stephy, a 35-year-old female, was able to identify oranges as the one and only allergen that affected her. She complained that she was developing additional allergies to foods such as bananas, grape juice and squash. During routine testing for allergies, it was discovered that an element found in fairly high concentration in oranges, was potassium. Because she had let the orange allergy go untreated, the potassium was untreated. Because the potassium was untreated, she began to react to other foods that contained potassium even though there was a lower concentration in these foods.

She is really fortunate that she did not run into a recipe that called for a large amount of cream of tartar. This food additive is commonly used as a stiffener in meringue for pies and candies and is potassium bitartrate.

We live in a highly technological age. New substances are being introduced to preserve color, flavor and extend the shelf life of foods. There are some additives used in foods as preservatives that have caused severe health problems. Some artificial sweeteners cause mysterious problems in particular people. They may mimic various serious diseases such as multiple sclerosis, acute prostatitis, trigeminal neuralgia, hyperactivity, fibromyalgia, attention deficit disorder, autism, ear infections, cardiac arrhythmia, skin problems, itching, hives, insomnia, vertigo, chronic dry cough, joint pains and sciatica, to name a few. The majority of these additives are harmless to most people, but can be fatal to those who react to these substances.

Statistics show that most sports injuries take place after food breaks or lunch periods. It is better to consume simple foods during sports sessions to avoid injuries. As you can see, great care must be taken to know exactly what is contained in each and every thing a person with allergies puts into his/her mouth.

If the allergic person could become proficient in MRT, the simple testing for energy compatibility before buying, preparing and eating foods, most hazardous reactions from food allergies could be prevented.

CONTACTANTS

Contactants produce their effect by direct contact with the skin. They include the well-known poison oak, poison ivy, poison sumac, cats, dogs, rabbits, cosmetics, soaps, skin creams, detergents, rubbing alcohol, latex gloves, hair dyes, various types of plant oils, chemicals such as gasoline, dyes, acrylic nails, nail polish, fabrics, formaldehyde, etc.

Allergic reactions to contactants can be different in each person, and may include asthma, skin rashes, hives, fainting spells, migraine headaches, coughing, joint pains, various kinds of arthritis, stomach aches, constipation, mental confusion, swelling of the body, frequent urination, mental irritability, insomnia, skin cancer, etc. An allergen contacted by the skin can produce symptoms as devastating to the patient as anything ingested or inhaled.

Natural or unnatural fabrics can also cause allergic reactions. Many people react to cotton. Cotton is used in numerous items. It is not easy to find one kind of material anymore. Many products seen in the market are a blend of many things. Cotton fibers are used in carpets, elastics, bed sheets, fleece material, cosmetic applicators, toilet paper, paper towels, etc. Wool may also cause allergies. We have seen people who cannot wear wool without breaking out in a rash. Some people who are sensitive to wool also react to creams with a lanolin base since lanolin is derived from sheep wool. Cotton, nylon or woolen socks can cause allergic reactions with symptoms of knee pain, etc. People can also be allergic to carpets and drapes, which can cause knee pains, joint pains, and pain in the sole and heel of the foot.

We had a few female patients who were allergic to their pantyhose and suffered from leg cramps, swollen legs, psoriasis, persistent yeast infections, and, in some cases, high blood pressure. Toilet paper and paper towels also cause problems, mimicking yeast infections in many people.

Many people are allergic to crude oils and their derivatives, which include plastic and synthetic rubber products as well as latex products. Can you imagine the troublesome difficulty of living life in this modern society, attempting to be completely free from products made of crude oil? You would literally be immobilized. The phones you use, the milk containers you drink from, the polyester fabrics you wear, most of the face and body creams you use…all are made from a common source—crude oil!

Kathy, one of the secretaries in our office, was attending a computer demonstration when she complained of feeling discomfort and heat sensation all over her body. She was working at the computer keyboard. Instantly, she began having blisters on her lips, rashes on her face and a sensation of lightheadedness. We found that the keyboard material (plastic) was the root of the problem. She was treated to overcome the special plastic keyboard allergy and sent home. The next day when she returned to work, she felt fine and has since worked on that computer keyboard without any further ill effects.

Food items normally classified as ingestants may also act as a contactant on persons who handle them constantly over time. Mike, a 59-year-old male baker, came in with severe skin rashes and itching of both hands and arms below the elbow. Cortisone cream kept his itching and weeping ulcers under control. He worked four days a week, Thursday through Sunday. By Sunday, his skin became raw and weeping. The next three days he used a cortisone cream, and by Thursday his skin looked better. This had been going on for 27 years when he came to us to be evaluated. He was found to be highly allergic to wheat flour, a substance he came in contact with all day—every day—as a baker. The itching and rashes on his hands cleared up after treating with NAET for wheat. Seven years later, he still remains symptom free.

Other career-produced allergies have been diagnosed in cooks, waiters, grocery-store keepers, clerks, gardeners, etc. Virtually no trade or skill is exempt from contracting allergens.

A writer by profession, Pete was completely disabled when he was diagnosed as having carpal tunnel syndrome. Pete was given an NAET treatment before he went for the scheduled surgery to free the pinched median nerve (the nerve that usually gets irritated in carpal tunnel syndrome). He was simply allergic to the paper he wrote on. Soon after he was treated by NAET, his carpal tunnel syndrome cleared up without the surgery. His carpal tunnel symptoms have never returned in the past nine years.

Another case of a paper allergy was observed during an interview with an attorney who complained that he always came away from his office with a headache. Drained of energy, he could only go home and immediately go to bed. This attorney was allergic to paper—but with a completely different reaction from that of the professional writer.

INJECTANTS

Allergens are injected into the skin, muscles, joints and blood vessels in the form of various serums, antitoxins, vaccines, childhood immunizations, and drugs. Injectants also include substances entering the body through insect bites. As with any other allergic reaction, the injection of a sensitive drug into the system creates the risk of producing dangerous allergic reactions. To the sensitive person, the drug actively becomes a poison with the same effect as an injection of arsenic. The seemingly harmless substance can become more allergenic for certain people over time without the person being aware of the potential risk. For example, take the increasing number of incidents of allergies to the drug penicillin. The reactions vary from hives to diarrhea to anaphylactic shock and death.

Such is the unique case of Anne, a 38-year-old female who manifested tremendous allergic reactions to a multitude of foods and objects in the environment. Her history revealed that when she was a year old, she suffered a severe reaction after a routine smallpox vaccination and almost died. For many years she suffered physical allergies such as asthma, hives, joint pains and migraines; gastrointestinal allergies such as indigestion, heartburn, intermittent chronic diarrhea or constipation; and emotional reactions such as depression, anger, crying spells, lack of interest in day-to-day   activities; and severe premenstrual syndrome, etc. When she was treated for smallpox vaccination by NAET, she was able to clear her allergic reactions to various items. Her physical, physiological and emotional symptoms improved and stabilized swiftly after the treatment.

Most of us do not consider an insect bite similar to an injection received from a physician—but the action is quite the same. At the point of the bite, a minute amount of the body fluid from the insect is injected into the body. These fluids may be incidental to the bite. They may be simply secretions normal to the salivary gland of the insect, or they may be a necessary part of the biting mechanism, such as the saliva of the mosquito, which is formulated to keep the host's blood from coagulating so blood extraction is not difficult.

This fluid may be specifically formulated to produce immobilizing pain, for either an offensive tactic or protective mechanism. An insect bites to secure food and inflict pain to defend its territory; the bee uses its sting for defense, while the scorpion employs its sting to obtain food.

Certain animal bites can also inject near-lethal toxins into the bloodstream of victims; the toxins are designed to protect the animal from its own predators or accidental harm from a clumsy neighbor. Examples include vipers and particular lizards as well as a number of fish and crustaceans that are capable of imposing painful stings or puncture-delivered poisons from their sharp spines and/or spinelike fins. Bites from mammals also fit into this category. They include children's bites, which can produce considerable infection at the site, and the injection of dreaded viruses from the bite of an infected animal.

The normal reaction to bites, other than the obvious lethal bites, include mild swelling and reddening around the site of the injection and, of course, a slight to moderate discomfort in the body from attempting to free the toxin that produces the itching. Rarely are these bites and stings lethal to a person of normal sensitivity.

However, for some people, a sting or a bite by an animal or insect is potentially lethal. Even a single mosquito bite may produce an extreme and sudden onset of edema (the abnormal collection of fluids in the body tissue and cells) and severe respiratory distress. There have been many cases of anaphylactic shock, respiratory and/or cardiac failure in sensitive persons following the slightest insect bite.

Many carcinomas result from various type(s) of allergies; if you could trace the specific allergen triggering the activity of a particular carcinoma, the allergen could be desensitized and many precious lives could be saved from the clutches of cancer. Same goes with other diseases arising from allergies as well. Good detective work is essential to find the basic root of the problem.

INFECTANTS

Infectants are allergens that produce their effect by causing a sensitivity to an infectious agent, such as bacteria. For example, an allergic reaction may result when tuberculin bacterium is introduced as part of a diagnostic test to determine a patient's sensitivity or reaction to it. A typical reaction to the tuberculin test may be seen as an infectious eruption under the skin. This type of reaction may occur with a skin patch, or scratch tests, performed in the normal course of allergy testing in the traditional western medical approach.

An infectant is a substance that is a known injectant and is limited in the amount administered to the patient. A slight prick of the skin introduces the toxin through the epidermis (as in vaccination) and a pox or similar harmless skin lesion will erupt if the patient is allergic to that substance. For most people, the pox soon dries up and forms a scab that eventually heals, without much discomfort. However, in some cases the site of the injectant becomes infected and the usual inflammatory process can be seen (redness, swelling, pain, drainage of pus from the site) for many days. Some sensitive individuals may experience fainting, nausea, fever, swelling (not only at the scratch site but also over the whole body), respiratory distress, etc., if left untreated.

In other words, the introduction of an allergen into a reactive person's system creates the potential risk of causing a severe response regardless of the amount of the toxic substance used. Great care must be taken in the administration of traditional allergy testing procedures in highly sensitive individuals. However, if NAET is administered correctly and immediately, it can stop such adverse reactions.

Various vaccinations and immunizations may also produce such allergic reactions. After receiving their usual immunizations, some children become extremely ill physically, physiologically and emotionally. Various neurological disorders, hyperactive disorders, attention deficit disorders, autism, mental retardation, manic disorders, Crohn's disease, chronic irritable bowel syndrome, tumors, cysts, etc., could manifest as a delayed reaction of a childhood immunization.

A 42-year-old man suffered from chronic irritable bowel syndrome since he was 9 years old. After all of his basic allergies were treated, he was evaluated and tested through NTT. His problem was traced down to a polio vaccine that he had received as an infant. Immediately, he was treated for polio vaccine. He had severe abdominal pains and watery stools for two weeks following the initial NAET treatment. During this time, he had to repeat the treatment for polio vaccine six times. When he finally completed the treatments, he said good-bye to his irritable bowel syndrome.

Carol, a 46-year-old woman, had complained of severe sinusitis for 28 years. Her history showed that she was admitted to a hospital when she was 18 years old and given a cortisone injection. She had a severe reaction to the cortisone injection that she received and went into a cardiac shock. It took hours before she recovered from that episode. When she returned home from the hospital, she began experiencing severe sinusitis and continued to do so for the next 28 years. When she successfully completed the treatment for cortisone in our office, she said good-bye to her 28-year-old sinusitis.

It should be noted that bacteria and virus are contacted in numerous ways. Casual contact with objects and people exposes you daily to dangerous contaminants and possible illnesses. When your immune system is functioning properly, you pass off the illness without notice. When your system is not working at maximum performance levels, you may begin to experience infections, fevers, and allergies.

From a strictly allergenic standpoint, however, contact with an injectant does not always produce the expected reaction. The intensity and type of reactions vary from individual to individual, depending on their immune system, age and the amount of injectant received. Usually, a typical reaction takes place in a specific individual as we saw in the tuberculin test. It is clear that the reaction to the test was not a case of tuberculosis, but rather a mild allergic response that resulted in an infectious eruption under the skin.

PHYSICAL AGENTS
Sensitive people can react to various physical agents:

■ Heat, humidity, cold, cold mist, dampness, drafts, dryness, heating and air conditioning, changes in barometric pressure and high altitude.

■ Radiation from the sun, computers, microwave ovens, X-rays, geopathic sources, electrical and electromagnetic fields, fluorescent lights, cellular and cordless telephones and power lines. Burns may also be included in this category.

■ Mechanical irritants like vibrations from a washer, dryer, hair dryer, electric shaver, electric massager, house alarm; sirens from fire engines, police vehicles and ambulances, etc. Motion vibrations from a moving automobile, motion sickness (car sickness, sea sickness), sickness while playing sports, roller coaster rides and/or horseback riding can also act as mechanical irritants. Airplane sounds, traffic noises, loud music and voices in a particular pitch may also cause allergic reactions.

■ Different colors (red, white, blue, black, etc.). Colored fabrics, household objects (toothbrush, hair brush, plastic cups or plates), toys, books, coloring books, just about anything in colors can be reactants.

When you suffer from more than one allergy, physical agents can affect you immensely. For example, if a woman wore a blue outfit, which she was allergic to (blue affects the lung meridian), had already eaten an allergic food—a cinnamon roll (cinnamon, a spice, affects the lung meridian), and then walked in the cold air (cold affects the lung meridian) with her boyfriend who often argued with her (sadness affects lung meridian), she might develop upper respiratory problems like a sore throat, cough, bronchitis, or even asthma by the time they reach their destination.

Although it is rare, some people are very sensitive to cold or heat whether or not they have eaten anything allergic. One of the young patients who came to our office had a history of canker sores whenever he walked in the sun. He turned out to be highly allergic to vitamin D (one of the vitamins produced in the body with the help of sunlight). After he was treated by NAET for vitamin D, the incidence of canker sores after exposure to the sun diminished.

Contrary to what people might think, the causative factor for skin cancer may not only be overexposure to the sun, but may also be due to allergies to suntan lotions, skin creams, shaving creams, razor blades (stainless steel), clothing or other allergenic products. Continuous use of these products could cause skin irritation, leaving it more susceptible to skin cancer.

Many patients' symptoms of arthritic pain, asthma, migraine, PMS, and mental disorders become exaggerated on cold, cloudy or rainy days. These patients could suffer from severe allergy to electrolytes, cold or a combination of both. Some people, especially people who suffer from mental imbalances, also react to moonlight or moon radiation.

Some patients with respiratory problems (such as asthma or emphysema) experience breathing difficulties when taking a hot shower, or visiting humid places like Hawaii or the Caribbean Islands. People can also react to high altitude, low altitude, wind, dampness, dryness, rainwater. Hypertension and asthma are the two major health problems we see among islanders. This may be due to an allergy to salt, which is unavoidable when one lives near the ocean. Even if one avoided the salt intake, breathing the salty air or being in the magnetic field of salt for a number of years is enough to cause these problems. Some patients react to heat or cold violently, suffering aches and pains during a cloudy day or experiencing icy cold hands and feet even if they are clad in mittens and warm socks. All of these problems can be treated successfully with NAET.

Exercise-induced asthma, migraines, anaphylaxis and death are seen more frequently since people are getting more and involved with fitness programs around the country. Endorphins and enkephalins are produced in large amounts during exercise. These are the brain enzymes that give a sense of well-being. It is possible for you to be allergic to your own endorphin and other hormones. People who get anaphylaxis during exercise may be allergic to their own endorphins. They should first get treated with NAET for their hormones and exercise motions before they begin a vigorous exercise program.

Yoga exercises are gentle, and can be practiced by anybody, weak or strong. These are specific exercises practiced to strengthen weak vital organs. Very weak patients should begin with one or two Yoga exercises until they are strong enough to add more into their schedule. Exercise is a good way to expel toxins from specific organs, to reduce stress and to bring overall calmness. Yoga shouldn't be practiced without proper knowledge or guidance. People with reactions to aerobics or other type of exercises should look into learning Yoga. It is taught in schools and universities. There are many Yoga centers around the country. Please find one near you and learn the exercises properly from a teacher.

GENETIC FACTORS

Discovery of possible tendencies toward allergies carried over from parents and grandparents opens a large door to achieving optimum health. Most people inherit the allergic tendency from their parents or grandparents. Allergies may also skip generations or can be manifested differently in parents and their children.

Polly, a 35-year-old female, had suffered from various allergies since she was an infant. When she was three weeks old, she broke out in a rash, which transformed into big heat boils and pustules. Her parents tried various medications in attempts to cure her, including allopathy, homeopathy and herbal medicines. Finally, herbal medicine brought the problem somewhat under control. Even with the herbal treatment, she still occasionally suffered from outbreaks of skin lesions. When Polly was ten years old, she developed a type of severe, debilitating arthritis that persisted until she was in her late teens. She then developed migraine headaches and severe insomnia along with the arthritis. She tried various medicines from different doctors without much relief.

After evaluation, she was found to be reacting to malaria parasites. It was discovered that both her parents were malaria victims before she was born. The effect of malaria from her parents transferred to her and was manifested in her body in the form of skin and joint problems. After she was treated successfully with NAET for malaria, her health took a quantum leap. She was freed of migraines and arthritis after she was treated for malaria parasites. After 13 years, she still remains symptom-free.

Many people with various allergic manifestations respond well to the treatment of various agents that cause hereditary diseases. A woman who suffered from bronchial asthma was cleared of her asthma following her treatment for pneumococcus, (the bacterium responsible for pneumonia). Both her parents had died of pneumonia soon after her birth.

Parents who have had rheumatic fever may transmit the disease to their offspring, but in the children the causative agent for rheumatic fever may not be manifested in its original form.

Carcinomas can also be a result of various allergies, sometimes as offshoots of inherited allergies from parents or as an allergy acquired from one's own life-style. Various chemical agents around us are carcinogenic, but in cases of diagnosed cancer it is better to check out all the possibilities of genetically transmitted allergenic offshoots if the cancer does not respond to western traditional treatment.

MOLDS AND FUNGI

Molds and fungi are in a category by themselves because of the numerous avenues through which they can come into contact with people in everyday life. They can be ingested, inhaled, touched, or even injected as in the case of penicillin. They can also come in the form of airborne spores, making up a large part of the dust we breathe or pick up in our vacuum cleaners; in fluids such as our drinking water; and the dark fungal growth in the corners of damp rooms. They can appear on the body as athlete's foot and in particularly fetid vaginal conditions, commonly called "yeast infections." Molds and fungi, which also grow on trees and in damp soil, are a source of food (truffles and mushrooms), disease (ringworm and the aforementioned yeast infections) and even of medicine (penicillin).

Reactions to these substances are as varied as the reactions to other kinds of allergies because they are a part of one of the largest known classifications of biological entities. The number of reactions is multiplied considerably because of the number of ways they can be introduced into the human anatomy.

Fungi are parasites that grow on both living and decaying organic matter, including some forms which grow in the human anatomy. Athlete's foot is a prime example; it is a human parasite fungus that grows anywhere in the body that is fairly moist and unexposed to sunlight or air. It is particularly difficult to eliminate, even with attentive treatment consisting of a topical preparation, multiple daily cleansing of the area, a medicinal powder, and wearing light cotton socks to avoid further infection from dyes in the material.

Athlete's foot is contacted from person to person from anywhere there is high potential for contact with the fungus: gymnasium, shower, locker rooms and other areas where people share facilities or walk barefoot. If it is a real case of athlete's foot, it will clear with NAET treatment, but certain allergies, like reactions to socks made of cotton, Orlon, or nylon, etc., can mimic athlete's foot. In such cases, you should treat for fabrics like cotton, nylon, polyester, wool, etc., to clear the symptoms. In these instances, athlete's foot may not respond to medications.

Mike, a 31-year-old man, came to the clinic for treatment of athlete's foot. In the interview he disclosed that he has suffered from athlete's foot for years. He was unsuccessful to help his feet using numerous treatments that he had tried for years. The infection was not only distracting and painful, but was also destroying his toenails. The problem was increasing to the point that it started to interfere with his passion for tennis. During allergy testing, it was discovered that he was allergic to the cotton in his socks. He also mentioned that he dried his feet with cotton towels. After treatment for cotton, his athlete's foot cleared up.

Allergies to cotton, orlon, nylon, or paper could result in the explosion of infections, including Ascomycetes fungi (yeast) that women find so troublesome. Allergies to feminine tampons, toilet papers, douches, and deodorants also cause yeast-like infections. One of the patients reacted to everything she ate from her freezer. More investigation proved that she was allergic to the fungus and molds found in the freezer.

Another patient complained of frequent angina pain, sinus problems, arrhythmia, frequent eye inflammation, etc., which were completely relieved after treating for fungus. Although the cause wasn't frozen foods, she contracted it from a source that was equally unrelated—her dog. Her dog was suffering from some unknown, fungus-related skin problem. In this case, the dog was also treated for fungus. Both the dog and his owner's skin problem improved.

One patient knew that she had a reaction to elm trees since childhood. While she was treated for elm trees, her condition worsened. Huge hives broke out all over her body. She needed repeated treatments for elm trees for a full week. By the end of one week, not only had her skin cleared up, but most of her other allergies were greatly diminished as well.

EMOTIONAL STRESSORS

Many times, the origin of physical symptoms can be traced back to some unresolved emotional trauma. Each cell in the body (meridians) has the capability to respond physically, physiologically and psychologically to our daily activities. When the vital energy flows evenly and uninterrupted through the energy pathways (acupuncture meridians), the body functions normally. When there is a disruption in the energy flow through the meridians (an increase or decrease), energy blockages can occur, causing various emotional symptoms in those particular meridians. According to Oriental medical theory, there are seven major emotions that can cause pathological health problems in people: sadness (lung), joy (heart), disgust (stomach), anger (liver), worry (spleen), fear (kidney), depression (pericardium).

For example, a 65-year-old man who struggled financially his entire life bought one California lottery ticket. After hearing the winning numbers in the newscast, his granddaughter announced that he had the winning ticket worth 87 million dollars. The man couldn't believe it. He stood up from his chair, took his ticket out of his pocket and matched the numbers that his granddaughter had written down on a paper. When he realized that he had won the lottery, overwhelmed with joy, he fell back into his chair holding on to the winning ticket, staring wide-eyed. Those eyes never closed again. A sudden surge of excess energy flowed into the heart meridian and caused his heart to stop.

More explanation on emotional stressors can be found in Chapter 18, Allergy and the Body, Mind and Spirit.

CHAPTER 3

DIAGNOSIS OF ALLERGIES

Allergic conditions occur much more frequently than most people realize. Every year there are more and more recognized cases of allergies in the United States. Statistics show that at least 50 percent of the population suffers from more or less acute forms of allergy. Most people are interested in understanding the differences and/or the similarities of the methods of diagnosis, the effectiveness and length of treatment between traditional western medicine and Oriental medicine. Since the purpose of this book is to provide information about the new treatment method of NAET, more attention will be given to Oriental medicine.

With NAET, it is extremely important for the patient to cooperate with the physician in order to obtain the best results. It is my hope that this chapter will help bring about a clearer understanding between allergists and their patients because, in order to obtain the most satisfactory results, both parties must work together as a team.

The first step in diagnosing an allergy is for the allergist to take a thorough history of the patient, including, among other things, a record of any allergic symptoms in the patient's family. The patient will be asked whether either of his or her parents suffers from asthma or hay fever, ever suffered from hives, reacted to a serum injection (such as tetanus antitoxin, DPT), or experienced any other type of skin trouble. Additionally, the allergist will ask whether the patient's parents were unable to eat certain foods;

complained of sinusitis, runny nose, frequent colds or flu; had dyspepsia, indigestion or any other conditions where an allergy may have been a contributing factor (although not recognized as such at the time).

The same questions are asked about the patient's relatives: grandparents, aunts, uncles, brothers, sisters and cousins. An allergic tendency is not always inherited directly from the parents. It may skip generations, or manifest in nieces or nephews rather than in direct descendants.

The careful allergist will also determine whether or not such diseases as tuberculosis, cancer, diabetes, rheumatic or glandular disorders exist or have ever occurred in the patient's family history. All of these facts help give the allergist a more complete picture of the hereditary characteristics of the patient. Allergic *tendency* is inherited. It may be manifested differently in different people. Unlike the tendency, an actual allergic condition, such as asthma, is not always inherited. Parents may have had cancer or rheumatism, but the child can manifest that allergic inheritance as asthma.

When the family history is complete, the allergist will need to look into the history of the patient's allergic attacks. Some typical preliminary questions include: "When did your first attack occur?" Did your allergy first occur when you were an infant or a child, or did you first notice the symptoms after you were fully grown? Did it occur after going through a certain procedure? For example, did it occur for the first time after a dental procedure like a root canal?" One of my patients reported that her asthma occurred for the first time 4 hours after root canal work. She was allergic to Gutta Percha tissue that was used in the root canal work.

Once a careful history is taken, the allergist often discovers that the patient's first symptoms occurred in early childhood. He or she may have suffered from infantile eczema, but never associated it with the asthma, which may not have appeared until middle age.

Next, the doctor will want to know the circumstances surrounding and immediately preceding the first symptoms. Typical questions will include: "Did you change your diet or go on a special diet? Did you eat something that you haven't eaten lately (perhaps for two or three months)? Did you eat one type of food repeatedly, every day, for a few days? Did the symptoms follow a childhood illness (whooping cough, measles, chicken pox, diphtheria) or any immunization for such an illness? Did they follow some other illness, such as influenza, pneumonia or a major operation? Did the symptoms first appear at adolescence or after you had a baby? Were they first noticed after you acquired a cat, a dog, or even a bird? Did they appear after an automobile accident or any major physical or mental trauma? Did they appear after a lengthy exposure to the sun, a day at the beach or 18 holes of golf?"

Chronic Cough Eliminated!

S.R. had coughed continually for over a year. After treating for BBF (an NAET sample called Brain-Body-Balancing Formula), she stopped coughing and has had no more coughing for the last six months. NAET is wonderful.

Dr. Margaret A. Owens
105 Medical Parkway #202-204
Austin, TX 78756
Mowers3108@msn.com
www.allergyeliminationclinic.com

Any one of these factors can be responsible for triggering a severe allergic manifestation or precipitate the first noticeable symptoms of an allergic condition. Therefore, it is very important to obtain full and accurate answers when taking the patient's medical history.

Other important questions relate to the frequency and occurrence of the attacks. Although foods may be a factor, if the symptoms occur only at specific times of the year, the trouble most likely is due to pollens. Often a patient is sensitive to certain foods but has a natural tolerance that prevents sickness until the pollen sensitivity adds sufficient allergens to throw the body into an imbalance. If symptoms occur only on specific days of the week, they are probably due to something contacted or eaten on that particular day.

The causes of allergic attacks in different patients can, at first, appear to be random. Regular weekly attacks of sneezing and nasal allergy were caused in one patient after he read the Sunday newspaper. The ink caused a severe allergic reaction. Another patient reacted similarly to the comic section of the newspaper. A man always had a gastrointestinal allergic attack on Sunday morning. The cause was traced to eating a traditional pizza

NAET Helped to Clear Cyst in The Breast!

Mary was a 58 year old woman, who was recently put on medications, due to fibrocysts in her breast tissues. One month later she developed a large fluid filled cyst on her thyroid gland. After successful NAET treatments for her prescribed medications, her cyst reduced by more than ½ size and after approximately 2 more months her cyst is completely gone. Thanks to Dr. Devi and NAET, Mary does not have to have her Thyroid gland removed.

Dr. Ron Arconati, D.C.
St. Louis, MO 63129
(314) 846-2100

every Saturday night with his family. He was allergic to the tomato sauce on the pizza. Still another patient had an allergic attack of sneezing and runny nose on Saturdays. I traced the allergy to the chemical compounds in a lotion she used to set her hair on Friday afternoons.

The time of day when the attacks occur is also of importance in determining the cause of an allergic manifestation. If it always occurs at night, it is quite likely that there is something in the bedroom that is aggravating the condition. It may be that the patient is sensitive to feathers in the pillow or comforter, wood cabinets, marble floors, carpets, side tables, end tables, bed sheets, pillows, pillow cases, detergents used in washing clothes, indoor plants, shrubs, trees, or grasses outside the patient's window.

Many patients react violently to house dust, different types of furniture, polishes, house plants, tap water and purified water. Most of the city water suppliers change the water chemicals only once or twice a year. Although, this is done with good intentions, people with chemical allergies may get sicker if they ingest the same chemicals over and over for months or years. Contrary to traditional western thinking, developing immunity can be the exception rather than the rule.

Occasionally, switching the chemicals around gives a change of allergens to the allergic patients and a chance for him to recover from the existing reactions. In this way, repeated use of the same chemicals can be avoided.

Drinking water comes from different sources. The major sources are ground water and surface water. The ground water supply includes underground aquifers, wells and springs. Most aquifers get their water supply from surface water, which includes lakes, ponds and rivers. Dumping contaminants onto the soil contaminates both sources. They are carried either throughout the soil to the underground source (such as wells and springs), or through the runoff of the contaminated soil into lakes and rivers.

Contamination may also be caused by natural degradation of vegetation, animal matter or pollutants in the air and rain. Surface water is also tainted via contaminated lakes, rivers and ponds through direct dumping of pollutants from accidental spills, pesticides, septic tank cesspools, landfills, dump or refuse spills, gasoline or diesel spills, industrial disposals, bacteria, virus and parasites (roundworms, hookworms and tapeworms).

Across the United States, chlorination is used as the primary disinfectant in water systems. Although chlorination will kill most of the bacteria, viruses are not destroyed by any of these cleansing processes. Trihalomethanes, which are a by-product of chlorine, are also used to clean the water. Ozone is used as a disinfectant for drinking water. Some of these chemicals are known to cause cancer, birth defects, nervous system disorders, damage to body organs and many other irreversible sicknesses.

The amount and strength of the pollutants and disinfectants in the water varies. In any given region, after a heavy rain or flood, many of these pollutants become mixed with the water. After the first heavy rain, we usually see an epidemic of influenza in that area.

Tina, age 54, had complained of having frequent dizzy spells and light-headedness for the last four years. On certain days, she experienced as many as six or seven dizzy spells. She also had experienced severe joint pain accompanied by a tingling sensation all over her body. At times, she felt extreme fatigue, suffered from severe insomnia and frequent migraine headaches. She was examined by many specialists, undergoing various X-rays, CAT scans and MRI of the brain, head and neck. Psychiatric evaluations were also done on her. Tina's doctor prescribed hormone and iron supplements, but nothing gave her relief. Her unsuccessful search for a proper diagnosis and cure cost her thousands of dollars.

Finally, she was referred to our office. Her history did not disclose anything significant. Kinesiological tests revealed that her entire problem was caused from something she was drinking every day. Further questioning revealed that Tina had installed a water filter throughout her house four years ago. We soon discovered she was extremely allergic to the chemical in the filter. She used the filtered water for drinking, washing and bathing. After following our advice to disconnect the filter system for a while, her health improved dramatically. Her symptoms did not completely disappear until she was treated for the particular water-filter chemical with NAET. After NAET, she began using the water filter without any adverse reactions. Two years later, she was still in excellent health without any trace of her previous problems.

The doctor should ask the patient to make a daily log of all the foods he/she is eating. The ingredients in the food should be checked for possible allergens. Certain common allergens like corn products, MSG (monosodium glutamate or Accent), citric acid, etc., are used in food preparations.

Allergy to corn is one of today's most common allergies, especially in asthmatic and arthritic patients. Unfortunately, cornstarch is found in almost every processed food and some toiletries and drugs, too. Chinese food, baking soda, baking powder and toothpaste contain large amounts of cornstarch. It is the binding product in almost all vitamins and pills, including aspirin and Tylenol. Corn syrup is the natural sweetener in many of the products we ingest, including soft drinks. Corn silk is found in cosmetics and corn oil is used as a vegetable oil.

People react severely to various gums used in many preparations: acacia gum, xanthine gum, karaya gum, etc. Numerous gums are used in candy bars, yogurt, cream cheese, soft drinks, soy sauce, barbecue sauce, fast food products, macaroni and cheese, etc.

Mary, 43, came to us with severe pain in her right breast. She had a history of repeated breast abscesses, including seven incisions and drainage treatments within the last two years. She was on antibiotics throughout the year. When questioned, it was revealed that the present problem started after she ate a piece of cheesecake. When we examined the ingredients, we discovered that gum in the cream cheese was one of the major ingredients in her recipe for cheesecake. She was consuming a lot of gum in various forms every day. After being treated for gum, she has not experienced another abscess in 18 months.

Carob, a staple in many health food products, is another item that causes many common diseases among allergic people. Many health- conscious people are turning to natural food products in which carob is used as a chocolate and cocoa substitute. It is also used as a natural coloring or stiffening agent in soft drinks, cheeses, sauces, etc. We discovered that some of the causes of "holiday flu" are allergies to carob, chocolate and turkey.

Helena, 37 years old, came to the office during the first week of March. Her history consisted of severe, excruciating pain under the left breast at the level of the sixth and seventh ribs. Her spleen was enlarged and tender. The usual laboratory work showed no abnormalities other than a slightly enlarged spleen. Upon questioning her in detail, we discovered that she had eaten some carob-covered cherries during the Christmas period. In fact, she had eaten about 25 of these particular treats within three to four days' time. She worked as a distributor for a nutrition company and used their protein drink and milk shakes, which had carob as a flavoring agent. By muscle response testing, we found that Helena was highly reactive to carob. After successful treatment by NAET she was relieved of her nagging pain. Her spleen became normal size again. She was soon back on the nutrition products without any further discomfort.

After completing the patient's history, allergists should examine the patient for the usual vital signs. A physical examination is performed to check for any abnormal growth or condition. If the patient has an area of pain or discomfort in the body, it should be inspected. It is important to the type and area of pain, and its relation to an acupuncture point. Excluding traumas, most pain in the body usually occurs around some important acupuncture point.

There are 12 major acupuncture meridians in the body. These energy pathways (meridians) are like rivers beginning from the source and flowing to a destination. Many different channels and branches join the flowing river throughout its journey. The starting point of the meridian is usually an end point of a limb, a hand or a foot. The meridians usually travel through to the other end of the body.

Acupuncture meridians also have various channels and branches. Twelve meridians combined with their channels and branches cover almost every part of the human body. An acupuncturist is trained to understand the exact location of the pathways of these meridians. For this reason, the location of the pain is very important. By identifying the location of the pain, you can identify the area of the energy blockage. From this location, the experienced acupuncturist can detect the meridians, organs, muscles and nerve roots associated with the blockage. The acupuncturist will then be able to make an appropriate diagnosis by evaluating the presenting symptoms (read Chapter 10 for possible pathological symptoms) and determine what particular allergen is causing the specific problem. When the source of the problem is identified, treatment becomes easier.

CHAPTER 4

NAMBUDRIPAD'S TESTING TECHNIQUE

Our brain is analogous to a highly evolved computer, surpassing man-made computers in its range of functional levels. Vast amounts of data can be entered into it. Our brain needs to be reprogrammed in the manner we want it to function. If we do not reprogram it, it cannot respond appropriately.

Our human computer can be reprogrammed for our benefit. We are born with a brain like a *pre-wired computer.* If we are happy with our existing program, we don't have to make any changes. We just need to take good care of it. However, if we are unhappy with the existing program, we can modify or rewrite it. As in making corrections on the computer screen, we may have to delete every incorrect entry one by one and replace it with a more desirable entry. The more corrections to be made, the longer it takes to input the correct data. Referring back to allergic reactions, if you have many allergies it may take months or years before they all can be treated and corrected.

Nambudripad's Testing Technique, or NTT, includes the following evaluation methods:

1. History

■ A complete history of the patient is taken.

- A symptom survey form is given to the patient to record the level and type of discomfort he/she is suffering.

2. Physical examination

- Observation of the mental status, face, skin, eyes, color, posture, movements, gait, tongue, scars, wounds, marks, body secretions, etc.

3. Vital signs

- Evaluation of blood pressure, pulse, skin temperature and palpable pains in the course of meridians, etc.

4. SRT

- Skin Resistance Test for the presence or absence of a suspected allergen is done through a computerized electro-dermal testing device; differences in the meter reading are observed (the greater the difference, the stronger the allergy).

5. MRT

- Muscle Response Testing is conducted to compare the strength of a predetermined muscle in the presence and absence of a suspected allergen.

6. Dynamometer Testing

- Hand-held dynamometer is used to measure finger strength (0-100) in the presence and absence of a suspected allergen.

In order to achieve a particular goal or way of life, you must make sure that your computer is programmed correctly to fit your needs. You should open up the database and inspect it carefully for any self-damaging type of information that may exist in any part of the program. If you find such information, it should be deleted or rewritten. Using MRT, you can open up your computer and inspect it for a sabotaged program. Once inspected, the program can be fixed. It may be time consuming, but it is worth doing if you want to live a healthier life. You can input the "program" in your brain in many ways. MRT is one way to *recall,* and NAET is a way to *reinstall* the program with the correct message or data.

Another possible way to alter the program is through affirmation. If the affirmation is positive, part of the brain (subconscious) will rewrite it positively; for example, *I want to be healthy, I want to be spiritual, I want to be rich,* etc. If you input the affirmation negatively, the brain will encode negatively. Negative and positive input takes place all the time in your daily lives without thinking about it. You may hear it in the lyrics of songs you listen to, the TV shows you watch, in overheard conversations, in your own dialogues between friends, anywhere. When the brain is constantly bombarded with negativity, the negative message gets encoded firmly in the subconscious mind. The subconscious mind does not have the ability to separate the good from the bad, or negative from the positive.

Upon careful examination, you may be surprised to discover that some of our cultural habits are pointing towards self-sabotaging programming. Some of the everyday conversational words and common slang expressions add to this list. For example, "If you break your promise, I will kill you!" "She is dressed to kill." "I love you to death!" "No matter how hard I try, I can never make it," or "I will fall on my knees . . ." etc. By consciously watching your negative words and thoughts carefully, you can avoid self-damaging types of programming in our master computer.

POSITIVE INPUTS

We subconsciously alter the data positively when someone compliments another for doing good work: a teacher rewarding a student with a gold star sticker for each correct homework assignment; when you make a positive comment when your spouse makes a good pot of coffee, a delicious dinner or a thoughtful gift. All these gestures of warmth and love will implant in the subconscious part of the brain as positive and inspiring messages.

MRT TO DETECT ALLERGIES

Muscle Response Testing is the body's communication pathway with the brain. Through MRT, the patient can be tested for various allergens. MRT is a standard test used in applied kinesiology to compare the strength of a predetermined test muscle in the presence and absence of a suspected allergen. If the particular muscle (test muscle) weakens in the presence of an item, it signifies that the item is an allergen. If the muscle remains strong, the substance is not an allergen. More explanation on MRT will be given in Chapter 7.

SRT (ELECTRO-DERMAL TEST-EDT)

After the MRT, the Skin Resistance Test (SRT) is administered. The patient is tested on a computerized instrument that is designed to painlessly measure the body's electrical conductivity at specific, electrically-sensitive points on the skin, particularly on the hands and feet. The computerized operation is based on two theories that have been shown to be clinically valid.

The first theory comes from biomechanics and acupuncture. More than 40 years ago, acupuncture researchers determined that the body's electrical characteristics measured at specific acupuncture points are predictive of the health of organs and organ systems along corresponding acupuncture meridians. The computer applies this theory by challenging the body with a very small current and then measuring the body's response. The computer records these resistance measurements to provide data that is helpful in recognizing the intensity and severity of the energy blockage in the body.

The second theory is based on quantum physics and science. It postulates that the body's functions are controlled and coordinated by a very intelligent part of the body. This intelligent "Master Computer" understands and speaks a number of languages and has the ability to keep track of an incredible amount of information at every moment of the day.

Today, there are different types of man-made computers for accessing our master computer and receiving biofeedback information from this "Master Computer" in the form of changes in galvanic skin responses. These changes occur in a meaningful, consistent manner that can be interpreted by trained doctors. This computerized tester is a non-invasive Class III investigational medical device. In conjunction with MRT, the computerized tester can provide rapid, painless allergy testing to determine the allergens that affect the body and immune system. Foods, inhalants, animal epithelial, drugs, chemicals, vitamins, amino acids, pollens, trees, wood, weeds, grasses, molds, fabrics, metals and other materials can be tested for allergies by the computerized tester.

The computerized tester also helps to determine the various intensities of the allergies based on a 0 - 100 scale. This is probably one of the most accurate tests available today to determine allergies. The machine is designed to test food, environmental and chemical allergies, as well as allergies to molds, fungi, pollens, trees, grasses, proteins, vitamins, drugs, radiation, etc. It can be used to test allergies and their intensities before and after treatment so that we are able to compare and show the body's response to the treatment.

The procedure does not involve breaking or puncturing the skin. There is no pain or discomfort. Hundreds of allergies can be tested on the patient in minutes. Since the testing probe only touches the skin for less than a second for each allergy tested, this method can be used for infants and children as well as adults. Another advantage of this machine is that it has a TV/computer monitor where the patient can read his own allergies as they are being recorded. A printout is produced and the data is saved for future comparison.

DYNAMOMETER TESTING

A hand-held dynamometer is used in this testing. The dynamometer is held with thumb and index finger and squeezed to make the reading needle swing between 0-100 scale. Initial baseline reading is observed first, then with contact with an allergen. The finger strength is compared in the presence of the allergen. If the second reading is more than the initial reading, there is no allergy. If the second reading is less than the initial reading, then there is an allergy. For example—if the initial (baseline reading) is 40 on a scale of 1-100, and if the reading in the presence of an allergen (apple) is 28—the person is allergic to the apple. If the second reading is 60- or 70- there is no allergy. Another benefit of dynamometer testing is that the degree of the weakness/strength is measured in numbers. This gives us some understanding of the degree of allergy.

OTHER STANDARD ALLERGY TESTS

ALCAT TEST

One of today's most reliable and effective tests to detect allergies and sensitivities to food, chemicals, and food additives is the ALCAT test. This system is designed to measure blood cell reactions to foods, chemicals, drugs, molds, pesticides, bacteria, etc. The methodology of this simple test includes using innovative laboratory reagents allowing accurate cell measurement in their native form. Individually processed test samples, when compared with the "Master Control" graph, will show cellular reactivity (cell count and size) if it has occurred. Scores are generated by relating these effective volumetric changes in white blood cells to the control curve.

SCRATCH TEST

Although other available methods of allergy testing are plentiful, traditional methods of testing have never been very reliable. Western medical allergists generally depend on skin testing (scratch test, patch test, etc.), in which a very small amount of a suspected allergic substance is introduced into the person's skin through a scratch or an injection. The site of injection is observed for any reaction. If there is any reaction at the area of injection, the person is considered to be allergic to that substance. Each item has to be tested individually.

This manner of testing is more dangerous, painful and time consuming than SRT. Some patients can go into anaphylactic shock due to the introduction of extremely allergic items into the body. This painful procedure can cause soreness for several days. The patient must wait for a few days or weeks between tests because only one set of allergens can be tested at a time. This method is not very effective in identifying allergies to foods. Since it is not normal to inject foods under the skin, it is not surprising that there usually isn't a significant reaction.

PROVOCATIVE / NEUTRALIZING TECHNIQUE

This test evaluates cellular immunity by determining patient response to the intradermal injection or topical application of one or more antigens. A minute amount of allergen (a weak dilution) is injected skin deep. It is strong enough to provoke the allergic symptoms in a person. The dilution and the amount of allergen used are noted. The allergen can produce skin erythema and/or wheal around the injected site. A record is kept of the amount, dilution and time injected. After a period of time, the size and shape of the wheal is observed. If the patient feels any reaction (dizzy spells, nausea, etc.), the tester will inject a smaller dose (weaker dilution) of the allergen that is capable of neutralizing the provocative action. This usually takes away the unpleasant symptoms or allergic reactions the patient felt from the initial injection. This is called the neutralizing dose. The neutralizing dose is used to relieve the allergic symptom and keep the patient under control for days.

INTRADERMAL TEST

The intradermal test is considered to be more accurate for food allergies than a plain scratch test. The name comes from the fact that a small portion of the extract of the allergen is injected intradermally, between the superficial layers of skin. Many people who show no reaction to the dermal or scratch type of testing show positive results when the same allergens are applied intradermally.

As in scratch tests, some patients can go into anaphylactic shock when extremely allergic items are injected into the body. The painful procedure can cause soreness for several days. The patient must wait a few days or weeks between tests, because only one set of allergens can be tested at a time.

RADIOALLERGOSORBANT TEST (RAST)

The radioallergosorbant test, or RAST, measures IgE antibodies in serum by radioimmunoassay and identifies specific allergens causing allergic reactions. In this test, a sample of the patient's serum is exposed to a panel of allergen particle complexes (APCs) on cellulose disks. Radiolabeled anti-IgE antibody is then added. This binds to the IgE-APC complexes. After centrifugation, the amount of radioactivity in the particular material is directly proportional to the amount of IgE antibodies present. Test results are compared with control values and represent the patient's reactivity to a specific allergen.

ELISA

Another blood serum test for allergies is called the "ELISA" (enzyme-linked immuno-zorbent assay) test. In this test, blood serum is tested for various immunoglobulin and their concentrations. Previous exposure to the allergen is necessary for this test to be positive in the case of an allergy. Elisa can identify an antibody or antigen, and replaces or supplements radioimmunoassay and immunofluorescence. To measure a specific antibody, an antigen is fixed to a solid phase medium, incubated with a serum sample. Then it is incubated with an anti-immunoglobulin-tagged enzyme. The excess unbound enzyme is washed from the system and a substrate is added. Hydrolysis of the substrate produces a color change, quantified by a spectrophotometer. The amount of antigen or antibody in the serum sample can then be measured. This method is safe, sensitive, and simple to perform and provides reproducible results. For this test to show some positive results, the patient must be exposed to particular foods within a certain amount of time. If the patient has never been exposed to certain foods, the test results may be unsatisfactory.

EMF TEST (ELECTRO MAGNETIC FIELD TEST)

The electromagnetic component of the human energy field can be detected with simple muscle response testing. The pool of electromagnetic energy around an object or a person allows the energy exchange. The human field absorbs the energy from the nearby object and processes it through the network of nerve energy pathways. If the foreign energy field shares suitable charges with the human energy field, the human field absorbs the foreign energy for its advantage and becomes stronger. If the foreign energy field carries unsuitable charges, the human energy field causes repulsion from the foreign energy field. These types of reactions of the human field can be determined by testing an indicator muscle (specific muscle) before and after coming in contact with an allergen. The electromagnetic field of the humans, or the human vibrations, can also be measured by using the sophisticated electronic equipment developed by Dr. Valerie Hunt, Malibu, California. This genius researcher, a retired UCLA professor of physics, has proven her theory of the Science of Human Vibrations through 25 years of extensive research and clinical studies. Her book, "Infinite Mind" explains it all.

SUBLINGUAL TEST

Another prevalent allergy test, which is used by clinical ecologists and some nutritionists, is called a sublingual test. It involves the instillation of a tiny amount of allergen extract under the tongue. If the test is positive, symptoms may appear very rapidly. The symptoms may include dramatic mental and behavioral reactions in addition to physical reactions. Some kinesiologists also use sublingual testing, but only for food items. A tiny amount of the food substance is placed under the tongue, and the patient is checked by muscle response testing.

CYTOTOXIC TESTING

Cytotoxic testing is a form of blood test that was developed a few years ago. Many nutritionally oriented practitioners use this test. In this method, an extract of the allergic substance is mixed with a sample of the person's blood. It is then observed under the microscope for changes in white cells. Since foods and other allergic substances do not normally get into the blood in this manner, cytotoxic testing does not give reliable results.

PULSE TEST

Pulse testing is another simple way of determining food allergy. This test was developed by Arthur Coca, M.D., in the 1950's. Research has shown that if you are allergic to something and you eat it, your pulse rate speeds up.

Step 1: Establish your baseline pulse by counting radial pulse at the wrist for a full minute.

Step 2: Put a small portion of the suspected allergen in the mouth, preferably under the tongue. Taste the substance for two minutes. Do not swallow any portion of it. The taste will send the signal to the brain, which will send a signal through the sympathetic nervous system to the rest of the body.

Step 3: Re-take the pulse with the allergen still in the mouth. An increase or decrease in pulse rate of 10% or more is considered an allergic reaction. The greater the degree of allergy, the greater the difference in the pulse rate.

This test is useful to test food allergies. If you are allergic to very many foods, and if you consume a few allergens at the same time, it will be hard to detect the exact allergen causing the reaction just by this test.

BLOOD PRESSURE TEST

This test is similar to the pulse test. The systolic blood pressure reading is checked for changes in reading before and after the contact with the allergen.

Step 1: Establish your baseline by checking the systolic blood pressure.

Step 2: Put a small amount of the suspected allergen in the mouth, preferably under the tongue. Taste the substance for two minutes. Do not swallow any portion of it. The taste will send the signal to the brain, which will send a signal through the sympathetic nervous system to the rest of the body.

Step 3: Re-take the systolic blood pressure with the allergen still in the mouth. An increase in systolic blood pressure rate of 10% or more is considered an allergic reaction. The greater the degree of allergy, the higher the blood pressure change will be.

THE ELIMINATION DIET

The elimination diet, which was developed by Dr. Albert H. Rowe of Oakland, California, consists of a very limited diet that must be followed for a period long enough to determine whether or not any of the foods included in it are responsible for the allergic symptoms. If a fruit allergy is suspected, for example, all fruits are eliminated from the diet for a specific period, which may vary from a few days to several weeks, depending on the severity of the symptoms. For patients who have suffered allergic symptoms over a period of several years, it is sometimes necessary to abstain from the offending foods for several weeks before the symptoms subside. Therefore, the importance of adhering strictly to the diet during the diagnostic period is very important. When the patient has been free of symptoms for a specific period, other foods are added, one at a time, until a normal diet is attained and the offending foods are discovered.

ROTATION DIET

Another way to test for food allergy is through a "rotation diet," in which a different group of food is eaten every day for a week. In this method seven groups of food are eaten each week, with something different each day. The rotation starts again the following Monday. This way, reactions to any group can be traced and eliminated. All of these diets work better for people who are less reactive. The inherent danger in any of these methods is clear: if you are highly allergic to a certain food item, you can become very sick if you eat that particular food during testing, even if you have not touched it for years.

LIKE CURES LIKE

There are other allergy treatment methods in practice. Homeopaths believe that if an allergen is introduced to the patient in minute concentrations at various times, the patient can build up enough antibodies toward that particular antigen. Eventually, the patient's violent reactions to that particular substance may reduce in intensity. In some cases, reactions may subside completely and the patient can use or eat the item without any adverse reaction.

This is a fairly safe method to most people since with this method, usually, a patient may not react violently. In this procedure, a minute amount of the suspected allergen (usually one part per million parts or less amount of dilution) is used to prepare the sublingual drops (remedies). Extremely sensitive people break out in hives and rashes even with this diluted remedy. The rashes disappear in a couple of days in most cases and the patient will begin to feel better and healthier as time goes by. Some of these reactions are called a "healing crisis." If you are highly allergic to a certain food item (in cases with a history of anaphylaxis), you can react severely even with this harmless procedure, too. The patient should inform the doctor about any history of anaphylaxis so that the doctor can be prepared for any such emergency and appropriate steps can be taken by the doctor and the staff to prevent such situations.

SIT WITH THE ALLERGEN IN YOUR PALM

NAET patients are taught to test the allergen in another easy and safe way. Place a small portion of the suspected allergen in a baby food jar and ask the person to hold it in her/his palm, touching the jar with the fingertips of the same hand for 15 to 30 minutes. An allergic person will begin to feel uneasy when holding the allergen in his/her palm, giving rise to various unpleasant symptoms: begin to get hot, itching, hives, irregularities in heart beats (fast or slow heart beats), nausea, lightheadedness, etc. Since the allergen is inside the glass bottle, when such uncomfortable sensation is felt, the allergen can be put away immediately and wash their hands to remove the energy of the allergen from the fingertips. This should stop the reactions immediately. In this way, the patient can find out the allergens easily.

All of the above methods work on a certain percentage of people. Curiously, people who had undergone all of these treatments were still found to be allergic to their identified allergies when they were tested again by muscle response testing. They still had to be treated by NAET to make them non-reactive.

CHAPTER 5

THE LIVING MAZE

The nervous system is without a doubt the most complex, widely investigated and least understood system in the body known to man. Its structures and activities are interwoven with every aspect of our lives: physical, cultural and intellectual. Accordingly, investigators of many different disciplines, all holding their own methodologies, motivations, and persuasions, converge in its study. Depending on the context, there are many appropriate ways of embarking upon a study of the nervous system. For example, the approach could be from the developmental point of view or from a variety of other philosophies including, but not limited to, phylogenetic, physicochemical, energetic, structural (gross or cellular), cybernetic or even behavioral standpoint.

One of the primary functions of the human nervous system is gathering and processing of information. Even as you read this page, conscious gathering and processing of information is taking place. In terms of homeostasis (maintaining a balance within the organism), you who can read this page and find it challenging, or hopefully interesting, will continue to read it or put it aside to read later. Similarly, if you cannot read it, you will make a conscious decision about it, or perhaps seek a translator to read it, or simply put it down as a useless exercise. No matter which response is chosen, it is one of consciousness.

These simple responses to reading this page are transmitted along millions of nerve cells to the area in the brain where memory is stored. From there, the information may be recalled either on command or at the whim of the subconscious mind. For the reader, both conscious recall of the experiences and the effects of the subconscious are possible as a result of contact with this printed page. It is inescapable, for you are constantly in the process of "becoming" in response to your life experiences.

Just as the total human being consciously senses and responds according to the stimuli presented by the environment, millions of minor adjustments are constantly being made automatically without our conscious decision-making. For instance, when you are hot, you consciously move yourself away from the sun, or turn on the air conditioning. But the body is already unconsciously making several hundred minor adjustments that trigger changes in the blood flow and the heart rate, expanding and contracting the blood vessels near the skin surfaces, activating the lymph glands, turning on the sweat glands, and so on. These actions of the autonomic nervous system are re-programmed into the very cells of the body that respond to conscious activity. The autonomic responses are constantly readjusting to respond appropriately to the changing environment.

Consider the human body's reaction to fear. When we sense a potentially dangerous situation, the autonomic nervous system prepares for a *fight or flight* reaction. Both are appropriate responses to danger. Within seconds, our body adjusts physically by displaying signs of fear, which include the onset of sweating, clammy hands and beads of perspiration forming on our forehead. In addition, the biochemical reaction reduces the blood flow to the head, limiting our thinking and reducing our ability to hear. Meanwhile, blood flow to the heart, lungs, and motor muscle tissue increases. Again, these are all appropriate responses for the body to make in the presence of immediate danger.

Often the body is unable to differentiate between physical and physiological or emotional danger. Consequently, you respond involuntarily to a potential mugging in much the same way as you would to a job interview; or to a confrontation with an angry dog as you would to a public speaking assignment. In essence, the brain confuses us because it has developed patterns of responses that are inappropriate to the situation at hand. This is not just an idle philosophical discussion of consciousness, but a foundational premise upon which the understanding of allergies is based; the muscle response testing detects allergies and NAET eliminates allergies.

The conscious and the unconscious functioning of the central nervous system has been discussed, but it is extremely important to recognize the body's attempts to maintain a homeostatic state (balance within the organism). The total balance takes place in various steps, utilizing assistance from a number of functional units. These functional units are large bodies of tissues composed of many microscopic cells, each having a specialized job in the body. These special tissues provide assistance in creating homeostasis at the lowest levels within the individual's cells themselves.

The process through which this occurs is very complex, requiring considerable understanding of the biochemical and bioelectrical properties of the cells. Simplified, it can be said that all cells are surrounded by a plasma membrane similar to a microscopic plastic bag. The walls of this membrane are thick enough to contain the intracellular materials while maintaining the cell shape and size. It is also strong enough to protect the cells from invasion of the intercellular materials that surround each and every cell. Conversely, it is thin enough and permeable enough to allow the free flow of nutrients. The ionic or magnetic properties of the atoms that make up the fluids inside the cell differ from the fluids surrounding the cells. Because of the differences in ionic composition, there are differences in their electrical properties. This makes the cells electrical. The disparity in electrical energies can be measured in laboratory experiments on various kinds of tissues. But more importantly, it can assess the individual cell's responses to the electrical charges, which add up to millions of measurements per minute.

As a stimulus is applied at some point on the organism, it sets up a sequence of events that is eventually transmitted to the surfaces of the excitable cells, which in turn redistributes the ions across the surface. This becomes a transient, reversible wave of change which presumably affects the permeability of cell membranes, allowing fluids to penetrate. The transfer of fluids changes the cell shape, size and function until it turns back to its original or homeostatic state.

In some primitive multicellular and all unicellular life forms, individual cells are capable of reacting to stimuli; whereas most complex life forms (that make up the processing nervous system) consist of a system of specific cells to accept and interpret stimuli. Thus, in the human body we have highly specialized receptor cells whose total function is to receive stimuli. These receptor cells work in accord with other neurons (nerve cells), for the integration and conduction of information; the effector cells (the contractile and glandular cells) operate the action of the responses.

Neurons are stepping stones in the neural pathways. They interact through the use of axons (which carry impulses to neurons) and dendrites (which carry impulses away from the cell body). The ends of various dendrites and axons do not connect together to create a wire link; rather, they are interlaced, without touching. The space between the ends of the threadlike axons and dendrites are called synapses. The electrical impulses, or energy impulses, jump these spaces in their journey to the brain and back.

Enzymes on the surface of the neurons act as mediators (like cholinesterase) and complete the circuit. These enzymes are known as neurotransmitters and are extremely important in making intercommunication possible among the cells, neurons, tissues, organs and different body parts. These neurotransmitters vary among neurons, depending upon the specificity of tissue. Although vastly different in chemical composition, all these enzymes share a common origin. They are produced by the neurons, then released into the synapses as the nerve impulse arrives. This sets off the response in the next cell. Lately, much interest has been shown in these enzymes. They may hold the key to a natural means of controlling pain, addiction to chemicals, aging, disease, the healing mechanism and controlling and eliminating allergies.

The actions and neurological functions of these enzymes in our bodies are still not completely understood, primarily because of the wide distribution of such enzymes throughout the body. These enzymes include mono-amino acids, known as noradrenalin, serotonin, histamines, (all of which have an excitatory affect on the body's nervous system) and dopamine, which has an inhibitory effect.

The ability of the central nervous system to react almost instantaneously to a stimulus (such as the sensation of heat, cold, smell, etc.), even on the most remote part of the extremities, is probably the result of the common origin of the nervous system. The body is made up of trillions of individually well-equipped cells. Each cell has the memory to reproduce any number of chemicals and functions in the body. When the cell duplicates, the duplicated cell takes over all the memory of the mother cell. This memory or duplicating effect is accomplished by deoxyribonucleic acid, or DNA, which controls the functions of the body through various sensory receptors installed in each cell surface. This DNA and the other characteristics of the individual cells were duplicated and carried over from the beginning of the unicellular life. Since the body formed from a single cell, identical memory through duplication of the memory in each cell is made possible.

The embryonic ectoderm gives rise to the whole nervous system, including the central, peripheral, and autonomic nervous system, and the sensory and touch receptors, etc. It is this origin that accounts for the body's ability to function as a unit (each part corresponding to another) through the central nervous system using the sensory receptors. When one of the sensory receptors senses something in the functional unit that is within the body, the message is passed on to the central nervous system. From there, the message goes to every cell of the body through the centrifugal or efferent nerve fibers. The whole body is then alerted to accept or reject the stimulus.

If the stimulus reaches the brain (providing it is not short-circuited by nerve damage, blockage, or missed chemical response due to some defect in the neurotransmitters), the brain accepts the message. It then formulates and transmits a response to all other receptors in the body. In turn, the receptors receive the message as either harmful or harmless. If the receptors receive the message as harmful, they repel it and confirm their findings to the brain. If more stimuli with negative reactions reach the brain, the brain accepts the rejection message from the majority of receptors. Since the brain's responses are impartial, the receptors corresponding to the area of the stimuli will react accordingly, setting in motion evasive actions. In the worst case scenario, where the body cannot effectively avoid or reject the stimulus, it will set up a reaction in an effort to cleanse the body of the stimulus.

For the most part, the nervous system that produces negative responses to a stimulus, especially to an allergic stimulus, is the automatic nervous system. It consists of two parts, the parasympathetic and the sympathetic, as we discussed earlier. Physiologically, parasympathetic reactions are localized. They slow down the heart rate and increase glandular and peristaltic action of the gut and other hollow organs. By contrast, sympathetic activities are exhibited as mass responses to stimuli. They include increasing the blood flow to the heart, lungs, muscles and brain by constricting the blood vessels under the skin. Other activities include accelerating the heart rate, increasing blood pressure and decreasing peristalsis (kneading action of the gut), etc.

Activities of the sympathetic system prepare the body for increased activities. Biochemically, the action of the sympathetic system is characterized by the formation of noradrenaline and adrenaline (along with some other basic enzymes) to prepare the body for reaction.

Chiropractors who specialize in the study of the spinal column can perform miraculous cures in certain patients without the use of any medications because the sympathetic nerves exit from the thoracic region of the spinal cord. Half an inch to one inch away from both sides of the spinal column are a group of important acupuncture points. They are directly related to the vital organs and organ functions. Correct stimulation of these points with acupuncture needles results in similar, positive responses in patients. Chiropractors and acupuncturists are stimulating the sympathetic and parasympathetic nerve activity, during that process, removing the nerve energy blockages from the energy pathways to reinstate the freeflow of nerve energy circulation in the body. These two groups of medical practitioners from East and West have learned to manipulate the autonomic nervous system to the patient's advantage and promote healing power within the body itself without the introduction of foreign chemicals.

Beyond this point, the nervous system becomes a matter of complicated medical study. It is sufficient to say, however, that even a very minor stimulus sensed by any receptor nerve cell located on the body, will set in motion the manufacturing process of hundreds of different kinds of chemicals. Each assists the nerves in producing appropriate responses to the particular stimulus.

CHAPTER 6

KINESIOLOGY AND ACUPUNCTURE

The word "kinesiology" refers to the science of movement. It was first proposed in 1964 by Dr. George Goodheart, a Detroit doctor of chiropractic medicine. As a function of his practice, Dr. Goodheart learned a great deal about a patient's condition by using isolated movements of various muscles. Isolation techniques, a chiropractic procedure, made it possible to test the strength of an individual muscle or muscle group without the help of other muscles. Dr. Goodheart, with the help of Dr. Hetrick and others, concluded after many experiments that structural imbalance causes disorganization of the entire body. This disorganization results in specific disorders of the glands, organs and central nervous system. His findings were similar to what pioneer Chinese doctors also had observed.

Kinesiology holds that when the body is disorganized, the structural balance or electrical force is not functioning normally. When this happens, the central nervous system sends out a signal that is directed to every cell of the body via it's network of sensory and motor nerve cells. Under the direct command of the brain, they are capable of conducting messages back and forth with the brain at all times. The electrical energy, or life force, flows through these nerve cells, which are energy channels. This energy has been called different names by different people: in Chinese it is called "Chi," in Sanskrit, "Prana," and in English, "life force" or "vital energy." Using a more simple term in NAET, we call it energy.

According to the Chinese, the free flow of energy is necessary for the normal functioning of the body. When your flow of energy gets blocked, you become ill. The messages both from and to the brain also pass through this energy channel. The energy - and the messages - travel from cell to cell in nanoseconds.

Many years ago, pioneer Chinese doctors and philosophers had studied these energy pathways and networks of the human body energy system by observing living people and their normal and abnormal body functions. The Chinese had learned to manipulate these energy pathways, or meridians, to the body's advantage. About 4,000 years ago, there was no scientific equipment available to feel or observe the presence of the energy flow and its pathways. Now, it is possible to study and trace the energy flows and pathways by using Kirlian photography and radioactive tracer isotopes. Although the existence of energy pathways in the human body has only been confirmed relatively recently, the Chinese doctors hypothesized and established their existence long ago.

According to Chinese medical theory, any obstruction in the energy flow in the pathways can cause imbalance in the body. Any imbalance can cause illness. To rid the body of the imbalance, the cause has to be removed. It follows that if energy blockage is the cause of the imbalance, then the blockage must be removed for the balance to be reinstated. When the body is in perfect balance, it cannot experience any illness. When acupuncture needles are placed at various points in the acupuncture meridians, energy blockages are removed temporarily and the state of balance is achieved. This is how acupuncture treats various ailments.

Chinese medical theory points out that free-flowing Chi through the meridians is necessary to keep the body in perfect balance. In the United States during the 19th century, the founder of Chiropractic medicine, Daniel David Palmer, said, "Too much or too little energy is sickness." Even though it is believed that Palmer may have had no knowledge of Chinese medicine, his theory corresponded with the ancient Chinese theory of "free flow of energy."

In late 1800, American chiropractic medicine developed under D. D. Palmer. Through him, doctors of chiropractic learned about the importance of stabilizing energy and manipulating the spinal segments and nerve roots to keep them perfectly aligned, bringing the body to a balanced state. In the East, acupuncture developed based on the ancient Chinese theory. Eastern acupuncturists tried to bring balance by manipulating the energy meridians at various acupuncture points, inserting needles to remove blockages and reinstating the "free flow of Chi" along the energy pathways. East and West, unaware of each other's findings, worked in a similar manner toward the same goal: to balance the energy and to free sick people from their pain.

Both groups realized that the overflow or underflow of energy, or in other words, too much or too little energy is the cause of an imbalance. When the flow is reinstated, the balance is restored.

HOW CAN WE REMOVE THE CAUSE OF A BLOCKAGE?

What do I mean by overflow or underflow—too much or too little energy? If we evaluate the energy circulation with the help of Chinese principles, we can equate energy to water, energy flow to water flow and an energy meridian to a water canal. Assume the water is flowing through the canal freely and smoothly. Suddenly a huge rock rolls over from the top of the hill and falls into the canal, obstructing the entire width of the stream and creating a temporary dam. We can imagine what could happen to the water flow now. One side of the stream fills up with the incoming water and gets ready to flood. The water, unable to move forward, has to find another route. It has a few options. It can back up into the small streams and tributaries where it came from; it can create new channels; or it can simply flow over the sides of the channel to the neighboring land. Now, what happens on the other side of the rock? The water does not get to the other side because the fallen rock has created a temporary dam. The canal on the opposite side of the dam dries up. The neighboring land and vegetation, which depended on the water supply, suffer from the water shortage.

Similar things happen in the human body too. When the energy channel that carries energy back and forth is blocked by an allergen (same like the rock), When the adverse energy enters the channel, the meridian creates a kink in the pathway (resulting in a muscle spasm, etc.), equivalent to the rock. It obstructs the energy flow and doesn't let it travel forward. So, the incoming energy will back up in the meridian or take a detour through the various branches of the meridians. It is easy for the energy to back up into other channels, branches and organs since they are connected so efficiently to all other energy meridians, related organs and tissues, unlike the man-made or nature-made water stream. The reversing energy will fill up the sharing channels, forcing them to accommodate the excess energy along with their existing energy flow, until they can unload into their target organs and tissues. This sometimes creates overflow or overabundance (too much energy, as D. D. Palmer stated) of energy in those channels and in their target organs. The other side of the block and its target organs will suffer from the lack of energy creating an underflow (too little energy, as D. D. Palmer stated), just as it is in the water stream.

Now, to evaluate this situation through acupuncture theory, when there is an energy blockage in the meridian, there will be stagnation on one side and poor flow on the other. The stagnation will lead to back flow and then overflow to various connecting meridians. All the meridians, or energy pathways, are associated with various major vital organs. Any back flow and overflow will affect these organs directly or indirectly. The stagnation of energy can cause localized aches, pains, or discomfort. Back flow or overflow can lead to malfunctions in the related vital organs, or create an "excess" syndrome. Underflow on the other side of the blockage, also affects another group of meridians and their related organs, which will create deficiency syndromes in those meridians, associated organs and tissues.

Evaluating the situation further through our western medical knowledge, you can understand why a health problem, if unsolved, leads to many other health problems. A person may begin with a minor health problem like a common cold, initiated by a virus, bacteria or an allergen. This creates an energy disturbance in the respiratory energy pathway and the body will try to remove the foreign body or energy blockage from the meridian by sneezing, having a runny nose, etc. The unsuccessful attempt to remove the blockage (struggle between the defensive forces of the body and the foreign substance to throw the blockage out of the body) will produce a lot of heat in the body that may lead to fever. The reversed energy flow will invade neighborhood tissues and cause lymph collection, leading to cough, chest congestion, bronchitis, pneumonia, asthma, water retention and congestive heart failure, etc. Low energy supply on the other side of the meridian will cause poor appetite, digestion, assimilation of essential nutrients, elimination of the toxin, kidney and liver failure, etc. All of these events will begin to affect the entire body, eventually leading to improper functions of all vital organs, or complete stoppage of all functions, causing death.

A trained acupuncturist can differentiate between the overflow and underflow of Chi, and its affected meridians and organs. When treatment is administered to strengthen the under flowing or hypo-functioning organ, while draining the overflowing meridians and the organs, balance is achieved faster. This is the practice of acupuncture. NTT and NAET are built on

> *NTT and NAET are built on acupuncture theory, but have taken it one step further...without using actual needle insertion, meridians can be unblocked, overflowing meridians can be drained and the excess energy can be rerouted through the empty meridians.*

acupuncture theory, but have taken it one step further. Using the ideas from acupuncture theory, without using actual needle insertion, meridians can be unblocked, overflowing meridians can be drained and the excess energy can be rerouted through the empty meridians and associated organs. Thus, the entire body reaches homeostasis. NAET is perhaps the missing link the various professionals have been searching for. NTT and NAET will be discussed in detail in later chapters.

To recap, energy blockage takes place due to some disturbance in the energy system. Even earth has its own magnetic energy: gravity. Every object, living or nonliving, has an electromagnetic field around it. Objects on earth are attracted to the earth so that they all can stay on the surface of the earth without flying away from it.

When one body of energy comes near another body of energy, the first energy will interact with the second by inviting it to enter the first object's body, run through the energy pathways, and exit without any obstruction. That is because they share the same interest and recognize and respect each other's energy fields. They can be friends with each other. There is no repulsion between the energies. Their energies are compatible or attracted to each other.

Sometimes, the energy of the first body does not recognize the energy of the second body. Energy meridians of the first body will not permit the energy of the second body to come near its energy field without alerting all other energy meridians and defense forces about the intruder. This type of reaction is called an energy disturbance.

Objects on earth have an attraction or repulsion among themselves. In theory, there should not be any repulsion between objects, because they are all part of the universe; objects are meant to interact together in unison. Likewise, humans should not have any repulsion towards any objects or other living beings around them. But, due to genetic mutation and changes in the environment over thousands of years, the energy field of humans has changed. This altered state makes us incompatible with particular objects. When we come into contact with one of those substances, an energy disturbance takes place. Energy disturbance in the energy pathways leads to energy blockage. This causes the body to fall into an unbalanced state and eventually disturbs the whole body, including meridians, vital organs and their associated muscle groups.

The central nervous system instantly responds to the presence of the intruder. It may be a toxic substance that is causing the blockage of an energy pathway. Any kinetic changes or movements in the cells are recorded instantly in the brain's computer. Later, whenever the body comes in contact with that particular object, the brain will perceive it to be toxic and harmful, calling its defensive forces into action. One of the brain's primary functions is to take care of the body's welfare. So, whenever the brain senses a harmful substance, it tries to eliminate it to protect the body.

Most of the time the responses are hidden, masked by hundreds of simultaneous responses taking place every instant. However, a particular response to the toxic substance is observable and definable if the contact with the toxin and the affected muscle groups and organs is isolated. Our brain registers every body cell movement. When the presence of an unsuitable item causes an energy disturbance in the energy pathway, the flow of energy is blocked, the body goes into an imbalanced state and the normal bodily functions do not proceed as they should. These changes and disturbances are directly sensed and recorded by the brain through its abundant sensory nerve fibers present at various parts of the body. The normal flow of energy regulates and controls all bodily functions, including the functions of the body's immune system. When there is an energy disturbance, all the bodily functions are alerted and the brain records the event.

As an example, when you are exposed to a substance perceived to be the cause of an energy disturbance, such as strawberries, it is recorded in the brain's computer instantly. The next time your body approaches a strawberry, your brain will sense the danger and summon its defense forces to help get rid of the energy disturbance-causing strawberry (which, in turn, caused an imbalance and sickness in your body). Most people who are allergic to strawberries react violently upon eating the berries. Sneezing and a runny nose represent an effort on the part of the affected organs to eliminate some irritant already inside the body. When giant hives occur, watery fluid is present in the tissue, and along with it, severe vomiting and diarrhea can also occur. This may be due to the action of various defensive forces working in the body to get rid of the trapped toxins.

As long as energy flows freely through the energy pathways, you cannot get sick. However, any physical, physiological and psychological trauma can cause a disturbance in the flow of energy along the meridians. The presence of any allergic substances, like food items, fabrics, animals or materials, can be included in the category of items that may cause physical disturbances and energy blockage. The aftereffects of ingesting allergic foods, alcohol, drugs, etc., may also be included in the category of physiological disturbances. For example, consumption of too much sodium chloride ion can cause fluid retention in the body. Fluid retention can cause swelling of the tissues irritating the nerves, causing pain and discomfort in the body. This will, in turn, disturb the physiological function of other organs and cause imbalance throughout the body.

The third category of items that produce imbalance is psychological or emotional disturbances. Extreme joy, anger, shocking or sad news, sudden loss of loved ones, huge financial losses and natural disasters (such as fire, earthquakes, etc.), can all cause energy disturbances and blockages, leading to imbalances in the meridians, organs, and associated muscle groups. If you use or eat any allergenic item while your body is in such an unbalanced state, your body experiences the pangs of allergic reaction in heightened degrees.

If the body did not experience a major trauma, the allergies would probably have remained hidden or less reactive. When the body is in balance, most of the allergies do not exhibit their usual reactions. That is why most of the allergic manifestations follow a major trauma or event in one's life, (such as an automobile or other accident, major illnesses, loss of a loved one, or financial or job loss, childbirth, surgery, etc.).

When you experience a major trauma, your body uses all of its defensive forces to overcome that predicament. The body exhausts its entire reservoir of strength while trying to save itself from the trauma. At this time, if an allergen enters the body, the body is unable to defend itself and becomes a convenient victim of an allergic attack. During this process, the immune system becomes exhausted, the blockages enlarge, the stagnation and the body's disturbed energy flow become exaggerated. Soon, the energy blockages start affecting the tissues and organs. Temporary changes turn into permanent changes. Various organs of the body are affected by various diseases and symptoms like migraine headaches, asthma, emphysema, arthritis, lung disorders, tumors, carcinomas, Epstein-Barr viruses, tuberculosis and other immune deficiency disorders. From this explanation, you can see how sickness starts with simple imbalances in the body due to blockages in the energy flow.

Acupuncture on specific points will help drain the blockages out of the body by creating an exit via the insertion of the needle. Adverse energy from the allergen that causes blockages in the meridians will turn into heat. Under pressure, this heat causes tension. When the needle is inserted, the heat under pressure will get a chance to exit because metal needles have the ability to transfer heat from highly heated areas to low heated areas; their insertion allows the heat under pressure to escape. Heat from inside the body will not exit through skin because of the skin's ability to provide strong insulation. That is why a needle is needed to draw out the built-up heat from the inside layers. Expulsion of heat can be seen immediately after insertion of the needle in the form of redness, red welts or a red pimple. The larger the red areas, the greater the amount of heat that has accumulated and has been emitted from the body.

Kinesiology and acupuncture have much in common because the development of the former was based on acupuncture theory. Chinese "I Ching" is the kinesiology of the Oriental medicine, which has been practiced in China for many years. Many of the pioneer Chinese doctors did not share all their knowledge with their peers or students for fear of losing their power and position. It's possible that this very important knowledge has been buried with the passing years. In any case, the Chinese scientists' knowledge of the structure of the nervous system and circulatory system is apparent in their placement of acupuncture points.

Herbs can cause similar healing. Electromagnetic forces of special herbs actually have the ability to enter selective meridians and push energy blockages out of the body to restore the energy balances. A well-trained herbologist can bring about the same result as an acupuncturist. A combination of acupuncture and herbs can produce excellent results.

Ignorance is the worst enemy of progress. Western medical doctors depend on the latest scientific tools and medicines. Most western doctors are not encouraged to look at the body and study its own power of natural healing. If given a chance, appropriate stimulation to the body and brain can produce substances within the body, including adrenaline, thyroxin, pituitropin, serotonin, dopamine, endorphin, dynorphin, enkephalin, interferon and immune mediators, that will heal many problems. The brain has the ability to create appropriate remedial secretions that release to the target tissue and organs, when needed, to heal infections, allergies, tuberculosis, immune deficiency diseases, etc., as long as the brain receives the right directions and demand. This has been demonstrated repeatedly and proven in many cases when treated by NAET. It is necessary to raise the level of the immune system, which provides the right ingredients to create the necessary antidotes for any situations. The brain needs the right instructions to create these antidotes. This is done through NAET. Then the full power of the brain gets into action to heal the body appropriately. When the immune system is functioning optimally, your body can form antibodies that will clear these unsolved health problems, leaving the body in optimum balance. If all medical professionals from different fields would join together to share and learn each others' different techniques and practice in conjunction, holistic, Oriental and western medical knowledge would complement one another. Millions of suffering people all over the world would see some light at the end of the otherwise "blocked" tunnel.

This new technique is a blessing, especially to the multitudes of allergy sufferers that have already been helped. Both kinesiology and acupuncture help people immensely by removing energy blockages from energy pathways. They also help healthy people maintain their vitality by preventing energy blockages. Both of these disciplines can be used to maintain good health by promoting good nutrition, sound living habits, strong mental attitudes and exercise.

CHAPTER 7

MUSCLE RESPONSE TESTING

M uscle response testing is one of the tools used by kinesiologists to test the kinetic imbalances in the body. The same muscle response testing can also be used in detecting allergens that cause allergic reactions and allergy-based disorders in the body.

When the allergen's incompatible electromagnetic energy comes close to a person's energy field, repulsion takes place. Without recognizing this repulsive action, we frequently go near allergens (whether they are foods, drinks, chemicals, environmental substances, animals or humans) and interact with their energies. This energy disturbance produce energy blockages in the energy meridians creating disorganization in the body function giving rise to various types of allergic reactions and diseases.

To prevent the allergen from causing further disarray after producing the initial blockage, the brain sends messages to every cell of the body to reject the presence of the allergen. This rejection will appear as repulsion, and this repulsion can be seen as different physical, physiological and psychological symptoms in the person, like weak limbs, tiredness, aches, pains, insomnia, constipation, anger, depression and many other such unpleasant symptoms.

Tina, a nine-year-old girl, was undergoing treatment for asthma by NAET. She was treated for various food items and she was able to eat all of them without provoking an asthmatic attack. One day, her parents took her to a Chinese restaurant. When the food was brought to the table, she immediately whispered to her mother that she thought she was allergic to some of the food items on the plate and that she might become ill if she ate the food. The girl's mother ignored her and forced her to eat the food, saying that she had been treated for all of them. Before she finished eating, she had an asthmatic attack. The confused mother brought a sample of everything the child ate to the office next day. She was found to be allergic to the mixed vegetables that contained a great deal of cornstarch. She had not been treated for the corn yet. The nine-year-old was able to recognize the allergen before she ate it. She said her throat started itching as soon as the food was placed in front of her, giving her a clue that she might be allergic to something on the plate.

Your body has a way of telling you when you are in trouble. When you go near allergens, your brain will begin to produce various symptoms in your body in varying degrees, such as: an itchy throat, watery eyes, sneezing attacks, coughing spells, unexplained pain anywhere in the body, yawning, sudden tiredness, etc. If you learn to understand your brain and its clues closely you may be able to avoid many unpleasant events in your life including many serious health disorders. Muscle response testing is a good tool that can be used successfully to identify the same allergens in your surroundings that you were warned by your brain before. In this muscle response testing procedure, you will compare the strength of a strong muscle in your body in the presence and absence of a suspected allergen. If a previously strong test muscle tests weak in the presence of a substance, the substance is an allergen. If the substance was not able to elicit a weakness in the previously strong test muscle, then the substance is not an allergen. So this type of muscle response testing can be used to identify the presence of all allergens around you.

MUSCLE RESPONSE TESTING

(See illustrations of Muscle Response Testing on the following pages.)

Muscle response testing can be performed in the following ways:

1. Standard muscle response testing can be done in standing, sitting or lying positions. You need two people to do this test: the person who is testing, the "tester," and the person being tested, the "subject."

2. The oval ring test can be used in testing yourself. This can also be used in testing a physically strong person. This requires two persons like in standard muscle response testing.

3. Surrogate testing can be used in testing an infant, an invalid person, a very strong or a very weak person, an animal, a plant or a tree. In this case, the surrogate's muscle is tested by the tester, and the subject maintains skin-to-skin contact with the surrogate while being tested and/or treated. The surrogate is not affected by the testing.

STANDARD MUSCLE RESPONSE TESTING

Two people are required to perform standard muscle response testing. The subject can be tested lying down, standing or sitting. The lying-down position is the most convenient for both the tester and the subject. It also achieves more accurate results.

Step 1: The subject lies on a firm surface with one arm raised (left arm in the picture below), 45-90 degrees to the body with the palm facing outward and the thumb facing toward the big toe.

Step 2: The tester stands on the subject's (right) side. The subject's right arm is kept to his/her side with the palm either kept open to the air, or in a loose fist. The fingers should not touch any material, fabric or any part of the table the arm is resting on. This can give wrong test results. The left arm of the subject is raised 45-90 degrees to the body. The tester's left palm is contacting the subject's left wrist (Figure 7-1).

Step 3: The tester, using the left arm, tries to push down on the subject's raised left arm toward the subject's left big toe. The subject resists the push of the tester on the arm with the arm muscle. The test muscle is called an "indicator muscle or predetermined muscle or PDM"for short. The PDM remains strong if the subject is well balanced at the time of testing. It is essential to test a strong PDM to get accurate results. Either the subject is not balanced, or the tester is performing the test improperly if the muscle or raised arm is weak and gives away under pressure without the presence of an allergen. For example, the tester might be trying to overpower the subject. The subject does not need to gather up strength from other muscles in the body to resist the tester. Only five to ten pounds of pressure needs to be applied on the muscle for three to five seconds. The tester will feel a sensation of "lock" at the arm if the he is testing the arm properly and if the the subject is resisting the push appropriately. If the muscle tests weak the tester will be able to judge the difference with that small amount of pressure (5-10 lbs of pressure) he/she is applying. It may sound very easy, but much practice is needed to learn the procedure properly. If you cannot test effectively the first few times, there is no need to get frustrated. Please remember that practice makes you perfect.

Step 4: If the indicator muscle remains strong when tested—a sign that the subject is found to be balanced—then the tester should put the suspected allergen into the palm of the subject's resting hand. The sensory receptors, on the tips of the fingers, are extremely sensi-

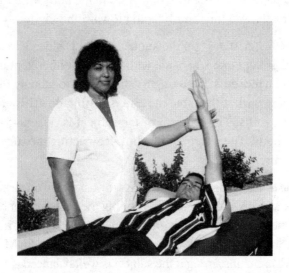

Figure 7-1
Standard Muscle Response Testing

tive in recognizing allergens. When the subject's fingertips touch the allergen, the sensory receptors from the fingertips sense the charges of the allergen and relay the message to the brain. The fingertips have specialized sensory receptors that can send messages to the brain and receive the replies in a nanosecond from the brain. If the charges are compatible to the body, the indicator muscle will remain strong. If it is an incompatible charge, the strong PDM will go weak. This way, you can determine the compatible or incompatible charges of the items you need to find out.

Step 5: This step is useful in balancing the patient if he/she is found to be weak on the initial testing without the presence of an allergen. You need to make the patient's test muscle strong before you can test and compare the strength of the muscle with and without the aller-

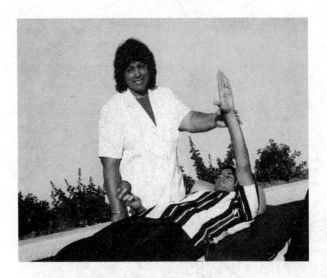

Figure 7-2
Muscle Response Testing with an Allergen in Lying Position

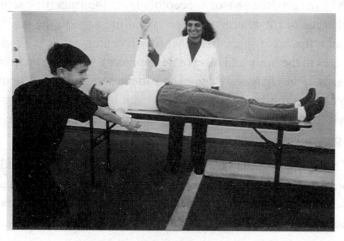

Figure 7-3
Testing a Hyperactive Child

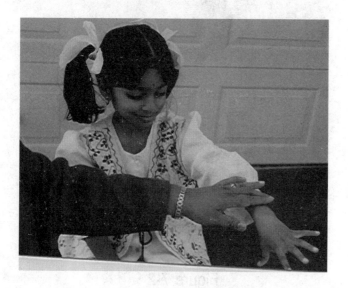

Figure 7-4
Testing an Allergen in Sitting Position

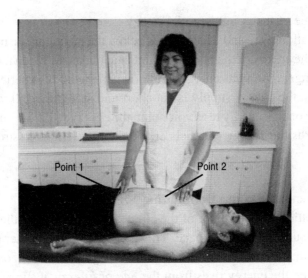

Figure 7-5
Balancing the Patient

gen. The tester places his/her fingertips of one hand at "point 1" on the midline of the subject, about one and a half inches below the navel at the conception vessel "6". The other hand is placed on conception vessel "17" (point 2), in the center of the chest on the midline, level with the nipple line. The tester massages these two points clockwise gently and simultaneously with the fingertips about 20 or 30 seconds, then repeats steps 2 and 3. If the indicator muscle tests strong, continue on to step 4. If the indicator muscle tests weak again, repeat this procedure several times. It is very unlikely that any person will remain weak after repeating this procedure two to three times.

Point 1:

Name of the point: **Sea of Energy**

Location: One and a half inches below the navel, on the midline. This is where the energy of the body is stored in abundance. When the body senses any danger around its energy field or when the body experiences energy blockages, the energy supply is cut short and stored here. If you massage clockwise on this energy reservoir point, the energy will flow out of the storage towards the energy channels and make the weak area strong again.

Point 2:

Name of the point: **Dominating Energy**

Location: In the center of the chest on the midline of the body, level with the fourth intercostal space. This is the energy dispenser unit. This is the point that controls and regulates the energy circulation, or Chi, in the body. When the energy rises from the *Sea of Energy*, it flows straight to the *Dominating Energy* point. From here, the energy is dispersed to different meridians, organs, tissues and cells as needed to help remove the energy blockages. It does this by forcing energy circulation from inside out. During this forced energy circulation, the blockages are pushed out of the body, balancing the body's state. You feel this through the strength of the indicator muscle.

OVAL RING, OR 'O' RING TEST

The oval ring test can be used in self-testing, and this requires one person to perform the test. This can also be used to test a subject if the subject is physically very strong with a strong arm and the tester is a physically weak person.

Step 1: The tester makes an "O" shape by opposing the little finger and thumb on the same hand. Then, with the index finger of the other hand, he/she tries to separate the "O" ring against pressure. If the ring separates easily, you need to use the balancing techniques as described in step 5 of the muscle response test.

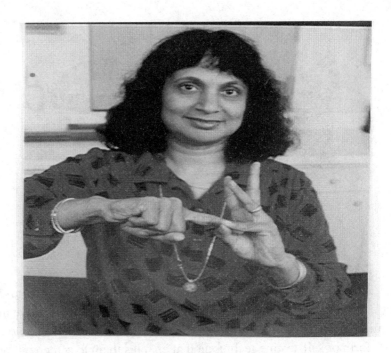

Figure 7-6
"O" Ring or Oval Ring Self-Test

Step 2: If the "O" ring remains inseparable and strong, hold the allergen in the other hand, by the fingertips, and perform step 1 again. If the "O" ring separates easily, the person is allergic to the substance he/she is touching. If the "O" ring remains strong, the substance is not an allergen.

The finger-on-finger test (Figure 7-7) is another way to test yourself. This also needs much practice to become good at testing. The strength of the interphalangeal muscles of two fingers of one hand is used here to test and compare the strength without and with holding an allergen. The middle finger is pushed down, using the index finger of the same hand, or vice versa, in the absence and presence of the allergen in the other hand.

Muscle response testing is one of the most reliable methods of allergy testing, and it is fairly easy to learn and practice in every day life.

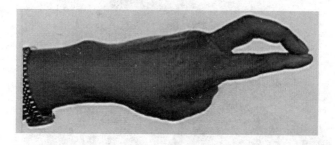

Figure 7-7
Finger-on-Finger Test

After considerable practice, some people are able to test themselves very efficiently using these methods. In order to have freedom to live in this chemically polluted world, it is very important for allergic people to learn some form of self-testing technique that enables them to screen out possible allergens before they contact them. This will help them to prevent allergic reactions. After receiving the basic 30-40 treatments from an NAET practitioner, you will be free to live wherever you like if you know how to test and avoid unexpected allergens from your surroundings. Hundreds of new allergens are thrown into the world daily by non-allergic people who do not understand the predicament of the allergic population. If you want to live in this world looking and feeling normal among normal people, side by side with the allergens, you need to learn how to test on your own. It is not practical for every allergic person to get treated for thousands of allergens from his/her surroundings or go to an NAET practitioner every day for the rest of his/her life. You will not be free from allergies until you learn to test accurately. It takes many hours (months in some cases) of practice. But do not get discouraged. I have given enough information on testing methods here. You need to spend time and practice until you reach perfection.

A TIP TO MASTER SELF-TESTING

Find two items, or ten items. one strong group of items (non-allergic, tested and determined by another person, then another group that you are allergic to. For example, a non allergic group of items consists of: an apple, book, polyester, plastic bag, and the car key; another groupf of allergic items consists of: a banana, lemon, orange, computer key board, and a potato. You are allergic to the apple group and not allergic to the banana group. Hold the apple group one at a time in your free hand and test with the other hand using the oval ring test or finger on finger test. The ring easily breaks or the muscle weakens easily when you hold the items from the allergic group and the muscle of the hand remains strong if you are testing with the items from the nonallergic group. When you test the allergic items, if the muscle didn't go weak, make it happen intentionally for the first few times. Now, hold the items from the nonallergic group and do the same test. This time, the ring doesn't break. Practice this procedure for a while. Rub your hands together for 30 seconds between changing the test samples to interrupt the energy at the fingertips of the previous sample. Practice this every day until your subconscious mind is able to recognize the strength of the allergen just by

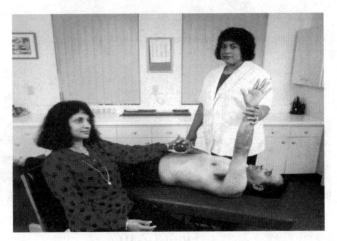

Figure 7-8
Testing Through a Surrogate

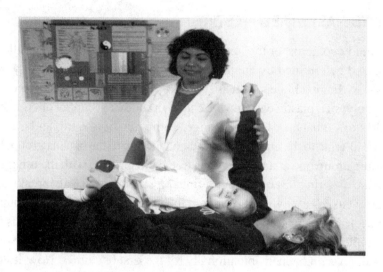

Figure 7-9
Testing an Infant Through a Surrogate

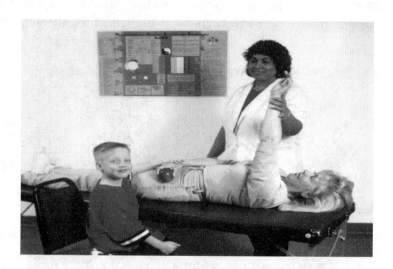

Figure 7-10
Testing a Toddler

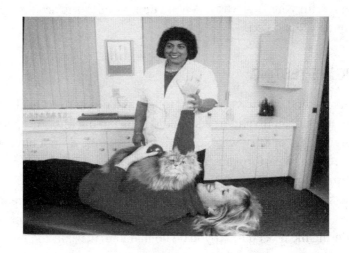

Figure 7-11
Testing an Animal

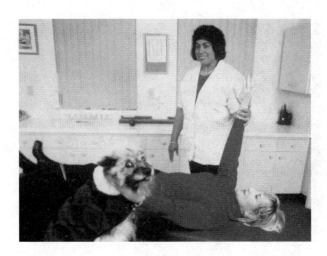

Figure 7-12
Testing Your Pet Through a Surrogate

touching it with your fingertips. When you master this procedure, you can test anything around you.

SURROGATE TESTING

This method can be very useful to test and determine the allergies of an infant, a child, an invalid or disabled person, an unconscious person, an extremely strong, or very weak person, because they do not have enough muscle strength to perform an allergy test. You can also use this method to test an animal, a plant, or a tree.

The surrogate's muscle is tested by the tester. It is very important to remember to maintain skin-to-skin contact between the surrogate and the subject during the procedure. If you do no maintain the skin-to-skin contact, then the surrogate will receive the results of the testing and treatment.

NAET treatments can also be administered through the surrogate very effectively without causing any interference to the surrogate's energy. The testing or treatment does not affect the surrogate as long as the subject maintains uninterrupted skin-to-skin contact with the surrogate.

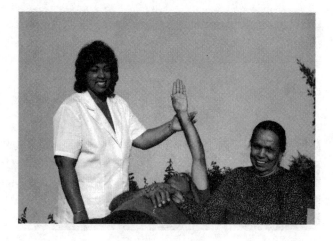

Figure 7-13
Testing Person-to-Person Allergy

Muscle response testing is practiced in this country since 1964. It was originated by Dr. George Goodheart and his associates. Dr. John F. Thie advocates this method through the "Touch For Health" Foundation in Malibu, California. Interested readers can write to "Touch For Health" Foundation, for more information and books on the subject.

You can test an allergy to anything around you using this technique. You can test your allergy to your pets, children, spouse, friends, and other family members using this method. When you test another person, the subject lies down and touches the other person (a suspected allergen) he or she wants tested. The tester pushes the arm of the subject as in steps 2 and 3. If the subject is allergic to the second person, the indicator muscle goes weak. If the subject is not allergic, the indicator muscle remains strong.

If people are allergic to each other (husband and wife, mother and child, father and son, patient and doctor, etc.), the allergy can affect a person in various ways. Husband and wife can be fighting all the time or if they do not have the nature to fight, their health can be affected. The same things can happen among other family members too. It is important to test the family members and other immediate associates for person-to-person allergy and, if found, they should be treated for each other to obtain health, wealth and happiness. More information on person-to-person allergy will be covered in Chapter 18.

HOW CAN "MRT" HELP YOU?

There are thousands of people all over the world who suffer from various mysterious health problems. They run from doctor to doctor, take medicine after medicine, go through surgery after surgery for their undiagnosed health problems. After exhausting their finances, interest and enthusiasm for life, they may receive the diagnosis as "incurable." Most of them may be suffering from undiagnosed allergies. If the medical professionals and the public alike could be taught the importance of allergies and the simple tools to locate them, you would not have to witness or suffer from so many "incurable" health hazards.

Many infants spit up or vomit milk after they drink it. Some infants have severe colic, crying spells, sleep disorders, constipation, etc. When this

---

An Allergy to Baby Formula!

Two month old Madeline stopped projectile vomitry of her formula after one NAET treatment for the formula. After her second treatment, her bowels started eliminating regularly for the first time in her life. Her mom and dad are eternally grateful.

Lisa Forsythe Michelson, AP
Acupuncture Pain Clinic
5600 Trail Blvd., #3
Naples, Fla. 34108
(239) 514-1922

---

happens, pediatricians usually change the milk formula until the infant gets better and does well with one that is suitable. In extreme cases, if the infant continues to throw up all the food, surgery is performed to tighten up the cardiac end of the stomach so the child can keep down what he/she ingests. In such cases, the child's misery is just beginning. Allergies build up and problems start, one after another. Eventually, the child spends his/her entire life with repeated corrective surgeries.

Such was the story of Nancy, 28-years old, who came to our office with complaints of severe migraine headaches. She suffered from headaches nearly once a week, which kept her in bed on medications. Also, she was frequently given pain shots. On examination of her history, we learned that she vomited every meal as an infant and a child. She had 32 surgeries during her 28 years of life. This included a hernia surgery when she was an infant, seven surgeries for gastric ulcers, six for her knees, two for her nose and two for her sinuses. She also had four surgeries on her shoulders, one to remove a cyst from her ovary, two on her ankle, two for the bladder, one for the ear and one for the throat to remove her tonsils. She had the feeling of a big mass on one side of her head whenever she had a migraine. Brain swelling was the cause of this pseudo-mass. Finally, she was advised to have brain surgery to prevent the severe debilitating migraine, when a friend referred her to us.

Muscle response testing revealed that she was highly allergic to almost every substance around her including food, drinks, clothings, carpet, bed linnen, and her pets. She was treated by NAET for nearly a year, at the rate of five treatments a week. Treatments included treating for all the basics, and every item she came in contact with in her everyday life. For the first few treatments, we concentrated on her regular food items. Then she was treated for her clothing, cosmetics, etc. By the end of three months, her migraines became less frequent and less intense. At the end of one year, she could almost live a normal life, not a life ruled by her sicknesses. If her parents had learned MRT to test allergies, she wouldn't have had 32 surgeries in her 28 years of life.

Incidentally, toward the end of the treatment, she met a young man and fell in love for the first time in her life. A year later, they got married. This is one of the happy endings to an otherwise miserable situation.

Muscle testing for allergies should be taught in every school and in every establishment. Everyone should learn to test to detect and avoid their allergies, even if the treatment is not available in your area. If you know your allergies, you can easily avoid them and that will alone help you a lot.

Let's look at the history of 6-year-old Ray, who suffered from severe allergies from birth. The second day of his life, he developed red, angry looking rashes all over his body. He began spitting up every meal, whether it was water or milk. He suffered from severe constipation, insomnia, irritability, colic pains and severe eczema. When he was 6 months old, his pediatrician suggested purse-string surgery (tightening up the lower segment of the esophagus to prevent continuous vomiting). But he was luckier than Nancy. His mother learned MRT and tested everything before she gave him. She fed him non-allergic food items only every day for four years (cream of rice, nonfat Carnation dry milk and water). He did fairly well on the special diet. His eczema was under control. He slept better. His constipation was relieved. His colic pain diminished. He appeared happy and friendly. When he was four, he began treatment through NAET. In a year or so, after being treated for various allergies, he was able to eat normal food and was ready for school. He is a healthy teenager now.

Just by knowing MRT and the testing procedure, Ray's mother could prevent unwanted surgeries on Ray. Nancy's mother did not have a chance to learn the simple MRT testing technique. Nancy couldn't go to regular school. She couldn't go to college and couldn't get trained in any job due to her ill health. She lived on disability all her life. We know both Nancy and Ray; and we know their lives before and after NAET, and their lives now, many years after completed the NAET treatments. We want to prevent people getting to be like Nancy due to their allergies. If we can teach testing skills to the mass media, people can hope to have a life like Ray.

Medical professionals, as well as the public, should be educated to listen and look for various types of allergies when they cannot find the cause of a problem. Unless you are educated to know about the MRT testing, you do not know what to look for. As you have seen, the theory of energy blockages and diseases comes from Oriental medicine. Oriental medicine also teaches that, if given a chance, with a little support, the body will heal itself.

CHAPTER 8

CAUSES OF DISEASE

A s mentioned earlier, an imbalance is caused by the obstructions of energy circulation along the energy pathways. The obstruction of energy can be caused by either internal (endogenous) or external (exogenous) factors.

Internal factors arise within the body itself and may be due to dysfunction of vital organs (heart, liver, lung, kidney, digestive tract, genito-urinary, skin and brain disorders, etc.), resulting in asthma, emphysema abnormal growths, etc. They can be due to emotional disturbances such as excessive joy, grief and sad news, or nutritional deficiencies, such as eating allergic foods, consuming foods without adequate nutrients, overeating, eating unhygienic food, or uncooked foods, etc.

External factors causing energy blockages include eating contaminated foods and drinks, environmental materials like pollens, airborne bacteria, viruses or any other disease-producing agents, fabrics, clothing (wool, cotton, synthetic materials), insect bites, cosmetics, etc. If not taken care of immediately, the prolonged effect of external factors may not only turn into internal problems, but may also cause illness and disease.

Diseases caused by various allergens can enter the body in a variety of ways. They may enter through the mouth via ingestion, by nose via inhalation, by skin via injection, and by osmosis via local application. According to NAET theory, allergens can also enter the body as electromagnetic energy by conduction via transmission through nerve endings under the skin. All substances, like fabrics, jewelry, metals, etc., have an electromagnetic charge around them. Therefore, nearly all of these substances are capable of affecting the human body in a negative or positive way.

According to NAET theory, when an incompatible electrical charge or an allergen (whether it is food, drink, materials, fabrics, animals or another human being) comes near the body, a clash between their electromagnetic fields will occur. The large force of repulsion between the charges creates blockages of the meridians. The sudden blocking of the meridians is one of the quickest defense mechanisms of the brain in its attempt to stop the allergen from entering deeper into the body.

Repulsion between charges causes blockages in the meridians. The greater the difference in the charges, the greater the repulsion and, therefore, the blockage. This proportionately affects the imbalances and disorganization in the body. When severe disorganization takes place in the body, energy becomes stagnated, causing overflow, reversed flow and underflow of energy in certain areas of the meridians. At this point, body functions cannot proceed properly.

When body functions do not take place freely, the body begins to succumb to health problems: body aches, joint pains, sore throat, sensations of heat, sensations of cold, fever, chills, painful lymph nodes, muscle pain, weak limbs, fatigue, headaches, sleep disturbances, irritability, forgetfulness, confusion, depression, difficulty in thinking, poor concentration, phobias, crying spells, suicidal thoughts, feeling of loneliness even in crowds, sores in the mouth, indigestion, bloating, frequent urination, water retention, burning sensations on the skin and on the limbs (hands, feet, palms and soles), etc. The intensity of the symptoms will depend on the location of the blockage and the status of the immune system of the sufferer.

If you fail to eradicate the blockage immediately, the adverse energy eventually could take over the body and cause problems at deeper levels. For example: the aches and pains can turn into chronic arthritis, causing degenerative changes in the joints; a sore throat can turn into an infection or become enlarged, or an infected tonsil could require surgery; painful lymph nodes may turn into pus-filled abscesses; breast abscesses may turn into tumors and cancers; muscle weakness may turn into muscle wasting disorders; headaches can turn into severe migraines; mild sleep disorders may turn into severe insomnia; neuropsychological complaints, such as anger, irritability, confusion, depression, etc., may turn the sufferer into a psychiatric case, possibly leading to institutionalization.

Many practitioners and patients are probably familiar with the initial stages of these problems linked with blocked energy flows; but just as many people classify these symptoms as "chronic fatigue syndrome," a debilitating disease for which, up until now, no successful treatment has been found by Western medicine.

We treated Stan, a 28-year-old computer programmer who began to feel extreme fatigue a year after he started working with a well-known computer firm. He had a wife and two children. When he started experiencing incapacitating exhaustion, he began dreading his work. His output also started to slow down. He was diagnosed as having "chronic fatigue syndrome." His energy was drained to the point that he was unable to walk without assistance. Finally, he had to file for disability. His health improved when he was away from work for a while. Once he returned to work, his problems started all over—even though he was given regular physical therapy and supportive treatments.

After four years of illness, he was referred to our office and it was discovered that he was highly allergic to plastic products and his computer keyboard. He was also allergic to computer radiation. After he was treated by NAET for plastics, keyboard, and radiation, he was able to resume his regular work.

Robert, a 32-year-old computer analyst, had also suffered from chronic fatigue syndrome. He had been ill for seven years and was completely disabled for two years. He also experienced frequent headaches, joint pains, indigestion, pain in the abdomen, and insomnia. Robert had been working with computers for ten years, was married for eight years with two children, ages seven and five. He was found to be allergic to eggs, milk, fruits, sugar, wheat, carrots, salt, corn, dried beans, spices, polyester, synthetic fabrics, chemical fumes, trees, grasses, his dog, inks, ceramics, computer, plastics, keyboards, computer radiation, formaldehyde, his wife and one of his children.

Evaluating each allergen separately, we can see how it individually contributed toward his disability.

Eggs and dried beans (proteins): From the time he was born, his body could not tolerate animal or vegetable proteins, making him less resistant to various allergens. This, in turn, weakened his immune system. The human body depends on protein utilization and assimilation for normal everyday body functions, such as protein synthesis, and Kreb cycle.

Milk (calcium): Milk and other dairy products provide many essential nutrients, mainly calcium. Calcium is necessary to keep the body healthy. Allergy to milk and milk products causes poor absorption of calcium. Robert had a calcium deficiency.

Vegetables (vitamin C): Vitamin C is necessary to repair wear and tear of the body and to help maintain a normal immune system, growth and development. His allergy to vitamin C impaired his body's ability to repair itself.

Grains (B complex vitamins): Allergy to grains also caused him to be allergic to B complex vitamins. B vitamins are necessary for the normal functions of the nervous system. In the absence of B vitamins, Robert's various enzymatic functions were not able to take place in his body.

Sugar (fruits and other sugars): Sugar provides energy for body functions. If the body cannot absorb or utilize sugar, many of the body functions suffer as a result. Robert's inability to utilize sugar contributed to his fatigue.

Iron: A person gets iron from foods like raisins, nuts and meats, etc. When you are allergic to this group of foods, iron absorption is impaired. Lack of iron makes the person anemic. As a result of his inability to absorb iron, he was always tired.

Salt: Allergy to salt means allergy to your own body because every cell of the body contains sodium. Integrity of the sodium-potassium pump depends on the ability to absorb and utilize the salts. The sodium-potassium pump keeps the body electrical. This electricity keeps the body alive. His allergy to salt interfered with his body's ability to utilize salt effectively.

Spices: Allergy to spices causes retention of water and swelling of the tissue in various parts of the body. This causes affected tissue to suffer from pain or discomfort. Headaches can occur if water retention and tissue swelling affect the brain tissue. If other joints are affected, pain and swelling of the joints occur. Robert's headaches and joint pains were directly related to his allergy to spices.

Chemicals: If you are allergic to chemicals, the adverse energy could penetrate the body through the skin, thus blocking the energy pathways. Adverse energy from chemicals travels faster, producing tiredness, light-headedness, brain fog, sharp pains in the body, etc., within a few seconds of exposure to the allergens. The same applies to fumes, formaldehydes, radiation, fabrics, etc. Robert's headaches and tiredness could be traced to his allergy to chemicals.

Allergies to human beings and animals also work like a chemical allergy. When you are near the adverse energy of another person or animal, the body tries to protect itself by creating blockages.

In the case of Robert, he was surrounded by the adverse energies of various foods from the time he was born. When he began working with computers for hours on end, the allergy to the computer material, along with radiation, added to the blockage. Then, the adverse energy of his wife came along and caused more blockages. His child added more to his agony. His body was constantly fighting various energy blockages, whether he was at work or home, and whether he was aware of the blockages or not.

As a result of this constant fight for survival, his body lost the battle and became physically ill and, later, disabled. When he finally retired in his house, his wife and other allergens were around him all the time. His condition worsened as the days progressed. Since he was bombarded with equally strong allergens, it is difficult to say which one affected him the most. He always felt sick. The reason for his illness was blamed on chronic fatigue syndrome or some unknown viral attack.

When his allergies were removed one by one through NAET, his blockages lessened. He started feeling better most of the time. When most allergens were eliminated, his body began identifying other allergens promptly, reacting immediately to those allergens he had not yet been treated for.

At this point, some people might wonder if he was becoming allergic to new things or if he was getting more sensitive to existing allergens. It was neither of these two options. He learned to look at his chronic illness in a different way. Until now, he was made to believe that there was no known cure for his debilitating disease. He took it as his destiny to be sick. Now, he was taught to look at all his health problems as the result of allergies. His awareness became sharper. When he was living in the midst of allergens, he always felt sick and miserable. His attacks became less frequent after he was freed of several allergens. He began experiencing good hours and days more often. However, when he experienced an allergic attack, he felt the effect more. The strength of his remaining allergies continued to affect him. Eventually, he became normal again.

NAET treatment works with the entire body: the physical body (organs, brain, nervous system and tissues), physiological body (circulation of blood, fluids and nerve energy) and emotional body (mind, thoughts and spirituality). It helps to detoxify the system by clearing the adverse energies of the allergens from the entire body. Thus, it enables the body to relax, absorb and assimilate appropriate nutrients from the food that once caused allergies and support the proper growth of the entire body.

A 29-year-old housewife, who worked as a dressmaker in her spare time, began complaining of severe chronic fatigue and severe bursitis, calcification in the right shoulder joint and pain in the elbow joint. She was listless most of the time, with no energy or enthusiasm to do anything, and felt high-

> *NAET helps to detoxify the system by clearing the adverse energies of the allergens from the entire body. Thus it enables the body to relax, absorb and assimilate appropriate nutrients from the food that once caused allergies and support the proper growth of the entire body.*

ly irritated with her two children. She suffered from weakness in her limbs, preventing her from performing normal household chores. Her husband employed a part-time housekeeper. Even with help, she was becoming weaker and weaker. She started having severe, debilitating migraine headaches and became dependent on pain medications. After a while, even pain medications did not give her any relief.

When she was seen in our office, she told us that she enjoyed sewing in the afternoon. That led us in the right direction for our investigation into her mysterious sickness. When she was tested by NTT, she was found to be highly allergic to the sewing needle, sewing materials, and needlework frame. The frame was made up of wood, and the needle contained iron. She was very allergic to iron and wood. After being treated for the needle, stainless steel, iron and wood, she began recovering from her debilitating illness. It took a few more months for her to gain full strength back from her unusual sickness.

A 30-year-old nurse had a similar problem. She complained of a severe tenosynovitis (pain in the thumb and metacarpal joints) of both hands. The pain was more severe on the right hand; it progressed and radiated into the elbow and shoulder joints. She had nine months of physical therapy along with many analgesics, but nothing gave her relief. Her treating physician referred her to our office. When we saw her, she was on disability because of excruciating pain and an inability to perform her nursing duties. She had severe insomnia due to pain, and suffered from asthma. She was treated for various allergens with NAET. Her asthma improved considerably, she slept better at night and her energy increased. After two months of continuous treatments, her original problem of tenosynovitis and bursitis did not improve. During detailed questioning in a re-evaluation interview, it was discovered that she cooked every day for her husband and three children. While cutting the vegetables and meat, she often used a crude pig-iron knife (black and coarse), that she had brought especially from India because she liked its sharpness. She was asked to bring this knife in for testing and was found to be extremely allergic to it. It took seven consecutive treatments with NAET to clear the allergy for that crude iron knife. After successful completion of her treatment, the ache in her joints subsided. Seven years later, she continues to be symptom-free.

We have a 16 year old male patient with ADD. He was socially delayed and had behavioral problems. He was doing very poor in his school subjects. We found him highly allergic to his mother and one brother as well as a combination of MMR/ DPT and stainless steel. His symptoms resolved and his attitude and grades improved when he completed these treatments.

Stephanie Kennedy ND, CNT, MT
824 7th Ave. South, Nampa, ID 83651
(208) 466-3517

A 33-year-old woman was seen in our office with a peculiar allergic reaction. Shortly after her marriage 12 years ago, her left hand went numb. Later she began experiencing severe shooting pains in her left arm and joints. Numerous orthopedic and neurological doctors saw her to no avail. Finally, she found a chiropractor who gave her temporary relief from the pain and discomfort. However, the numbness soon turned into excruciating pain in her left fingers, elbow, forearm and both shoulders.

Ultimately, the pain started affecting her upper back and right arm. She became a regular visitor to the chiropractor's office, sometimes twice a day. She started to use a sling to support her left arm. She also started getting severe bronchitis and regular attacks of pneumonia. She was in very poor physical condition when she was seen in our office in 1985. She was first treated for various food allergies, which eliminated her chronic upper respiratory infections and bronchitis, but the pain in her left arm remained. She said acupuncture sometimes helped her.

During one of her usual office visits, the doctor palpated her painful points at the elbow and followed the pain to determine the points to insert the acupuncture needles. To her surprise, the radiation of the pain was traced to the ring finger. Immediately, she was asked to remove her large, single-stone diamond ring to test for allergies. She felt guilty taking off the ring as she had made a vow never to remove her wedding ring. She was slightly superstitious, but with coaxing, she reluctantly took it off to perform the test. The woman was highly allergic to this "diamond ring to be worn forever." Diamond is a stone with a powerful electromagnetic force around it. After this discovery, she stopped wearing it. In two days the pain stopped in the left arm and upper back. She tried to wear the ring a few more times, but every time she tried, the excruciating pain in the left arm returned. Finally, after 17 days of consecutive treatments, she was able to successfully wear it without pain.

A 44-year-old woman came to the office complaining of severe pain all along her left leg down to her ankle. She had already been suffering for a year and three months. During that time, she had seen two neurologists, an orthopedic doctor, a chiropractor and a Rolfer. She received massages at least once a week in the hope that they would increase her circulation and rid her of the pain. During this period, she had to go to the emergency room four times, because the pain had become unbearable. Pain pills could no longer control her pain. Her X-rays and other examinations showed signs of osteoporosis. She was taking hormone therapy to reduce the presumed osteoporosis. In our office, she was tested through NTT and   evaluated thoroughly via her history, physical examination, and allergy tests for foods, chemicals and environmental materials. She was wearing a large diamond ring on her left ring finger. When she was tested for the ring, she was found to be highly allergic to the diamond. Through kinesiological examination, it was found that the allergy to the diamond was causing an energy blockage in the left leg. Even though she had completely recovered from having polio as a child, her history pointed out that her left leg had been affected. She also told us that she regularly wore another huge, single-stone diamond ring since her marriage.

Upon questioning her further, we discovered that she had received these two diamond rings from her husband when they married a year and four months earlier. Soon after the marriage, she was sick for three weeks with a severe bladder infection and flu-like symptoms. When she recovered from the infection, she developed the muscle spasm and pain in the leg. Energy blockage due to allergy always affects the weakest area of the body. Her left leg was the weakest area in her body due to her previous polio attack.

Motion Sickness

  I am so thrilled to report to you about one of my patients, Mary Ruth Piper McGee. This is regarding to the treatment I gave her for her inability to tolerate any sort of motion whatever from riding in a car to running a vacuum cleaner. I used a small hand-held vibrator as her allergen while giving her NAET treatment. When the 20 minute treatment time was up, she returned the vibrator to my receptionist and went into a fainting spell. After performing the usual emergency measures, she revived completely and finally was able to go home. However she had to walk the 3 kilometers to her home because she could not travel by car. when she arrived home she cancelled her work commitment for the week and went to bed. After 2-3 days of intense nausea even aggravated by the moving curtains from breeze, she recovered and reported to me the following week that she had travelled in the back seat of a subcompact car for a journey of approximately 200 kilometers. She states that this clearing has given her a new lease on life and that over the past two years there has never been any return of her previous symptoms. We watched her closely for the past two years now.
  You may use this letter in any way you wish to help others.

Dr. B.A. Hayhoe, D.C., N.D.
123 Hazen Street
Saint John, NB, CANADA (506) 6652-1778

The pain and discomfort of her leg disappeared after she was treated for the diamond by NAET.

Diamond has one of the strongest energy fields, extending up to 60 feet in radiation. If you have a sensitivity to diamonds and come within its energy field, you may experience an allergic reaction.

If the energy of the diamond is perceived as compatible by the brain, the energy from the diamond would add to the body's energy and enhance the energy flow through the meridians. This strengthened energy might even help remove possible energy blockages, leading to better health for the wearer. Many people believe in wearing birthstones for health, happiness and success. This may explain why the phenomenon is a possibility. However, compatibility with the stone is absolutely necessary for positive enhancement of energy. If you are surrounded by suitable energy fields from many different items in a room, the energy from all the products will flow through you and you will feel energetic and happy. The energy pathways open wide for free flowing energy to circulate through the body without any obstruction. This will improve the circulation of the blood, supplying plenty of oxygen and nutrients to all the cells and tissues of the body, keeping you healthy and strong. If you can find suitable precious stones and wear them daily, your health will improve. When you are in good health, your mind will experience happiness and your body will like to be active. You will work hard and good results will come out of your work, bringing good fortune. Thus, if you wear the right, compatible, precious birthstone, you will be rewarded with health, wealth and happiness. Now, you know the secret behind wearing the birthstone.

On the other hand, if you are surrounded by unsuitable charges from many objects around you that cause energy blockages in your meridians, no amount of massages, therapies or medications will benefit you. Your discomfort will only increase with no relief in sight.

From some of these case studies, you can understand how strongly the electromagnetic energies of substances can influence the health of humans (and probably other living beings) by causing energy blockages. We spoke of their adverse affects on the body. They also can exert good influences.

The unique case of a 24-year-old woman who met a man whom she married two weeks later is worth mentioning here. Her husband was very much into clean living and good eating habits. He only ate complex carbohydrates and unprocessed foods. This was a new type of diet for her. A couple of weeks after their marriage, she became very ill with chronic bronchitis. Antibiotics did not relieve the symptoms. She complained of severe and constant body aches and pain in her joints. She felt depressed and suffered from severe insomnia. Her concerned husband took her from doctor to doctor in the hope of some relief for his new wife.

One of the doctors asked her what events made her feel better and what made her feel worse. Her answer was that the only time she felt relief from her pain was when she had her husband's arm around her. At all other times, she hurt in spite of taking many analgesics daily. The doctor shook his head and referred her to a psychiatrist for the treatment of psychosomatic ailments. The psychiatrist agreed with her previous doctor and advised her to go to Hawaii for a vacation. The doctor believed she was seeking more attention from her husband. They tried the vacation and went to Hawaii and Tahiti for a few weeks, but her condition remained the same.

It turned out that she was highly allergic to the B complex family, which included all the healthy and unprocessed foods. When she started eating whole-wheat products and a high fiber diet, her body began building up toxins that caused her all that physical and mental agony. Nobody suspected that allergies were the cause of her problems. She was not allergic to her husband, nor was he to her. When she sat next to him, his strong energy field enhanced and improved her energy circulation, just like wearing a compatible precious birthstone, which helped to open up her blockages temporarily. When the energy circulated freely through the energy meridians, the aches and pains left her and she felt happy. She was right in saying that she felt better in her husband's arms. A regular psychologist or psychiatrist could not understand this woman's strange health problem. It took an NAET practitioner to recognize her health problem. After many NAET treatments, the woman received freedom from her constant pain and now lives a happy, healthy life with her husband and their healthy son.

CHAPTER 9

DISCOVERY OF NAET

Allergic conditions occur much more frequently than you might realize. Visit any multifunction clinic and you will find a large number of allergy patients anxiously filling the waiting room. Every year, more and more allergy cases are reported. There are several reasons for this. People are developing more allergic symptoms than ever before due to the increase in the population of our large cities, where certain industrial dust, chemicals, fumes and environmental pollutants, pollens, etc., are proliferating. We live in a techno-chemical age where researchers and scientists are competing to get better products into the market place faster, creating new products daily. The continuous discovery of various chemical compounds used to manufacture clothing and fabrics create new allergens. Many people quickly develop sensitivity to these compounds. Physicians are becoming more allergy conscious, recognizing and diagnosing allergies more frequently.

It is important to recognize that allergies, like people, do not exist in a vacuum. They are a part of a complex interrelation between the allergen and the central nervous system. The central nervous system controls the proper function of the various organs and systems in the body (the digestive, circulatory, skeletal, urogenital, integumentary, and lymphatic systems). Each of these complex systems, under the direction of the central nervous

Multiple Chemical Sensitivities!

A 27 year old female presented with severe symptoms of Multiple Chemical Sensitivities causing symptoms of dizziness, brain fog, disorientation, muscle spasms, overall weakness, eyes swelling shut, throat closing up, and blackouts. She often fainted when exposed to chemical smells and was in danger of concussion from hitting her head during these sudden episodes of loss of consciousness. Smells that triggered this did not even have to be especially noxious. She had fainted at the local health food store simply from turning down the aisle where supplements and shampoos were stored. She had been experiencing these symptoms for approximately one year. She stated that: "Since the onset of MCS I have become more and more sensitized to an increasing number of chemicals. I have become virtually housebound and have great difficulty leaving without an exacerbation of symptoms." She was unable to pursue her profession because of it. This patient treated all the basics and many other food allergies. In addition, she treated parasites, chemicals, viruses, pesticides, hormones, perfumes, mercury, plastics, formaldehyde, mold, leaf mold, and the smell of mold. She had to treat for many smells: perfumes, air freshener, bleach, fabric softener, ammonia, household cleaning products. She also treated propane, car exhaust, carpets, paint, and gasoline. We also worked on body parts: lung, adrenals, liver, gall bladder, bile, and muscles. Sometimes she didn't pass her treatments on the first try but would usually pass the next time. This patient made considerable progress. Her fainting stopped and she was able to go out in the world again. She was able to take several long trips on airplanes. At the point she moved out of state, she was much stronger and able to function much more normally again. I know she could not have made these improvements without NAET.

Sue Anderson, D.C.
Ann Arbor, MI.
Tel. (734)-662-9140

system, is capable of ignoring or reacting to a given stimulus. This happens either in concert with all other systems, producing a massive shutdown of the human machine, or separately, producing weakness and malfunction of any single part or all parts of the total system.

The exact reason the central nervous system chooses to react to or to ignore a given stimulus is so far unknown.Large areas of the brain are always under investigation to identify their multiple functions. One reaction, which has undergone intensive observation, is asthma. Strangely asthma sufferers do not experience attacks when they are frightened. In such situations, it is believed that the body prepares for *fight or flight*. The theory states that in this hyper-chemical state, the allergens are totally ignored. The adjustment has been made as though a switch was suddenly thrown. I utilized this idea when I developed NAET as a treatment to permanently eliminate allergies. Every time a patient is tested for an allergen, the central nervous system is alerted to the presence of the approaching danger. When the patient is then treated for the allergen, an intentional hyper-chemical state or a temporary *fight or flight* reaction is created in the body, forcing it to produce the appropriate neuro-chemicals to overcome the oncoming danger: the presence of the known allergen. Tapping at the specific nerve roots will alert the entire nerve pathway, from its origin in the brain to the nerve ending somewhere in the periphery, about the dangerous situation. This will inform the nerve about the adjustment the body is making by releasing appropriate neuro-chemical-antidotes (endorphins, enkephalins, etc.) to neutralize the threat. During the hyper-chemical state, the allergen is once again totally ignored. At a later time, whenever that particular allergen comes in contact with the body, the body will automatically go into a hyper-chemical state by releasing the particular chemical and will no longer react adversely to the allergen. The same allergen can trigger different individual allergic reactions in people, depending upon the number of energy pathways affected by the allergen's invasion. The different reactions of eight people to a common allergen such as chocolate can be compared. In every case, the standard scratch test and blood serum analysis did not identify chocolate as an allergen for that patient.

Case 1: Patient exhibited hyperactivity and insomnia upon eating chocolate (blockage in the Heart and Liver energy meridians).

Case 2: Patient's symptom was acute asthmatic distress (blockage in the Lung meridian).

Case 3: Chocolate resulted in the patient having a vascular frontal headache approaching the magnitude of migraines (blockage in the Stomach meridian).

Case 4: Patient experienced extreme fatigue and was unable to keep awake (blockage in the Spleen and Heart meridians).

Case 5: Whenever the patient ate chocolate, she became extremely emotional and often depressed (Liver, Lungs and Heart meridians).

Case 6: Patient experienced severe indigestion, bloating, belching and muscle ache (Stomach, Liver, Spleen and Small Intestine meridians).

Case 7: Patient had severe pain in the joints of the extremities, similar to that of arthritis (blockage in the Kidney meridian).

Case 8: Patient had severe diarrhea minutes after she consumed chocolate (blockage in the Large Intestine meridian).

Most of these patients, in spite of medical test results to the contrary, knew by instinct and experience that they should not eat chocolate. How the body reacted to contact with the allergen was not consistent with every patient; rather, each patient's body reacted at the "perverse whim" of the central nervous system.

The expression of the allergic reaction seemed to be centered in one or more of the organs alerted to the presence of the substance located in or near the body. The observation is consistent with traditional Oriental medicine; treatment for most diseases should begin by making adjustments to the central nervous system, the center of balance between all bodily functions. Offending elements introduced into the system trigger imbalances. This adversely affects the essence of the body, or *Chi*, further manifesting the problem in pathology of the various tissues and organs, or the *Zang Fu*.

The pathology can then be clearly demonstrated initially as a kinetic weakness observable through standard muscle response testing techniques, borrowed from applied kinesiology. In fact, each of the chocolate allergy sufferers, exhibited weakness when given a muscle response test. This fact becomes the pivotal premise in the foundation of the *NAET* therapy model. Kinetic weakness, or muscle weakness, makes diagnosis possible. Muscle weakness is the body's way of signaling to the patient and the doctor potential negative reactions to allergens. Since a simple and effective diagnostic tool is now available, it becomes a relatively simple matter of good detective work to identify all the substances that may be responsible for the presenting symptoms.

When Oriental medicine was introduced to the western world about three decades ago, many western medical minds were amazed that many so-called psychosomatic illnesses responded nicely to acupuncture treatment. They were even more amazed when they began to unlock the secrets of the central nervous system; how it controls the body's overall functions and the functions of its individual organs. They also knew that by stimulating the trunk of the central nervous system (and its branches or meridians that form the complex link between the brain and various body parts), one could receive temporary relief from pain. Although they did not understand the reason, they proceeded to develop methods to provide healing benefits to their patients.

For NAET to be effective, it is not necessary to follow the Chinese theory every step of the way. We can adapt the best of what Chinese medicine can offer and combine it with the best of what western science can render us. Putting both sources of knowledge together is like putting two heads together to better solve a problem. Both of these medical disciplines definitely help to better establish our need to understand ourselves and our brain functions. In my opinion, we can help ourselves and solve a lot of mysterious, *incurable* health problems by learning to strengthen our brain and nervous systems.

As previously discussed, all-living and nonliving substances, and the earth itself, have a magnetic energy around them. All the substances on the surface of the earth also are attracted to each other by each substance's own magnetic force. We are all products of the same universe, interrelated to each other. This may have been the state of the world when it began. Over the years, due to genetic mutation, genes of all living things have changed slightly, or have been altered from the original creation. Replication usually creates these differences, some noticeable and some not, from generation to generation, in any given life form.

When humans are replicated, the genes are altered, depending upon the circumstances of the replication. That is why some children may not look like their parents while others look very similar. If some of the energy channels were blocked during the time of replication or during the transfer of the genetic message, the reproduced gene will carry all the messages except that of the blocked area. When this partial replication is repeated over and over, transferred genes may lose the ability to recognize certain items that caused the blockage during the time of replication. In other words, the brain does not have the ability to recognize some of the energies around it. It repels what it does not recognize.

From this assumption another hypothesis can be formed. Allergic sensitivities are nothing but the signals to the central nervous system gone awry. The product of these signals, which create repulsion between the central nervous system and other substances, has little to do with the toxic or nontoxic properties of the substances. Instead, they are the result of the way the central nervous system perceives the substance and how it decides whether or not the substance is a compatible field. It is nontoxic or toxic according to how the brain perceives it. If it is perceived as toxic, it will cause blockages in the energy channels; if perceived as nontoxic, it will aid the energy flow in the channels, helping to clear any blockage present. The extent of the clearance will depend upon the strength of the substance's compatible field.

This brings us to a concept that is totally revolutionary to most people. Allergic reactions are the result of messages received and acted upon by the central nervous system and are not the result of the inherent properties of the substances we come in contact with.

The quest of every patient and, indeed, of the whole healing profession, is to discover the method that will change the signals from "danger" to "harmless." Of course, every medical philosophy has developed its own treatment concept, and each has its own following. The adherents of different philosophies cling to their particular treatment modalities and procedures, tenaciously directing patients to attain whatever levels of healing are possible through them.

Still, at best, real relief and comfort come only when the allergen is totally avoided, which is more often, impossible. Even then, as is often the case, new allergies replace those that are successfully avoided, leaving the patient in the same miserable condition or even worse than before. So the question still remains: Is a permanent cure possible for allergies? Can the central nervous system, which has been conditioned to respond in rebellion against the body for a long time, perhaps for a millennium, be reprogrammed and brought under submission? Can the central nervous system be trained to send positive signals that can attract anything around it to benefit the body, instead of conflicting with these fields of force and damaging the body balance? Can our own nervous systems help us to become free from the damaging effects of allergies? Is a permanent cure for allergies possible? At last, the answer to these questions is a definite "YES."

The central nervous system has the ability to ignore or reject a substance's force field and create a large variety of physical, physiological and psychological problems in the body as a result of its repulsive nature. The same nervous system has the ability to accept or approve other forces around us and make us feel good and comfortable. The brain acquired the ability of attraction, from the beginning, before it lost its ability (of attraction), due to cell mutation. This means that the brain was once aware of the ability of attraction and now has forgotten it. You need to retrain the body to go back to its original function so you can make the nervous system accept the presence of other rejected items without creating blockages or unpleasantness in the body. This can be accomplished. The treatment produces a permanent result, and the sufferers from allergies, once treated, will be free at last.

In previous chapters, you have seen that the allergen, or adverse charges of a substance, clearly can be demonstrated as a kinetic weakness observable through standard muscle response testing techniques from applied kinesiology. This fact then becomes the pivotal premise in the foundation of NAET therapy model. Kinetic or muscle weakness makes diagnosis possible.

Acupuncture stimulates the central nervous system, provides temporary relief from pain and promotes healing. Recently, many articles have been written about allergies in publications from both holistic and western medical writers. In every case, there is a message of hope along with a treatment methodology that includes a strict diet and/or some other careful behavior regimen. In every case, there are warnings to the patient about the potential for a relapse if the maintenance doses are not taken or if certain foods are not completely eliminated from the diet. In no instance of treatment is there hope for a total and irreversible cure. These practitioners are right to be cautious, because in order to achieve permanent relief from allergic reactions, the central nervous system must be reprogrammed to sense allergens differently than before treatment. The question is: Is this possible? Can NAET offer a solution? The answer is a resounding *YES*.

DISCOVERY OF NAET

The answer to this question was discovered quite by accident on Friday, November 23, 1983, at about 2:00 p.m. I was being treated by acupuncture for the relief of a severe allergic reaction to raw carrots. During the treatment, I fell asleep with the carrots still on my body. After the acupuncture treatment (and a restful nap during the needling period), I woke up and experienced a unique feeling. I had never felt quite that way following other similar acupuncture treatments in the past. I realized that I had been lying on some of the carrot. A piece was also still in my hand. I knew that some of the needles were supposed to help circulate the electrical energy and balance the body. If there is any energy blockage, the balancing process is supposed to clear it during the treatment and bring the body to a balanced state. I had studied this concept at school.

I asked my husband, who was assisting me in the treatment process, to test me for carrots again. The carrot's energy field had interacted with my own energy field, and my brain had accepted this once deadly poison as a harmless item. The two energy fields no longer clashed. This was an amazing NEW DISCOVERY. Subsequent tests for carrots by MRT confirmed that something phenomenal had happened. We repeated testing every hour for the rest of that day. I continued eating carrots the next day without any allergic reaction. This confirmed the result. My central nervous system had learned a different response to the stimulus, and I was no longer reactive to it. In some mysterious way, the treatment had reprogrammed my brain. What followed was a series of experiments treating my own allergies and those of my family. I cured most of my allergies in a year's time. The method was finally extended to my practice. In every case, allergies were "cleared out," never to return. After treating thousands of patients for a wide variety of allergens, the procedure is no longer experimental or of questionable value. It is a proven treatment method and the premise of NAET methodology.

Physical contact with the allergen during and after a treatment (which consists of stimulating certain specific points on the acupuncture meridians, thus stimulating the central nervous system) produces the necessary immune mediators or antidotes to neutralize the adverse reaction coming from the allergen held in the hand. This produces a totally new, permanent and irreversible response to the allergen. It is possible, through stimulation of the appropriate points of the acupuncture meridians, which have direct correspondence with the brain, to reprogram the brain.

The success of the NAET procedure confirms that a major portion of the illnesses we observe result from allergies. This includes the experience of a 65-year-old man who complained of a hacking cough during the day, but not when he went to bed at night. It was found that he was allergic to the cough drops he used to chew during the day. It also includes a 5-day-old infant with cardiac arrhythmia (a rapid and irregular heartbeat without any physical heart problem) that occurred after feeding. It was discovered he was allergic to his mother's milk.

For people like an 11-year-old Little League baseball player who accidentally ate a cookie made with peanuts and died within minutes from an allergy-produced shock, this breakthrough in treatment technique is too late. But for many others, the prognosis is bright. Coincidentally, the treatment procedure already has been used in helping another Little League player who reacted much the same way to a rice cereal. Testing has assured his parents that their boy will never have to worry about an accidental encounter with the once deadly rice cereal-filled snack after a baseball game. And what would the prognosis be for the little girl who was the victim of a similar accidental allergic poisoning from peanuts, which resulted in stroke, coma and paralysis for three months? If she had not been given a long series of NAET treatments for the specific type of peanut butter found in the cookie she ate at her friend's house, would she be walking around today a bright, happy, energetic kid? Probably not.

Yes, the prognosis is bright. The evidence suggests a convincing argument can be made that a significant number of patients suffering from latent, undiagnosed allergies, normally treated by traditional western medical practitioners for temporary relief, are going to experience a cure from holistic health practitioners. Freedom from allergies is becoming a fact for many patients formerly presenting a wide range of symptoms, from chemical dependency and stroke to eczema and asthma.

This is an age of instant solutions to everything and medicine is no exception. We want to be well, and we want to be well now! In many ways we suffer from a syndrome that says, "I don't care how much the medication costs as long as it will make me feel better in a couple of minutes." Then we are disappointed when we have to wait for months and sometimes years for relief, or in many cases, never get any relief at all. It is no wonder then that patients are not prepared to take charge of their own health care. They have not learned what it means to be sufficiently informed to be in charge.

Thus, the first lesson to be learned about taking charge of your own health care is *to be informed*—not only about your obvious health care needs, but also about the processes that take place within the body which result in poor health. When you are chronically ill and symptoms persist or recur shortly after treatment and after completing medications, you must learn as much as possible about the problem. You must make an effort to make decisions about health care alternatives. The public must be educated, particularly in these instances, that allergies should not be lightly dismissed as a possible root cause of these seemingly incurable or recurring symptoms. The public should be educated to find the cause of the problems. If the problem can be traced, you can easily avoid contact with the causative agent. If contact is unavoidable, you can go to any of the thousands of NAET medical professionals who have learned to eliminate the problem using NAET.

CHAPTER 10

ACUPUNCTURE MERIDIANS

The human body is made up of bones, flesh, nerves and blood vessels, which can only function in the presence of vital energy. Without this energy, the body cannot function. Like electricity, vital energy is not visible to the human eye.

No one knows how or why the vital energy gets into the body or how, when or where it goes when it leaves. It is true, however, that without vital energy, none of the body functions can take place. When the human body is alive, vital energy flows freely through the hypothetical energy pathways. The blood will be circulating through the blood vessels and distributing appropriate nutrients to various parts of the body. For experienced Chinese doctors, these meridians are real. Trained experienced hands are able to trace each meridian, point by point, and make the appropriate evaluation of the physical, physiological and emotional condition of a person with 99-100% accuracy.

The blood helps to exchange oxygen and carbon dioxide by cleaning up the impurities of the body. When blood receives proper nutrients, the body and bones grow, and the flesh and nerves, in turn, can protect the body. All body parts will work as a unit, like an efficient factory with all functions taking place as scheduled. When vital energy stops flowing through the energy pathways, the human machine ceases to function and the person is pronounced dead.

Acupuncture meridians are located throughout the body. They contain a free-flowing, colorless, noncellular liquid. (Note: this liquid is not the energy described above.) There are many specific acupuncture points along these meridians. Most of them connect or inter-link with branches from other meridians. These points, which consist of small oval cells called *Bonham corpuscles,* are electromagnetic in character, surrounding the capillaries under the skin, as well as the blood vessels and organs throughout the body. The Chinese have named these meridians by the life functions with which they seem to be associated. In most cases, these names are similar to the names of organs that we are familiar with. Careful study of the course of the channels and a knowledge of the most commonly seen pathological symptoms may help the reader isolate the specific area of the specific meridian that has a blockage. Energy blockage in the respective organs gives rise to specific symptoms that are unique to those meridians. Allergens can block a meridian at three levels: physical, nutritional (a.k.a. chemical, biochemical, or physiological) and emotional (a.k.a. psychological, mental, or spiritual). Each cell in the body holds three levels of memory and functions.

Step 1: Physical level — Each cell remembers any need/discomfort at the physical level. This is supposed to be the superficial level.

Step 2: Physiological level — Each cell remembers function or non-function at the physiological (functional) level. This is the middle layer, deeper than physical. Most people who are sick will fall in this group.

Step 3: Psychological level — The cell remembers the minute details of past events. It is the deepest layer, holding mainly all vague or strong memories of past events, substances, thoughts or incidents. This level will need NAET emotional treatment to clear. We often see a mixture of these various levels. It is hard to find someone with just one level quality.

PHYSICAL BLOCKAGE

Traditional pathology distinguishes symptoms appearing along the external course of the channels from those affecting internal organs associated with the channels. We can identify the blocked areas of the meridians by studying these symptoms. Manual manipulation, massages, exercise, hot bath, sauna, simple acupuncture treatments, etc., can give temporary relief to physical blockages.

A 54-year-old woman came in with a severe stiffness and neck pain that began when she woke up that morning. NTT revealed that her stiff neck was from eating some vegetables the night before. Questioning her, it was discovered that she had eaten cooked green beans for dinner. If she had been treated with chiropractic or straight acupuncture, physical therapy, massage or even given some pain pills, she may have received relief in a couple of days. Since we traced her problem to green beans, she was treated for beans with NAET. She became symptom-free in less than 10 minutes. During the past ten years she has never had any adverse reactions when she has eaten green beans.

> *Most medical practitioners do not look into the cause of the pain because they do not know how to find it.*

NUTRITIONAL (CHEMICAL) BLOCKAGE

Nutritional or chemical blockages affect mainly the internal pathways of acupuncture meridians. These types of blockages can take many office visits and intense treatments when manipulation, acupuncture, physical therapy, etc., is used but can be effectively removed by NAET in a shorter period of time. Left untreated, the chemical or nutritional level blockages can lead to acute or chronic allergic symptoms. Unpleasant or uncomfortable symptoms felt within 24 hours of contact with an allergen are known as "acute, allergic symptoms." Unpleasant physical, physiological or emotional symptoms continuing after 24 hours of exposure to the allergen, which last for days, months or years, are called "chronic allergic symptoms."

Tony, a 64-year-old farmer, complained of pain in his shoulders for the past 16 years. He was a regular chiropractic patient for years. He also tried acupuncture, massages, herbs, vitamins, detoxification programs and physical therapy with no success. Finally, he began taking prescription pain medications. He felt better for several days, but the good feeling did not last long.

After a few days, even the medication did not give him any relief from his constant pain. One day he met an old friend who referred him to our clinic.

In our clinic, through NTT, it was discovered that he was highly allergic to spices, which caused his shoulder and joint pains. Then he told us that he grew Jalapeno peppers and various other kinds of peppers for a living. He pickled and packed them daily to ship to his customers. He liked pickled peppers and ate them everyday. After being treated for the peppers with NAET, his 16-year-old pain said good-bye to him. He still remains symptom-free after three years.

In his case, the allergy to peppers caused blockage in the internal pathways of the small intestine meridian. Blockage in this meridian caused his constant shoulder pains since the shoulder and the shoulder joint were in the external pathway of the small intestine meridian. The blockage generated by the chemical reaction began in the internal pathways of the small intestine. Then the blockage was transmitted through all the associated tissues of the small intestine meridian, its network of nerves, muscles, bones, joints, tissues and other associated organs. Usually the blockage affects the weakest tissue of the meridian's travel pathway. In this case, Tony used both of his shoulders a lot when he worked in his garden, picking, pickling and preparing the peppers for sale. This made his shoulder joints weak. If the pepper caused the blockages only in the external course of the meridian, treatments like manipulation, acupuncture, massages or physical therapy, etc., would have given him relief. All the treatments, including the pain medication, helped him initially but failed to give him lasting results because they concentrated on treating the physical symptom without removing the cause. He always went right back to the irritant, the peppers! If he had moved away from the constant irritant, the pepper business, he may not have continued to have the pain for as many years as he did. Most medical practitioners do not look into the cause of the pain because they do not know how to find it. NAET treats the cause. When he was treated for peppers through NAET, he got relief from his chronic shoulder pain. He took about 20 office visits to remove the allergy to the pepper and the combination allergies that surfaced with the pepper allergy. Even though he did not eat or touch peppers during the 25-hour avoidance period, he was continually coming in close proximity with them in his house and yard by smelling them constantly, which caused him to lose his treatment. The electromagnetic interactions of the peppers with his body reduced in small increments. Finally, after 20 separate NAET treatments, the electromagnetic energy from the peppers was compatible with his body's energy. If you can avoid the EMF for 25 hours after the treatment, you will clear. Otherwise, it can take many office visits to clear completely. When he was successfully treated for peppers and combinations, he was able to continue in his business without further discomfort.

A man, age 32, was forced to run to the bathroom whenever he consumed food containing eggs. Curiously, he could cook for others and touch eggs and even chicken without any problem. He only became sick when he ate them, even as a tiny fraction in a cookie or pudding. He was treated for eggs by NAET 15 years ago. Now he eats as many eggs and egg-based foods as he wants, without any digestive problems.

EMOTIONAL BLOCKAGE

Allergens can cause energy blockages at the emotional aspect of the meridian. This can be treated very effectively using NAET. Of course, psychiatrists and psychologists using traditional Western treatments and therapies can also treat emotional allergies. But NAET is different from their treatments.

One day, Mary, a 45-year-old female patient, was brought into the office accompanied by her husband. She was holding a basin under her chin and appeared to be nauseated. Upon questioning her husband, he revealed that she began throwing up at about 8 p.m. the night before, shortly after she had eaten a peach. Her abdomen was very distended. She was unable to urinate, move her bowels or pass flatus the whole night. She was unable to keep anything in her stomach due to vomiting and complained of a knot at the solar plexus.

Her husband took her to the emergency room at about 5 a.m. She went through a series of tests. Radiological examination showed that she had an intestinal obstruction. She was advised to go to surgery immediately to remove the obstruction. Fortunately, because she had been treated for migraines and a few other complaints in our office, she was familiar with our treatment methods. When the emergency room doctor suggested surgery, she immediately thought of us and asked her husband to bring her to our clinic. Finally, when she arrived at our clinic, she appeared very tired her skin was cold and clammy and she was perspiring profusely. She also complained of tightening of the chest and pain while breathing. To keep her from fainting, a few acupuncture needles were inserted on selected points. She was too weak to undergo NTT by herself, so her husband was used as a surrogate. With the help of NTT, her problem was traced to an emotional blockage to the peach. When I mentioned "emotional blockage," her husband related the following story. The woman's 17-year-old son was on a cross-country tour. He was on the phone with her from New Hampshire about 8 p.m. the night she was eating the peach. In the middle of the conversation, she heard some loud noises and gunshots from the other end of the phone. The phone went dead. She suddenly came to the conclusion that someone had shot and killed her son. She panicked. She was so frightened she almost passed out. Coincidentally, she had been holding a half-eaten peach in her hand while talking to him.

The allergy to the peach, which caused the intestinal blockage, was further simplified to an emotional allergy to peaches. When the gunshots and sudden termination of the call frightened her, the confused mind had no time to sort out what had actually occurred. Her brain paired the eating of peach with the sudden fright. The brain continued to caution and warned her not to put any more peaches into her stomach, or even come close to them. Her brain identified the peach as a life-threatening item for her body.

In our office, she was immediately treated for the emotional allergy to the peach by NAET. In two minutes, her ailing body became alive again. She was able to breathe without pain. Her color came back. Her body became warm and dry. She was no longer nauseated. She drank some water without any problem and was able to instantly urinate, relieving the distention of the abdomen. Her dramatic instantaneous recovery amazed her family and our office staff as well.

By the way, her son had called her from a public telephone. When he reached his hotel room, he had called home again to let his mother know that everything was okay. When he heard the shots (which turned out to be a truck backfiring), surprised, he swung around and accidentally disconnected the phone call. He called back from his hotel room where he would not have to contend with noise disturbances. Of course, by the time he phoned again, his mother's brain was misguided by the wrong assumption. In this case, knowledge of her son's safety alone was not enough to assure her brain that the danger had been removed.

RELATED MUSCLES

Meridians, their channels, sub-channels and/or branches travel through various routes in the body including muscles and tissues. Therefore, the effect of the blockage can also be felt at the muscles and tissues. Each meridian is capable of affecting a group of muscles in the body. The weakness or strength of the particular muscle can give information about the status or integrity of that meridian.

For five years, a 32-year-old woman had been suffering from a dull constant pain on the lateral part of the left thigh. The tensor fascia lata muscle was just under the area of her chronic pain. Tensor fascia lata is related to the large intestine meridian. She did not have any other complaints. At the time of her symptoms, she had been married for five years. She wore a thick gold chain around her neck, a gold wedding band on her left ring finger and a gold nose ring on her right ala nasi (the flared up area of the nose is pierced and adorned with gold or a precious stone ornament to make women look beautiful) ever since the marriage. She was found to be allergic to gold, which caused energy blockages in the large intestine meridian (the end point of the large intestine meridian is the base of ala nasi.) The blockage of the large intestine meridian was felt as a dull pain on the related muscle, tensor fascia lata. When the allergy to the gold was eliminated, the muscle pain was relieved.

RELATED TIME

An energy molecule takes 24 hours to travel through the body, completing its circulation through all 12 major meridians, their branches and sub-branches. It takes two hours to travel through one meridian. According to Oriental medical principles, the Chi follows the flow of the meridian. The flow begins at the lung meridian and takes two hours to complete its journey. Likewise, each meridian takes two hours for the energy molecule to pass through it. Each meridian is very strong during its meridian time. Allergic reaction to an allergen will be strong when the allergy molecule is passing through that particular meridian, if the allergen is affecting it. For example, if a person has asthma and is allergic to an apple, if the apple is causing the blockage in the lung meridian, the patient can have a strong asthmatic attack during the lung meridian time between (3:00 a.m. and 5:00 a.m.). The meridian is at its strongest at the beginning of its meridian time and less effective near the end; so the asthma can be severe just after 3:00 a.m and taper off by 5:00 a.m.

How does this information affect the allergy treatments? When the allergy is treated through NAET, the patient has to wait 24 hours to let the energy molecule carrying the new information pass through the complete cycle of the journey. If the allergen has caused blockages in one or two meridians, when the energy molecule passes through those affected meridians without disturbance, the patient may not experience adverse symptoms or undo the treatment after that time. With this knowledge, after each NAET treatment, a competent practitioner may be able to test the exact number of hours a patient must avoid a particular allergen. You may not have to avoid the allergen for the full 24 hours after each treatment in such cases. This information may be helpful while treating certain cases like diabetes, where the patient cannot avoid eating food for long hours, and with heart patients as well. Most infants and children do not need to wait 24 hours. They usually have good energy circulation in their energy pathways and the desensitized (treated) energy molecules complete the journey in less time.

DENTAL CONNECTION

Some of the small branches of the major meridians pass through the gum and dental area. This knowledge helps us to understand why certain teeth hurt or become diseased when we eat certain foods or when we come in contact with certain chemicals, etc. When a particular tooth gives you discomfort, you should test the related major meridian and organ for an allergy. Immediate correction of that particular allergy and strengthening of that particular meridian may save you a trip to the dentist for unnecessary, painful, time-consuming and expensive dental work.

NUTRITIONAL NEEDS OF THE MERIDIAN

Meridians are part of our body. Our body is made up of flesh, bones and blood; so are the meridians. Our body needs proper nutrition for growth and development and to repair wear and tear, as do the meridians and their related organs and tissues. When you are allergic to nutritional elements, you cannot absorb or utilize nutrition from food. The body then suffers from nutritional deficiencies, impairing its normal function. After you go through the allergy elimination treatment, you need to take nutritious products to eliminate the deficiencies in the body. You also need to supplement your diet with appropriate nutritional supplements to strengthen the meridians and/or related organs and tissues. After NAET treatments, your body will begin to assimilate the necessary nutrients from your daily food. Since most of us do not usually eat high quality food daily, it may take years to correct your nutritional deficiencies if you just wait to get them from your food alone. If you can find the right non-allergic nutrients and assimilate them, you will reach your optimum level of health quickly.

If the blocked areas and the causative agents can be identified at an early stage of the disease process (blockage), the allergic reaction can be eliminated easily and the energy blockage can be removed immediately. Thus, the human body can be protected from any possible major pathology. For example, you began coughing when you drank a glass of orange juice. You tested and found out that you were allergic to the juice you drank. You took a sample and went to your NAET practitioner immediately and got treated for the juice that was causing the blockage in the lung, and the large intestine meridians. In a few minutes you would be normal, without any cough. If you neglected to treat the juice right away, in a few minutes to an hour you would have a sore throat, runny or blocked nostrils, flu-like symptoms, fever, dizziness, cough, later leading to bronchitis (especially if you drank that juice repeatedly), pneumonia, antibiotics, hospitalization, etc.

During Christmas time, Rinu, a five-year-old girl, one of our recent patients (who had a few basic treatments) accompanied her mother to her hair salon and ate a piece of candy cane given to her by the lady hair stylist. On the way home, she began coughing. In the evening, she complained of a sore throat. She began to have fever and chills at night. She was wheezing by 3:00 a.m. and developed severe asthma by 4:00 a.m. Her frightened parents called the ambulance and took her to the hospital. She was treated with a special breathing apparatus and medication. She was sent home with instructions to continue the medication. The next day she had several severe asthma attacks. Her nervous parents rushed her to the emergency room each time. Finally, on her fourth visit within 48 hours, she was admitted to a special care unit. She continued to suffer severe attacks of asthma in spite of all the medication and cortisone she received. Her mother was puzzled by her response to the hospital treatment. After two days of struggling in the hospital, her mother remembered NAET and contacted me by phone. Using surrogate testing through NTT, I traced the causative agent to the candy cane she ate at the hair salon. Her mother immediately went to the salon and luckily found a piece of the same kind of candy. Rinu was treated with NAET for the candy cane in the hospital. Within 45 minutes she stopped coughing, her breathing became normal and she began eating food. She went home the next day with a big smile, ready to greet Santa Claus. If the mother had known to check the candy for an allergy before Rinu ate it, they would not have had to spend a week in the hospital just before Christmas.

Allergy often affects the weakest area of the body. If you suffered from repeated attacks of cold, flu, bronchitis, pneumonia, etc., as a child, you may have weak lungs when you grow up. Any allergen you come in contact with can affect your lungs and give you continuous lung meridian related problems. At the same time, if you repeatedly use an allergen for days, months or years, it can make the area of contact with that allergen the weakest area in the body.

Maxine, a 64-year-old female suffered from severe bladder infection for years. She took antibiotics week after week. Her bladder infection started as soon as she stopped the antibiotics. She and her treating physician both were at their wit's end.

Her physician referred her to me to try acupuncture. When she was tested by NTT, her problem pointed towards an allergy to cotton. Of course, she always dressed in cotton underpants. Cotton underpants touched her bladder organ and caused a continuous bladder infection. When she was treated successfully for cotton, she said good-bye to repeated bladder infections.

Traditional Chinese medicine describes the meridians or energy pathways in detail, as well as the symptoms of each of the primary channels and secondary channels. In this chapter, each of the 12 primary channels, their distribution and symptoms will be discussed according to the levels of blockages. Overcharged and underactive energy pathways can also cause health problems. Meridian balancing can help to reduce some of the health problem. You are encouraged to read or refer to any of the respective acupuncture text books named in the bibliography to maximize your knowledge about this Oriental medical concept.

OVERCHARGED MERIDIAN

Malnutrition, undernourishment, or overwork, etc. can cause a meridian to become exhausted or overcharged. Overwork can be from physical or mental abuse. Physical abuse can be caused by too much exercise, exhausting physical work or by constant thinking without any rest. Becoming violently enraged and angered with someone without being able to express it outwardly is a form of mental abuse. For example, your father, mother, older sibling, or your teacher repeatedly insults and humiliates you in front of strangers. Out of respect, you don't return their treatment; but, following each incident, over a period of time, you spend many hours tormenting yourself with rage and anger, overcharging your heart and liver meridians.

UNDERCHARGED MERIDIAN

Inactivity, sluggishness, clumsiness, laziness, poor nutrition, poor blood and energy circulation, etc., can cause a meridian to be undercharged. Too much physical and mental abuse in childhood can also create undercharged meridians. Using the same example as above, your father, mother, older sibling, or your teacher, etc., repeatedly insults and humiliates you in front of strangers. Out of respect, you don't return their treatment; but, following each incident, you learn to suppress your rage and anger, creating multiple internal blockages. Eventually, this type of behavior from others will not enter the meridians through the previously established blockages, but create a general numbness towards everything. This is one of our defense mechanisms to protect us from pain. You will soon learn to ignore such stimuli coming from others. It becomes a habit to ignore things. When you begin to ignore things, you learn to lose sensitivity, causing loss of interest, lack of motivation, lack of enthusiasm, procrastination, laziness, coldness towards everything, even life itself.

LUNG CHANNEL (MERIDIAN)

The lung channel begins in the region of the stomach (middle burner or warmer) and passes downward to connect with the large intestine. Returning, it follows the cardiac orifice, crosses the diaphragm and enters its associated organ, the lung. Emerging transversely from the area between the lung and throat, the channel descends along the anterior aspect of the upper arm, lateral to the heart and pericardium channels. Reaching the elbow, it continues along the anterior aspect of the forearm to the anterior margin of the styloid, at the wrist. From here it crosses the radial artery at the pulse, and extends over the thenar eminence to the radial side of the tip of the thumb.

A branch splits from the main channel above the styloid process at the wrist and travels directly to the radial side of the tip of the index finger. This channel is associated with the lung and connects with the large intestine. It crosses the diaphragm and is joined with the stomach, the kidney and other organs.

Lung meridian is one of the most important meridians among the energy pathways. This is the beginning point of the energy cycle, not only in humans, but even in the universe itself. The energy of the universe begins to get active at about 3:00 a.m. in the morning after a long night's rest. When the energy becomes active in the universe, it vibrates through other living things demonstrating the energy vibration by activating the early morning breeze, making the trees, plants and creepers bathe and dance in the breeze, stimulating the circulation of energy in the neighborhood. The birds will wake up sensing the fresh energy vibration and begin to chirp; flower buds will open up by taking fresh energy and releasing the old energy into the atmosphere (fragrance); animals will wake up by breathing the fresh energy; humans will wake up by taking a deep breath and yawning, swallowing a big dose of fresh, rejuvenating energy and pushing old, stale energy out of the body. The vibrant energy, which enters the lung through the first morning breath, initiates new energy circulation making the lung the first meridian in the energy cycle. The first yawn helps the energy circulation to be a successful event by moving the diaphragm upward to help squeeze the deoxygenated air from each and every alveoli. It jump-starts the energy movement in the stomach meridian also by stimulating the peristalsis in the digestive tract. The activation of peristalsis helps to throw out the stale and

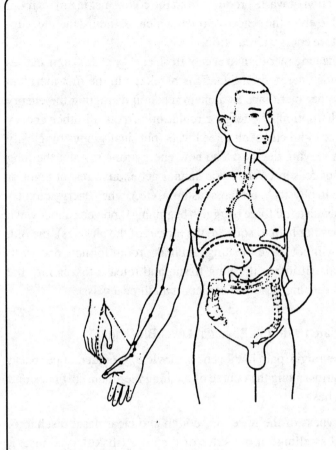

Lung Channel (Lu)
Figure10-1

unwanted accumulation of waste products from the colon, making more room for nutritious food to enter the digestive tract, which maintains the fuel supply to continue future energy circulation.

Inability of the lung meridian to accept fresh energy at 3:00 a.m. causes problems in the lung energy meridian. This blockage in the first meridian transmits into all other meridians as a chain reaction disrupting the energy circulation. The disruption of energy circulation affects all other energy pathways directly or indirectly at all three levels (physically, physiologically or emotionally) in varying degrees. The new energy fails to enter the lung meridian for various reasons. When you cannot get enough rest at night or breathe deeply due to physical problems (asthma, etc.), when energy circulation does not begin with a full force (sluggish beginning) and you cannot yawn (the diaphragm does not help to squeeze the air out of the air bags), the old, deoxygenated air will not leave the lung and make room for new energy to enter. The materials sit inside the lung tissue and release toxins into the energy circulation, causing various disorders at all three levels.

Symptoms Associated with the Physical Level Blockage

- Intercostal neuralgia, pain in the: chest, clavicle, shoulder, upper back, upper teeth, arms, along the course of the lung meridian, stiff neck and sinus headaches.

- Sneezing, dryness of the nose, dry cough and clear nasal discharge, and pain and swelling on the sides of the nose (maxillary sinuses), general body ache, dryness of the nose, hives, itching, and skin rashes.

Symptoms Associated with the Physiological Level Blockage

- Abscess, growth, or infection anywhere in the tract, afternoon fever, aphonia, asthma, bad breath, bad taste, blood in the sputum, bronchitis, burning in the eyes, burning, tingling and pain around the nose, inside the upper gum and teeth; chills and fever, congestion, cough, difficulty in breathing, painful breathing, dry throat, dysphagia, dysphonia, emphysema, epistaxis (nose bleed), fever, fullness in the chest, hay fever, headaches between eyes, internal trembling, laryngitis, mucous production, nasal discharge, nasal polyp, pharyngitis, pneumonia, post nasal drip, shortness of breath, sinusitis, sneezing, sore throat, tearing from the eyes and tonsillitis.

■ Abdominal bloating, nausea, poor appetite, loose stools, fever with or without excessive thirst, constipation, hot palms and/or changes in the color of urine.

■ Dizziness, irritability and insomnia.

Symptoms Associated with An Overcharged Meridian

Heaviness of the chest, shortness of breath, heavy cough with or without production of excessive mucus.

Symptoms Associated with an Undercharged Meridian

Low immune system, feel like coming down with a cold, frequent sneez ing, sniffles, cough, general fatigue, lack of motivation, silent weep ing, and internal trembling.

Acute Allergic Symptoms

■ Pain in the: maxillary sinuses, between third and fourth thoracic vertebrae, anterior fontanel, chest, and/or clavicle, first interphalangeal joint, intercostal area, thumb, upper back, upper first cuspid, second upper bicuspid, arms along the course of the lung meridian and tenosynovitis.

■ Afternoon fever, acute bronchial asthmatic attacks, cardiac asthma, asthma worse after 3:00 a.m., shortness of breath, burning in the eyes and nostrils, chest congestion, cough, coughing up blood, dry mouth and throat, emaciated look, fever; itching of the nostrils, headaches between eyes, nasal congestion, nose bleed, postnasal drips, runny nose with clear discharge, red or painful eyes, sneezing, and throat irritation.

■ Fatigue, lethargy, flu-like symptoms, general body ache and insomnia, cradle cap, generalized dry skin, urticaria, scaly skin, itching: of the body, scalp, and along the course of the lung meridian.

Chronic Allergic Symptoms

■ Arthritis of the thumb, tennis elbow, frozen shoulder, tendonitis of the shoulder, tenosynovitis, pain in the first interphalangeal joint, chronic toothache of upper cuspid and upper second bicuspids.

■ Afternoon fever, asthma, blood in the sputum, bronchitis, bronchiectasis, cardiac asthma, asthma worse after 3:00 a.m., chronic cough with or without sputum, dry mouth, nose, eyes, and throat, emaciated look, emphysema, fullness in the chest, generalized body ache, hay fever, excessive perspiration in some cases and lack of perspiration in others, husky voice, infection in the respiratory tract, influenza, irritability, low voice, lack of desire to talk, laryngitis, nasal polyps, night sweats, other chest infections, pleurisy, pneumonia, poor growth of hair and nails, post nasal drips, red cheeks, red eyes, pain in the eyes, runny nose with clear discharge (viral infections), runny nose with yellowish discharge (bacterial infections), shortness of breath between 3-5:00 a.m., sinus infections, sinus headaches, stuffy or runny nose, swollen throat, swollen cervical glands, throat irritation, tuberculosis and unable to sleep after 3:00 a.m.

■ Abdominal bloating, nausea, vomiting, constipation or loose stools, body ache and restlessness between 3-5:00 a.m.

■ Acne, atopic dermatitis, chronic hives, cradle cap, eczema, excessive sweating, skin rashes, chronic skin problems, tags, moles, warts, scaly and rough skin, heat sensation with hot palms, hair loss, thinning of the hair, poor growth of hair and nails, rough ridges on the nails, and brittle nails.

Symptoms Associated with the Emotional Level Blockages

Lung meridian dysfunction affecting the emotional aspect usually evolves from a childhood experience with an older person, a parent, older sibling, a guardian or someone else who repeatedly berated the child and criticized the child's thoughts and opinions. If the child learns to verbally or subconsciously fight back at the authority figure, an overcharged lung meridian can develop during the child's maturation into adulthood. If the child gives up the fight and accepts the bullying authority by suppressing the anger, then an undercharged lung meridian will result. When you experience grief or deep sorrow and fail to cry, your sadness will settle in the lungs and eventually cause various lung disorders.

Main Emotion: GRIEF

Related emotions: a tendency toward humiliating others, abandonment, addiction or craving onion, always apologizing, anguish, cloudy thinking, comparing self with others, contempt, dejection, depression (early morning), despair, early morning depression, emotionally super sensitive, expressions of over-sympathy, false pride, hopelessness, innability to express grief, insulting others, intolerance, low self-esteem, meanness, melancholy, over demanding, peppers, prejudice, craves pungent and spicy foods, Sadness, seeking others' approval, self-pity and weeping frequently without much reason, and yearning.

Lung Meridian - Related Muscles

Serratus anterior, coracobrachialis, deltoids and diaphragm.

Lung Meridian - Related Time

3 - 5:00 a.m.

Lung Meridian - Dental Connection

Upper first and second cuspid.

Lung Meridian - Essential Nutrition

Clear water, proteins, vitamin C, bioflavonoids, cinnamon, onions, garlic, B-2, citrus fruits, green peppers, black peppers and rice.

LARGE INTESTINE CHANNEL (MERIDIAN)

This channel begins at the radial side of the tip of the index finger and proceeds upward between the first and second metacarpal bones of the hand. It then passes between the tendons of the extensor pollicis longus and brevis at the wrist, and continues along the radial margin of the forearm to the lateral side of the elbow. From here, it rises along the lateral aspect of the upper arm, to the shoulder, following the anterior margin of the acromion, before turning upward. Just beneath the spinous process of the seventh cervical vertebra, the channel enters directly into the supraclavicular fossa and connects with the lung, before descending across the diaphragm to the large intestine.

A branch separates from the main channel at the supraclavicular fossa and moves upward through the neck, crosses the cheek and travels through the lower gum. From here it curves around the lip and intersects the same channel, proceeding from the opposite side of the body at the philtrum. The branch finally terminates at the side of the nose.

Another branch descends to the stomach at acupuncture point St 37, the lower uniting point of the large intestine. This channel is associated with the large intestine and connects with the lung. It also joins directly with the stomach.

The large intestine is the receiver of waste products produced as a result of various chemical and enzymatic reactions that happens at all three levels (physical, physiological and emotional) in the body. The body expects the colon to throw out the waste products as it is produced. In some people, the colon refuses to do its job. It allows stale products to remain in the colon and between the intestinal folds, releasing toxins from three levels into the energy and blood circulation, giving rise to various physical, physiological and emotional ailments.

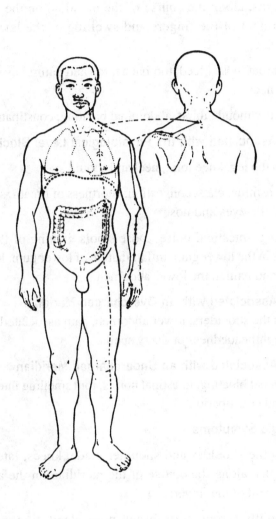

Large Intestine Channel (LI)
Figure 10-2

Symptoms Associated with the Physical Level Blockage

- Pain in the shoulder and shoulder blades, knees, lateral aspects of the thighs, along the course of the meridian on the arm and motor impairment of the fingers and swelling of the lateral part of the knee joint.

- Sore throat, nose bleed, toothache, red and painful eyes, and swelling of the neck.

- Fever, dry mouth, thirst, abdominal bloating, constipation or diarrhea.

Symptoms Associated with the Physiological Level Blockage

- Pain in the leg, knee joint, heel and shoulders.

- Latent asthma, chest congestion, shortness of breath, sinus headaches around the eyes and nose.

- Belching, intestinal noise, loose stools, itching of the body, hives, blisters in the lower gum, inflammation of lower gum, lethargy, bloody stools and pain in the lower abdomen.

Symptoms Associated with an Overcharged Meridian

Pain in the shoulders, lower abdomen, pain associated with constipation, lightheadedness or dizzy spells.

Symptoms Associated with an Undercharged Meridian

Abdominal bloating, intestinal noises, foul smelling intestinal gas, dry lips and constipation.

Acute Allergic Symptoms

- Pain in the shoulder and shoulder blade, knees, lateral aspects of the thighs, along the course of the meridian on the arm and motor impairment of the fingers.

- Dry mouth, throat, sore throat, nose bleed, toothache on lateral incisors, first lower and second lower bicuspid, red and painful eyes, swelling of the neck and of the lateral part of the knee joint.

- Lower abdominal cramps, constipation or diarrhea, spastic colon, spasms of the rectum and anal sphincter, itching of the anus, generalized hives, intestinal noise, flatulence, bleeding from the rectum, colitis and dizziness.

Chronic Allergic Symptoms

- Arthritis, muscle spasms of the lateral thigh and knee, pain in the shoulder, knee, wrist, index finger, lateral part of the elbow, lower back, heel, sciatic nerve and lateral aspect of the leg.

- Abdominal pain, bloating, bad breath, belching, chest congestion, shortness of breath and sinus headaches on the sides of the nose, between the eyes and over the eyes.

- Acne, blister / inflammation of the lower gum, dermatitis, feeling better or tired after a bowel movement, hair loss, hair thinning, hives, intestinal colic, itching, poor growth of the nail and hair, rough and/or bumpy skin, skin rashes and warts.

Symptoms Associated with Emotional Level Blockages:

Main Emotion: GUILT

Related Emotions: accumulates emotional junk, anxiety long period, bad dreams, compelled to neatness, crying spells, crying, defensive, defensiveness, dogmatically positioned, everything in present life reminds you of the past, extremely sentimental, feeling discomfort over a past memory, grief, guilt, haunted by past painful memories, holds emotional waste products in the intestinal folds, inability to recall dreams, nightmares, rolling restlessly in sleep, sadness, seeking sympathy, talking in the sleep, unable to forget the past, unable to throw unwanted things away, weeping, and worrying.

Large Intestine Meridian - Related Muscles

Tensor fascia lata, quadratus lumborum and hamstrings.

Large Intestine Meridian - Related Time

5 - 7 a.m.

Large Intestine - Dental Connection

The tensor facia lata is associated with the lower lateral incisor

The quadratus lumborum with the lower first bicuspid
The hamstrings with the first or second lower bicuspid.

Large Intestine - Essential Nutrition

Vitamins A, D, E, C, B, especially B-1, wheat, bran, oat bran, yogurt, and roughage.

A 60 year old female NAET and chiropractic patient of mine (Lynne) had come to see for sharp pains radiating into her left shoulder and arm. The pain had been gradually worsening over a period of weeks and now was reaching almost unbearable levels at times. Conventional chiropractic care and physical therapy gave her only brief remission from the daily pain and severe restrictions in her shoulder's range of motion. A visit to an orthopedic doctor informed her that the pain was caused by two degenerated discs in Lynne's neck and that a surgical replacement of the two discs was the only option. Full recovery could take up to a year. An appointment for the surgery was made. During the course of an advanced NAET seminar I learned from Dr. Devi that an allergy to urine can bring on arthritic symptoms. Lynne was one of my first patients on the Monday after the seminar and my first words to her were, "Let's check your urine!"

Lynne's shoulder pain disappeared half way through the first NAET session where a sample of her urine was used as the allergen.

After a few days of no symptoms Lynne started to experience the gradual resumption of her neck and shoulder symptoms, but at a much less intense level. The following allergens were then cleared on Lynne over the next 4 weeks:

Urine	CSF	Blood
Blood/CSF combo	Blood/urine combo	CSF/urine combo
Disc mix	Bone mix	Bone/blood combo
Bone/CSF combo		

During the course of these treatments the symptoms diminished to zero and stayed there. Three months later Lynne experienced a brief flare up of symptoms which quickly responded to combinations of Urine, Hypothalamus, Blood and CSF. That was 8 months ago and Lynne's symptoms have not returned.

NAET is a very powerful tool and I am grateful every day that I learned it from Dr. Devi and am able to pass it along to all my patients.

Dr. Roger Barnes, D.C., West Los Angeles, CA. (310) 441-9682

STOMACH CHANNEL (MERIDIAN)

This channel begins beside the nose, then ascends to the root of the nose where it intersects with the bladder channel. Descending along the lateral side of the nose, it enters the upper gum and joins the governing channel at the philtrum, then circles back around the corner of the mouth, meeting the conception channel at the mentolabial groove of the chin. From here it follows the angle of the jaw and runs upward in front of the ear. It proceeds along the hairline until it intersects with the gall bladder channel at gall bladder acupuncture point GB 6. Finally, it crosses to the middle of the forehead, parallel with the hairline, where it joins the governing channel.

One branch separates from the main channel, on the lower jaw and descends along the throat entering the supraclavicular fossa. From there, it travels posteriorly to the upper back, where it meets the governing channel internally at conception vessel channel acupuncture points CV 13 and CV 12 before entering its associated organ, the stomach, and communicating with the spleen.

Another vertical branch descends directly from the supraclavicular fossa along the mammillary line, passes beside the umbilicus and through the lower abdomen to the inguinal region, where it joins with the vertical branch just described. From here, the channel crosses to stomach acupuncture point St 31 on the anterior aspect of the thigh, and descends directly to the patella. It then proceeds along the lateral side of the tibia to the dorsum of the foot, terminating at the lateral side of the tip of the second toe.

Another parallel branch separates from the main channel at stomach acupuncture point St 36, three units below the knee and terminates at the lateral side of the middle toe.

Another branch separates at the dorsum of the foot at stomach acupuncture point St 42 and terminates at the medial side of the big toe, where it connects with the spleen channel at acupuncture point Sp 1. This channel is associated with the stomach and connects with the spleen. It is also directly joined with the heart, large intestine and small intestine.

Symptoms Associated with the Physical Level Blockage

■   Dry nostrils, nosebleed, sore throat, coated tongue, and sore tongue.

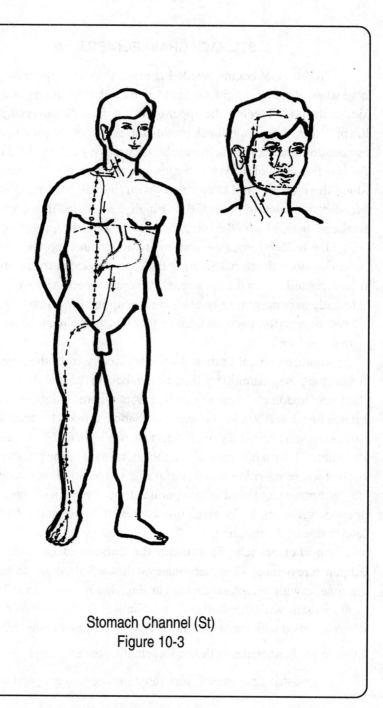

Stomach Channel (St)
Figure 10-3

- High fever, tidal fever, flushed face, fever blisters, sweating and delirium.

- Pain in the eye, chest pain, pain or distention along the course of the channel in the leg or foot, pain along the lateral aspect of the lower leg, pain in the middle back along T-8 vertebrae, swelling on the neck, facial paralysis, and coldness in the lower limbs.

- Acne, heat boils or blemishes along the channel, red rashes along the lateral aspect of the lower leg below the knee, black and blue discoloration below the knee, above the ankle, and along stomach channel.

Symptoms Associated with the Physiological Level Blockage

- Abdominal distension, fullness or edema, abdominal cramps, vomiting, nausea, discomfort when reclining, persistent hunger, yellowish coat on tongue and yellow urine.

- Insomnia, restlessness, mental confusion, personality changes, double personality, hyperactivity in children or adults, manic-depressive behaviors, schizophrenia, lack of concentration, and aggressive behaviors.

- Frontal headaches, migraine headaches on the forehead, seizures, toothache, pain on the upper jaw and upper gum diseases.

Symptoms Associated with Overcharged Meridian

Poor or no appetite, unhealthy weight loss, loss of taste and fatigue, overly attentive to the needs and wishes of others, neglecting themselves in the process; neglected or abused by others who take advantage of their pathologically willing generosity.

Symptoms Associated with Undercharged Meridian

Voracious appetite, excess weight and a lot of energy and pain along the stomach channel, very selfish, involved in excessive self-nurturing, tendency to lie, shop lift, steal, and gamble (kleptomaniacs fall into this group).

Acute Allergic Symptoms

- Dry nostrils, nosebleed, sore throat, coated tongue, and sore tongue.

- High fever, tidal fever, flushed face, fever blisters, herpes, sores on the gums, and inside of lips, red painful boils on the face, sweating and delirium.

- Pain in the eye, chest pain, pain or distention along the course of the channel in the leg or foot, pain along the lateral aspect of the lower leg, pain in the middle back along T-6 to T-10 vertebrae, swelling on the neck, facial paralysis, general body ache (fibromyalgia), and coldness in the lower limbs.

- Acne, heat boils or blemishes along the channel, itching and red rashes along the lateral aspect of the lower leg below the knee, black and blue discoloration below the knee, above the ankle, along stomach channel and hiatal hernia.

Chronic Allergic Symptoms

- Abdominal bloating, fullness or edema, abdominal cramps, vomiting, nausea, anorexia, bulimia, and discomfort when reclining.

- Yellow or white coat on the tongue, cracks on the center of the tongue and yellow urine.

- Insomnia, restlessness, mental confusion, personality changes, double personality, hyperactivity in children or adults, manic-depressive behaviors, schizophrenia, lack of concentration, and aggressive behaviors.

- Obsession, obsessive compulsive behaviors, panic disorders, frontal headaches, migraine headaches on the forehead, headache behind the eyes (dull, sharp, pressure or burning pain behind the eyes), nasal polyps, bad breath, fatigue, insomnia, seizures, toothache, pain on the upper jaw and upper gum diseases, fibromyalgia, and temporomandibular joint problems (TMJ).

Symptoms Associated with the Emotional Level Blockage

Main Emotion: DISGUST

Related emotions: Aggressive behaviors, alone, bitterness, butterfly sensation in the stomach, dependancy on others, deprived, despair, disappointment, disconnected, disgust, egocentric, emptiness, excessive thinking, expanded importance of self, fear of dying, fear of losing control, flightiness, greed, guilt, hyperactivity, lack of concentration, manic disorders, mental fog, nervous, nostalgic, obsession, obsessive compulsive disorders, oversympathetic, panic attacks, perceptual distortions, restlessness, seeks sympathy, stifled, terror (a sense that something unimaginably horrible is about to occur and one is powerless to prevent it), unable to move to new emotion, and unable to receive sympathy.

Stomach Meridian - Related Muscles

Pectoralis major clavicular, brachioradialis, sternocleidomastoideus, neck extensors, flexors, scalene muscle, and levator scapulae.

Stomach Meridian - Related Time

7 - 9 a.m.

Stomach Meridian - Dental Connection

The pectoralis major clavicular is associated with the first and second upper bicuspid.

The neck flexors and extensors are connected with the upper central incisors.

Stomach Meridian - Essential Nutrition

B complex especially B-12, B-6, B-3 and folic acid

SPLEEN CHANNEL (MERIDIAN)

The spleen channel begins on the medial tip of the big toe. From here, it follows the border between the dark and light skin of the medial aspect of the foot. It then passes in front of the medial malleolus and up the leg, along the posterior side of the tibia, crossing and then traveling anterior to the liver channel. From here, it crosses over the medial aspect of the knee and continues upward along the anterior, medial aspect of the thigh and into the abdomen. Then it crosses the conception channel at acupuncture point CV 3 and acupuncture point CV 4, its associated organ, the spleen, and communicates with the stomach. It then ascends across the diaphragm and intersects the gall bladder channel at acupuncture point GB 24, and the liver channel at acupuncture point Liv 14. Continuing upward beside the esophagus, it crosses the lung channel at acupuncture point Lu 1 and finally reaches the root of the tongue dispersing over its lower surface.

A branch of this channel separates in the stomach region and advances upward across the diaphragm, transporting Chi into the heart. This channel is associated with the spleen and connects with the stomach. It also directly joins with the heart, lungs and large intestine.

Symptoms Associated with the Physical Level

- Heaviness in the body or head, general body ache and feverishness, fibromyalgia, sluggishness, lethargy, fatigued limbs and emaciated muscles.

- Stiffness of the tongue, coldness of the leg and knee along the medial side.

- Edema of the foot and leg, generalized edema of the body, and overweight.

- Pain in the toes, and pain along the course of the meridian.

- Lack of enthusiasm, lack of interest in anything, moodiness, grumpy nature and inability to make any decision.

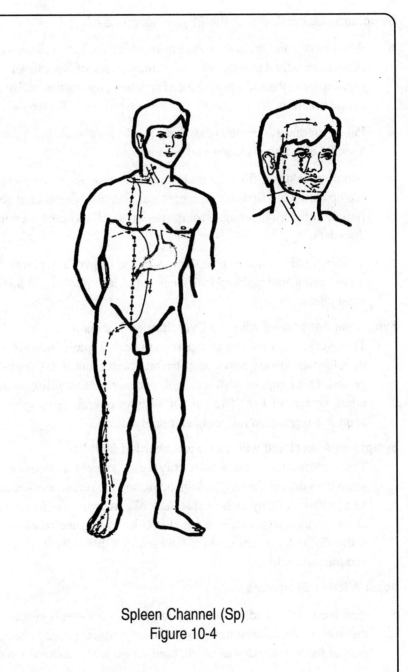

Spleen Channel (Sp)
Figure 10-4

Symptoms Associated with the Physiological Level

- Abdominal pain, fullness or distension, diarrhea, incomplete digestion of food, intestinal noises, nausea, vomiting, lack of taste, lack of smell, hard lumps in the abdomen, reduced appetite, constipation and hypoglycemic reaction.

- Pallor, tiredness, sleeplessness, dizzy spells, lightheadedness, jaundice, anemia, bleeding disorders and hemorrhoids.

- Scanty menstrual flow, irregular periods, absence of menstruation, cramps after the first day of menstrual periods, hormonal disorders, female infertility, premenstrual, menopausal and post menopausal disorders.

- Tingling, pain, numbness in the tips of the fingers and palms, carpal tunnel syndrome, pain and stiffness in the interphalangeal joints and wrist joints.

Symptoms Associated with the Overcharged Meridian

The overactive state causes a person to be extremely indecisive, continually swallowing new things before the present items are fully digested. This happens with food, job decisions, relationship and many other aspects of life. The person with an overcharged spleen may acquire a reputation for being extremely fickle.

Symptoms Associated with the Undercharged Meridian

The underactive state causes craving of sweets, loss of memory, sleepiness during the day, waking up during the night, bouts of depression, withdrawal, hypochondriac, lack of concentration, forgetfulness, absentmindedness, indifference, difficulty giving and receiving sympathy, difficulty reaching out to new sources, difficulty leaving the old and the past behind.

Acute Allergic Symptoms

- Heaviness in the head, abdominal pain, fullness or distension, incomplete digestion of food, intestinal noises, nausea, vomiting, lack of taste, stiffness of the tongue, lack of smell, hard lumps in the abdomen, reduced appetite, craving sugar, indigestion, loose stools, diarrhea constipation, hypoglycemic reaction, general feverishness and body aches.

- Pallor, tiredness, sleeplessness, sleepy in the afternoon, sleepy during the day, latent insomnia, dreams that makes you tired, dizzy spells, lightheadedness, jaundice, anemia, bleeding disorders and hemorrhoids.

- Scanty menstrual flow, irregular periods, absence of menstruation, cramps after the first day of menstrual periods, hormonal disorders, female infertility, premenstrual syndrome (PMS), menopausal and post menopausal disorders.

- Tingling, pain, numbness in the tips of the fingers and palms, carpal tunnel syndrome, pain and stiffness in the interphalangeal joints and wrist joints, coldness of the leg and knee along the medial side and edema of the foot and leg.

- Low self-esteem, procrastination, depression, intuitive and prophetic behaviors.

Chronic Allergic Symptoms

- Abdominal pain, fullness or distension, incomplete digestion of food, intestinal noises, nausea, vomiting, lack of taste, stiffness of the tongue, absence of the tongue coating, stripping of the tongue in patches or whole, lack of smell, hard lumps in the abdomen, reduced appetite, craving sugar, indigestion, loose stools, diarrhea constipation, hypoglycemic or hyperglycemic reaction, general feverishness and body aches, obesity, diabetes and chronic fatigue syndrome.

- Pallor, tiredness, sleeplessness, sleepy in the afternoon, sleepy during the day, latent insomnia, dreams that make you tired, dizzy spells, lightheadedness, jaundice, pedal edema, weak limbs, anemia, bleeding disorders and hemorrhoids.

- Scanty menstrual flow, irregular periods, absence of menstruation, cramps after the first day of menstrual periods, hormonal disorders, female infertility, premenstrual, menopausal and post menopausal disorders.

■ Tingling, pain, numbness in the tips of the fingers and palms, carpal tunnel syndrome, pain and stiffness in the interphalangeal joints and wrist joints, coldness of the leg and knee along the medial side and edema of the foot and leg.

■ Low self-esteem, procrastination, depression, intuitive and prophetic behaviors.

Symptoms Associated with Emotional Level

Main Emotion: WORRY

Related emotions: anxiety for the future, constant brooding, deprived, disappointment, dislikes crowds, distrust, easily hurt, pensiveness, excessive use of mind (study, thinking, concentrating, memorizing), gives more importance to self, helplessness, hopelessness, irritable, keeps feelings inside, lack confidence, lack of control over events, lack of self-confidence, likes loneliness, likes to be praised, likes to take revenge, lives through others, low self-esteem, mental listlessness, needs constant encouragement otherwise falls apart, obsessive-compulsive behavior, over-sympathetic, restrained, shy, talks to self, timid, unable to make decisions, and worried all the time.

Spleen Meridian - Related Muscles

Latissimus dorsi, middle trapezius, triceps, opponents pollicis longus, and lower trapezius.

Spleen Meridian - Related Time

9 - 11 a.m.

Spleen Meridian - Dental Connection

The latissimus dorsi is associated with the upper first molar;
Middle trapezius with the upper third molar.

Spleen Meridian - Essential Nutrition

Vitamin A, vitamin C, calcium, chromium, and protein.

HEART CHANNEL (MERIDIAN)

The Heart channel begins in its associate organ—the heart. Then it emerges through the blood vessel system surrounding the heart and travels downward across the diaphragm, where it connects with the small intestine. A branch of the main channel separates in the heart and ascends alongside the esophagus to the face, where it joins the tissue surrounding the eye. Another branch goes directly from the heart to the lung, then slants downward to merge below the axilla. From here the channel descends along the medial border of the anterior aspect of the upper arm, behind the lung and pericardium channels to the antecubital fossa where it continues downward to the capitate bone proximal to the palm. It then enters the palm and follows the medial side of the little finger to the fingertip. This channel is associated with the heart and connects with the small intestine. It is also directly joined to the lung and kidneys.

Symptoms Associated with the Physical Level

- Pain: in the eyes, along the back of the upper arm, along the scapula or medial aspect of the forearm.

- General feverishness, headache and dry throat.

- Hot or painful palms, coldness in the palms and soles of the feet.

Symptoms Associated with the Physiological Level

- Pain or fullness in the chest and ribs or below the ribs.

- Mental disorders, nervousness, emotional excesses (excessive laughing or crying); sometimes abusive, sad and irritable.

- Vertigo, nausea, dizziness or lightheadedness.

- Shortness of breath, excessive perspiration, insomnia, chest distension, palpitation, heaviness in the chest and sharp chest pain.

- Irregular or knotted pulse and discomfort when reclining.

Symptoms Associated with an Overcharged Meridian

Talkative, dry mouth and heaviness in the chest.

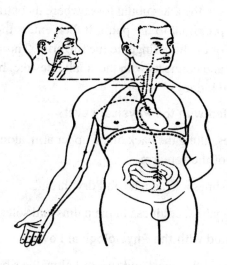

Heart Channel (Ht)
Figure 10-5

Symptoms Associated with an Undercharged Meridian

Extreme fatigue and heart palpitation.

Acute Allergic Symptoms

- Pain: in the eyes, in the shoulder, chest along the heart meridian, along the back of the upper arm, along the scapula or medial aspect of the forearm.

- General palpitation, poor circulation and dizziness, general feverishness, headache and dry throat.

- Hot or painful palms, coldness in the palms and soles of the feet.

Chronic Allergic Symptoms

- Pain or fullness in the chest and ribs or below the ribs.

- Mental disorders, nervousness, emotional excesses, sometimes abusive, and irritable.

- Vertigo, nausea, dizziness or lightheadedness.

- Shortness of breath, excessive perspiration, insomnia, chest distension, palpitation, heaviness in the chest and sharp chest pain and chest distention.

- Irregular or knotted pulse and discomfort when reclining.

Symptoms Associated with the Emotional Level Blockage

Main Emotion: Joy

Related Emotions: feeling of abandonment, abnormal (inappropriate) laughing, abusive nature, aggressive, agitation, anger, bad manners, compulsive behaviors, depression, dizziness and easily upset, does not make friends, does not trust anyone, dream disturbed sleep, ensuing sadness from breaking up of relationship, excessive crying, excessive expression of emotion, excessive joy, excessive laughing, fidgetiness, frightfully overjoyed, frustration, guilt, hostility, impulsiveness, insecurity, lack of insight, lack of emotions, lack of laughter, lack of understanding, meeting and parting of old and new, mental confusion (phlegm), mental dullness, mental restlessness (heart feels vexed), nausea, nervous laugh, overexcitement, prolonged anxiety, prolonged sadness, prolonged worry, propensity to be startled, rash behavior (phlegm), resentment, sadness, shock, talkative, type A personality, uncontrolled crying, uncontrolled laughter, uneasiness, and unforgiving.

Heart Meridian - Related Muscles
Subscapularis, abdominalis and supra spinatus.

Heart Meridian - Related Time
11-1 p.m.

Heart Meridian - Dental Connection
Subscapularis associated with upper lateral incisors.

Heart Meridianc
Calcium, vitamin C, vitamin E, and B complex.

SMALL INTESTINE CHANNEL (MERIDIAN)
The small intestine channel originates at the ulnar side of the tip of the little finger and ascends along the ulnar side of the hand to the wrist emerging at the styloid process of the ulna. From here, it travels directly upward along the posterior aspect of the ulna, passing between the olecranon of the ulna and the medial epicondyle of the humerus at the medial side of the elbow. It then proceeds along the posterior border of the lateral aspect of the upper arm, emerging behind the shoulder joint and circling around the superior and inferior fossa of the scapula. At the top of the shoulder, it crosses the bladder channel at acupuncture points B 36 and B 11, and the governing channel at acupuncture point Gv 14, where the channel turns downward into the supraclavicular fossa and connects with the heart. From here, it descends along the esophagus and crosses the diaphragm to the stomach. Before reaching its associated organ, the small intestine, the channel intersects the conception vessel channel, internally and very deep, at acupuncture points CV 13 and CV 12.

A branch of this channel travels upward from the supraclavicular fossa and crosses the neck and cheek to the outer canthus of the eye, where it meets the gall bladder channel at acupuncture point GB 1. Then it turns back across the temple and enters the ear at the small intestine acupuncture point SI 19.Another branch separates from the former branch on the cheek, ascends to the infraorbital region of the eye and then to the inner canthus, where it meets the bladder channel at acupuncture point B1. It then crosses horizontally to the zygomatic region. Another branch descends to stomach acupuncture point St 39, the lower uniting point of the small intestine. This channel is associated with the small intestine and connects with the heart. It also joins directly with the stomach.

Symptoms Associated with the Physical Level

Pain in the neck or cheek, along the lateral aspect of the shoulder and upper arm. Numbness of the mouth and tongue, sore throat and stiff neck.

Symptoms Associated with the Physiological Level

Bloating and pain in the lower abdomen, pain radiating around the waist or to the genitals. Abdominal pain with dry stool, constipation or diarrhea.

Symptoms Associated with an Overactive Meridian

Noisy intestinal movements, pain in the neck, and back of the shoulders.

Symptoms Associated with an Under Active Meridian

Odorless intestinal gas, unilateral headaches, pain around the ears and under the cheekbone.

Chronic Allergic Symptoms

■ Bloating and pain in the lower abdomen, pain radiating around the waist and to the genitals.

■ Abdominal pain with dry stool, constipation and diarrhea.

■ Knee pain, shoulder pain and frozen shoulder.

Symptoms Associated with the Emotional Level Blockage

Main Emotion: INSECURITY

Related emotions: absentmindedness, becoming too involved with details, daydreaming, easily annoyed, easily hurt, emotional instability, feeling of abandonment or desertion, introvert, Irritability, joy, lacking

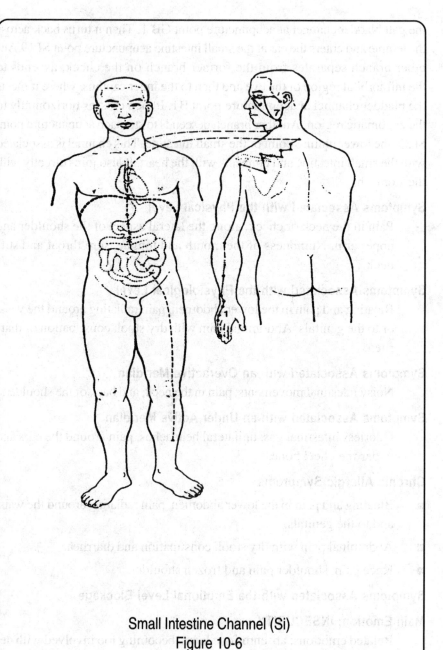

Small Intestine Channel (Si)
Figure 10-6

the confidence to assert oneself, over-excitement, paranoia and sighing, poor concentration, sadness, shyness, sorrow and suppression of deep sorrow.

Small Intestine - Related Muscles

Quadriceps, rectus abdominalis and transverse abdominalis.

Small Intestine - Related Times

1 - 3:00 p.m.

Small Intestine - Dental Connection

■ The quadriceps is associated with the first lower molar.

■ Rectus abdominalis is associated with the upper first molar.

Small Intestine - Essential Nutrition

Vitamin B complex, vitamin D and vitamin E.
Acidophilus, yogurt, fibers, wheat germ and whole grains.

BLADDER CHANNEL (MERIDIAN)

The bladder channel begins at the bladder channel acupuncture point B 1 at the inner canthus of the eye and ascends across the forehead, intersecting the governing channel at acupuncture point GV 24 and the gall bladder channel at acupuncture point GB 20. From here a branch descends to the area above the ear, joining the gall bladder channel at acupuncture points GB 7, GB 8, GB 12, etc. A vertical branch enters the brain at the vertex and intersects with the governing channel at point GV 17, before emerging and descending along the nape of the neck and the muscles of the medial aspect of the scapula. Here the bladder channel meets the governing vessel channel at acupuncture points GV 14, and GV 13, after which it continues downward parallel to the spine, to the lumbar region. The channel then enters the internal cavity via the para vertebral muscles, communicating with the kidneys and finally joins its associated organ, the bladder. Another branch separates in the lumbar region, crosses the buttocks and descends to the popliteal fossa of the knee. Yet another branch separates from the main channel at the back of the neck and descends parallel to the spine, from the medial side of the scapula to the gluteal region. Here it crosses the buttocks to intersect the gall bladder channel at acupuncture point GB 30, and then descends across the lateral posterior aspect of the thigh to join with the other branch of this channel in the popliteal fossa continuing downward through the gastrocnemius muscle.

The channel emerges behind the external malleolus, then follows the fifth metatarsal bone crossing its tuberosity to the lateral lip of the little toe at bladder acupuncture point B 67. The bladder channel connects behind the knee with its lower uniting acupuncture point B 54. This channel is associated with the bladder and connects with the kidneys. It is also joined directly with the brain and heart.

Symptoms Associated with the Physical Level

- Pain: in the lumbar region, along the back of the leg and foot and along the meridian.

- Alternating chills and fever, headache, nasal congestion, stiff neck, and disease of the eye.

Symptoms Associated with the Physiological Level Blockage

Pain in the lower abdomen, enuresis, and retention of urine, painful urination and mental disorders.

Symptoms Associated with an Overactive Meridian

Nagging low backache with radiculitis (sciatic neuralgia).

Symptoms associated with an under active meridian

Upper and middle backache, frequent urination, bed wetting in children and incontinence of urine.

Acute Allergic Symptoms

- Frequent, painful and burning urination, loss of bladder control and bloody urine.

- Chills, fever, headaches (especially at the back of the neck), stiff neck, nasal congestion and disease of the eye.

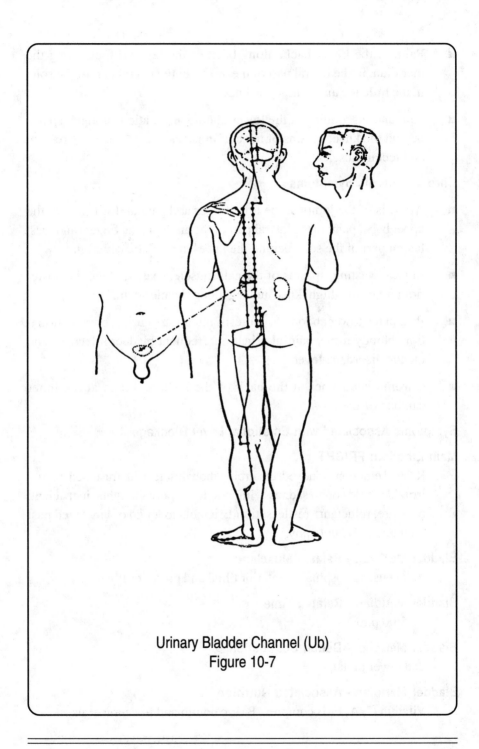

Urinary Bladder Channel (Ub)
Figure 10-7

- Pain: in the lower back, along back of the leg and foot, along the meridian, in the lateral part of the ankle, in the lateral part of the sole, in the little toe and behind the knee.

- Pain and discomfort in the lower abdomen, sciatic neuralgia, spasm behind the knee, spasms of the calf muscles, weakness in the rectum and rectal muscle.

Chronic Allergic Symptoms

- Arthritis of the joints of the little finger and pain and stiffness of the upper back, pain: in the lateral part of the ankle, in the fingers and toes, lateral part of the sole, behind the knees and sciatic neuralgia.

- Muscle wasting, spasms of the calf muscle, spasms along the posterior part of the thigh, knee and leg along the meridian.

- Pain in the lower abdomen, enuresis, retention of urine, burning urination, bloody urine, painful urination, frequent bladder infection, and mental disorders, fever,

- Chronic headaches at the back of the neck and pain at the inner canthus of the eyes.

Symptoms Associated with Emotional Level Blockage

Main Emotion: FRIGHT

Related emotion: annoyed, disturbing thoughts, fearful, frustrated, highly irritable, holds on to sadness, impatient, impure thoughts, inefficient, insecure, reluctant, restless, timid, unable to let go of unwanted past memories, and unhappy.

Bladder Meridian - Related Muscles

Peroneus, sacrospinalis, anterior tibial and posterior tibial.

Bladder Meridian - Related Time

3 - 5:00 p.m.

Bladder Meridian - Dental Connection

2nd lower molar.

Bladder Meridian - Associated Nutrition

Vitamin C, A, E, B complex, B-1, calcium and trace minerals.

KIDNEY CHANNEL (MERIDIAN)

The kidney channel begins beneath the little toe, across the sole of the foot and emerges at kidney acupuncture point K 2 on the inferior aspect of the navicular tuberosity at the instep. From here, it travels posterior to the medial malleolus, enters the heel and proceeds upward along the medial aspect of the lower leg, where it intersects the spleen channel at acupuncture point Sp 6. Continuing up the leg within the gastrocnemius muscle, the channel traverses the medial aspect of the popliteal fossa and the medial, posterior aspect of the thigh to the base of the spine, where it intersects the governing vessel channel at acupuncture point GV 1. Here, it threads its way beneath the spine to enter its associated organ, the kidney, and to communicate with the bladder. It intersects the conception vessel channel at acupuncture points CV 4 and CV 3.

A branch ascends directly from the kidney, across the liver and diaphragm, enters the lung and follows the throat to the root of the tongue.Another branch separates in the lung, connects with the heart and disperses in the chest. This channel is associated with the kidneys and connects with the bladder. It is also joined directly with the liver, lungs, heart and other organs.

Symptoms Associated with the Physical Level Blockage

Pain: along the lower vertebrae, in the low back, in the sole of the foot or along the posterior aspect of the leg or thigh and along the meridian. Motor impairment or muscular atrophy of the foot and coldness in the feet, dryness of the mouth and sore throat.

Symptoms Associated with the Physiological Level Blockage

Vertigo, facial edema, blurred vision, irritability, loose stools, chronic diarrhea or constipation, abdominal distension, vomiting and impotence.

Symptoms Associated with an Overactive Meridian

High energy, high stamina, high immune system, good appetite and high fertility.

Symptoms Associated with an Under Active Meridian

Timid, low fertility; lacking courage, self-assurance and sexual interest.

Acute Allergic Symptoms

- Pain: along the lower vertebrae, in the low back, in the sole of the foot or along the posterior aspect of the leg or thigh and along the meridian.

- Coldness in the back, coldness in the feet, spasms of the ankle and feet and swelling in the legs.

- Puffy eyes, bags and dark circles under the eyes.

- Motor impairment or muscular atrophy of the foot, dryness of the mouth, sore throat, pain in the sole of the foot and in the posterior aspect of the leg or thigh.

- Pain and ringing in the ears, lightheadedness and nausea.

- Nagging mild asthma, tiredness, excessive sleeping and excessive salivation.

- Frequent burning and painful urination.

Chronic Symptoms

- Fever, fever with chills, irritability, vertigo, facial edema, blurred vision, ringing in the ears, spasms of the ankle and feet, swelling in the legs, and swollen ankles.

- Loose stools, chronic diarrhea, constipation, abdominal bloating, vomiting, tiredness, dry mouth, excessive thirst, poor appetite, and poor memory.

- Lower backache, lack of concentration, poor memory and impotence.

- Pain: along the lower vertebrae, in the low back, in the sole of the foot or along the posterior aspect of the leg or thigh and along the meridian.

Symptoms Associated with Emotional Level Blockage

Main Emotion: FEAR

Related Emotion: anguish, anxiety, bad memory, caution, confusion, contemplated, droopy, easily provoked, fear, frustrated, impatient, indecision, lethargy, mental restlessness, profound long standing sadness, read, seeks attention, sexual indecision, shock, sleepy, terror, unable

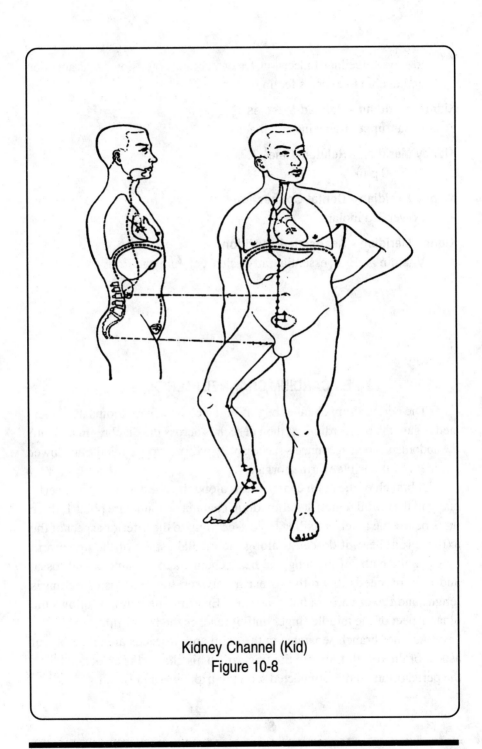

Kidney Channel (Kid)
Figure 10-8

to express feelings Indecision, terror, caution, confusion, seeks attention and unable to express feelings.

Kidney meridian - Related Muscles
Psoas, upper trapezius and iliacus.

Kidney Meridian - Related Time
5 - 7:00 p.m.

Kidney Meridian - Dental Connection
Lower 3rd molar.

Kidney Meridian - Associated Nutrition
Vitamin A, E, B, essential fatty acids, calcium and iron.

PERICARDIUM CHANNEL (MERIDIAN)

The pericardium channel begins in the chest where it joins its associated organ, the pericardium. It then descends across the diaphragm and into the abdomen, where it connects successively with the upper, middle and lower warmers of the triple warmer organ.

A branch of the main channel runs along the chest, emerging superficially in the costal region at pericardium channel acupuncture point 1, three units below the anterior axillary fold ascending to the inferior aspect of the axilla. From here, it descends along the medial aspect of the upper arm between the paths of the lung and heart channels to the antecubital fossa, and then proceeds down the forearm between the tendons of palmaris longus and flexor carpi radialis muscles. Entering the palm, it follows the ulnar aspect of the middle finger until it reaches the finger tip.

Another branch separates in the palm and proceeds along the lateral aspect of the fourth finger to the fingertip. This channel is associated with the pericardium and is connected with the triple warmer organ.

Symptoms Associated with the Physical Level

■ Stiff neck, spasms in the arm or leg, flushed face, pain in the eyes and subaxillary swelling.

■ Spasms and contracture of the elbow and arm, restricting movements, hot palms, and pain along the channel.

Symptoms Associated with the Physiological Level

■ Impaired speech, fainting, irritability, fullness in the chest, palpitations and chest pain.

■ Mental disorders, heaviness in the chest mainly on the left side, motor impairment of the tongue and heaviness of the chest due to extreme emotional changes.

Symptoms Associated with an Overactive Meridian

Dull headaches, heaviness in the head, upper abdominal distress and dream-disturbed sleep.

Symptoms Associated with the Under Active Meridian

Phobias, fear of heights (agoraphobia), fear of crowds, fear of closed areas (claustrophobia), insomnia, somnambulism (sleepwalking), continuous chain of thoughts and mental restlessness.

Acute Allergic Symptoms

■ Stiff neck, spasms in the arm, spasms in the leg, spasms of the elbow and arm, frozen shoulder, restricting movements, hot palms and pain along the channels.

■ Impaired speech, fainting spells, flushed face, irritability, fullness in the chest, heaviness in the chest and slurred speech.

■ Sensation of hot or cold, nausea, nervousness, pain in the eyes and subaxillary swellings.

Chronic Allergic Symptoms

■ Contractures of the arm, or elbow, sciatic neuralgia, pain in the anterior part of the thigh and pain in the medial part of the knee.

■ Motor impairment of the tongue, palpitation, chest pain and heaviness in the chest due to emotional overload.

■ Irritability, excessive appetite, fullness in the chest and sugar imbalance.

Symptoms Associated with Emotional Level Blockage

Main Emotion: HURT and/or EXTREME JOY
Related Emotion: agitation, anxiety, aphasia, day dreaming, delirium, depleted, difficulty in keeping up with relationships, fear of heights and various phobias, fidget, generous, happiness, heaviness in the head, hitting people, hurt, imbalance in the sexual energy, jealousy, Joy, lack of courage, lack of passion, lack of warmth, laughing uncontrollably, light sleep with dreams, manic behavior, manic disorders, mental confusion, mental restlessness, never having enough sex or no sexual desire, non emotive, non thinking, over-excitement, regret, remorse, severe deficiency of blood may lead to fear, sexual coldness, sexual frustration, sexual tension and stubbornness, shouting, sluggish memory, speechless, stubborn, Suppressed, talking incessantly, unable to protect emotions, uneasy, uninspired for joy or pleasure, and unworthiness.

Pericardium Meridian - Related Muscles
Gluteus medius, adductors, piriformis and gluteus maximus.

Pericardium Meridian - Related Time
7 - 9:00 p.m.

Pericardium Meridian - Dental Connection

■ The gluteus maximus muscles are associated with lower cuspid.

■ The gluteus medius are associated with lower central incisors.

■ The piriformis and adductors are associated with lower lateral incisors.

Pericardium Meridian - Essential Nutrition
Vitamin E, vitamin C, chromium, and trace minerals.

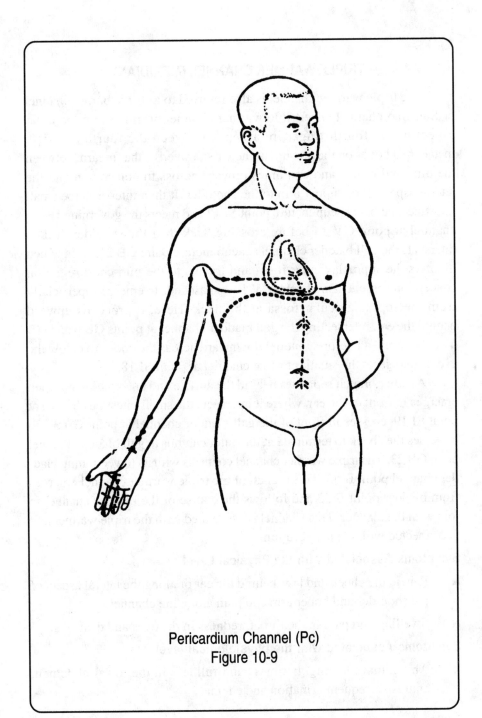

Pericardium Channel (Pc)
Figure 10-9

TRIPLE WARMER CHANNEL (MERIDIAN)

The triple warmer channel is also referred to as triple burner channel or San Jiao channel. The triple warmer channel originates on the ulnar aspect of the fourth fingertip, ascends between the fourth and fifth metacarpal bones on the dorsum of the wrist, traverses the forearm between the ulna and radius and continues upward across the olecranon and the lateral aspect of the upper arm to the shoulder. It then intersects the small intestine channel at acupuncture point SI 12 and meets the governing vessel channel at point GV 14 before crossing back over the shoulder. It then intersects the gall bladder channel at acupuncture point GB 21, from which it enters the supraclavicular fossa and travels to the mid-chest region at conception vessel channel point CV 17 and ascends to emerge superficially from the supraclavicular fossa at the neck. Here, it proceeds upward behind the ear, intersecting the gall bladder channel at points GB 6 and GB 4 on the forehead before winding downward across the cheek to below the eye. It intersects the small intestine channel at point SI 18.

Another branch separates behind the auricle and enters the ear. It then emerges in front of the ear, where it intersects the small intestine channel at point SI 19, crosses in front of the gall bladder channel at point GB 3 and traverses the cheek to terminate at the outer canthus at gall bladder channel point GB 23. The triple warmer channel connects with its lower uniting bladder channel point B 53. This branch of the triple warmer channel emerges from bladder point B 53 and follows the course of the bladder channel to join with the bladder. This channel is associated with the triple warmer and is connected with the pericardium.

Symptoms Associated with the Physical Level

- Pain in the cheek and jaw, behind the ear or along the lateral aspect of the shoulder and upper arm and pain along the channel.
- Swelling and pain in the throat, redness in the eyes and deafness.

Symptoms Associated with the physiological level

- Abdominal bloating, hardness and fullness in the lower abdomen, enuresis, frequent urination and edema.

■   Dysuria, excessive thirst, excessive hunger and vertigo.

Symptoms Associated with an Overactive Meridian

Loss of hearing, ringing in the ears, tingling on the lateral part of the forearm and heavy or tight feeling at the elbow.

Symptoms Associated with an Underactive Meridian

Sensation of cold all over the body, tips of the fingers and toes become too cold and even may turn blue (Raynaud's syndrome).

Acute Allergic Symptoms

Pain: in the cheek and jaw, behind the ear, along the lateral aspect of the shoulder, upper arm and along the channel. Excessive hunger, redness of the eye, deafness, swelling and pain in the throat.

Chronic Allergic Symptoms

■   Abdominal pain, bloating, hardness and fullness in the lower abdomen, enuresis, frequent urination and edema.

■   Dysuria, excessive thirst, excessive hunger, always feels hungry even after eating, vertigo, indigestion and constipation.

■   Pain in the medial part of the knee, shoulder pain and fever in the late evening.

Symptoms Associated with Emotional Level Blockage

Main Emotion: HOPELESSNESS

Related Emotions: depression, deprivation, despair, excessive emotion, emptiness, grief, and phobias.

The Triple Warmer Meridian - Related Muscles

Teres minor, sartorius, gracilis, soleus and gastrocnemius.

The Triple Warmer Meridian - Related Time

9 - 11:00 p.m.

The Triple Warmer Meridian - Dental Connection

Lower 1st molar.

The Triple Warmer Meridian - Associated Nutrition

Iodine, trace minerals, vitamin C, calcium, fluoride and water.

THE GALL BLADDER CHANNEL (MERIDIAN)

The Gall Bladder channel begins at the outer canthus of the eye and traverses the temple to the gall bladder channel point GB 22. It then ascends to the corner of the forehead where it intersects the stomach point S 8 before descending behind the ear. From here, it proceeds along the neck in front of the triple warmer channel, crosses the small intestine channel at point SI 17, then at the top of the shoulder, turns back and runs behind the triple warmer channel to intersect the governing vessel channel at point GV 14 on the spine. Finally, the channel turns downward into the supraclavicular fossa.

One branch of the main channel emerges behind the auricle and enters the ear at gall bladder point GB 17, emerging in front of the ear. This branch intersects the small intestine channel at SI 19 and the stomach channel at S 7 before terminating behind the outer canthus. Another branch separates at the outer canthus and proceeds downward to stomach point S 5 on the jaw. Then crossing the triple warmer channel, it returns upward to the infraorbital region before descending again to the neck, where it joins the original channel in the supraclavicular fossa. From here, it descends further into the chest, crossing the diaphragm and connecting with the liver before joining its associated organ, the gall bladder. Continuing along the inside of the ribs, it emerges in the inguinal region of the lower abdomen and winds around the genitals submerging again in the hip at gall bladder point GB 30.

Yet another vertical branch runs downward from the supraclavicular fossa to the axilla and the lateral aspect of the chest. It crosses the ribs and intersects the liver channel at point Liv 13 before turning back to the sacral region where it crosses the bladder channel points B 31 to B 34. This branch then descends to the hip joint, and continues down the lateral side of the thigh and knee, passing along the anterior aspect of the fibula to its lower end. Here, it crosses in front of the lateral malleolus and traverses the dorsum of the foot, entering between the fourth and fifth metatarsal bones before terminating at the lateral side of the tip of the fourth toe or gall bladder point GB 44.

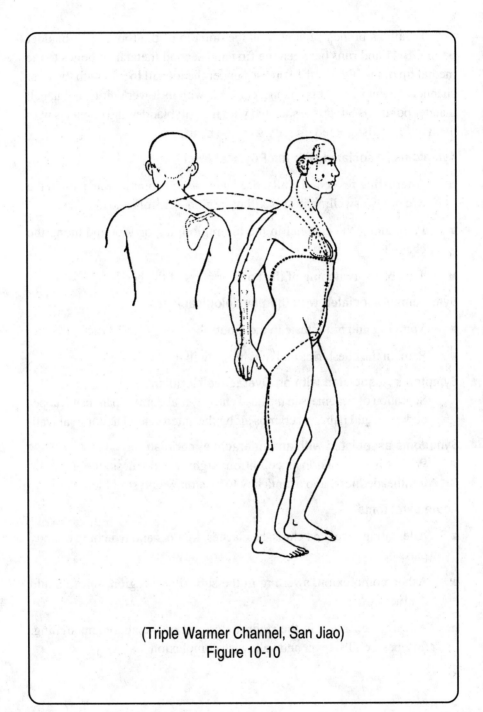

(Triple Warmer Channel, San Jiao)
Figure 10-10

Finally, a branch separates on the dorsum of the foot at gall bladder point GB 41 and runs between the first and second metatarsal bones to the medial tip of the big toe, then crosses under the toenail to join with the liver channel at point Liv 1. This channel connects with its lower uniting point, gall bladder point GB 34. It is associated with the gall bladder and connects with the liver. It is also joined directly with the heart.

Symptoms Associated with the Physical level

- Alternating fever and chills, headache, ashen complexion, pain in the eye or jaw, swelling in subaxillary region, scrofula and deafness.

- Pain: along the channel in the hip region, leg or foot and along the channel.

- Tremors or twitching of the body or parts of the body.

Symptoms Associated with the physiological level

- Vomiting and bitter taste in the mouth.

- Pain: in the chest, ribs and moving pain in the joints.

Symptoms Associated with an Overactive Meridian

Sensation of heaviness in the head and upper abdomen, pain in the upper abdomen and pain and cramps along the anterolateral abdominal wall.

Symptoms associated with an underactive meridian

Person is in an acidosis condition: sighing, dizziness, feeling cold, lightheadedness, and a tendency to be sloppy and stumble.

Acute symptoms

- Alternating fever and chills, headaches, tremors and twitching of body parts.

- Ashen complexion, swelling in the subaxillary region, scrofula and deafness.

- A heavy sensation in the right upper part of the abdomen, sighing, dizziness, chills, fever and yellowish complexion.

- Pain: along the gall bladder channel, in the hip, leg, foot, eye, jaw and cramps along the anterolateral wall.

Chronic Symptoms

- Pain: in the intercostal areas, in the right side of the abdomen, in the chest, pain along the channel and moving arthritis.

- Vomiting, bitter taste in the mouth, problem to digest fats and nausea with fried foods.

Symptoms associated with Emotional Level Blockage
Main Emotion: RAGE

Related Emotions: aggression, assertion, denied worthiness, depressed, easily startled, emotionally repressed, indecisive, Irrational, lack assertiveness, lack of courage, lack of initiative, prolonged accumulated anger, rage, (anger, frustration and bottled up resentment), resentment, shouting, sighing, nervousness, stubborn, talking loud, timidity, and unable to make decisions.

Gall Bladder Meridian - Related Muscle
Anterior deltoid and popliteus.

Gall Bladder Meridian - Related Time
11 p.m. - 1 a.m.

Gall Bladder Meridian - Dental Connection

- The popliteus is associated with the upper first bicuspid

- The deltoid is associated with upper cuspid.

Gall Bladder Meridian - Essential Nutrition
Vitamin A, calcium, linoleic acids and oleic acids (for example, pine nuts)

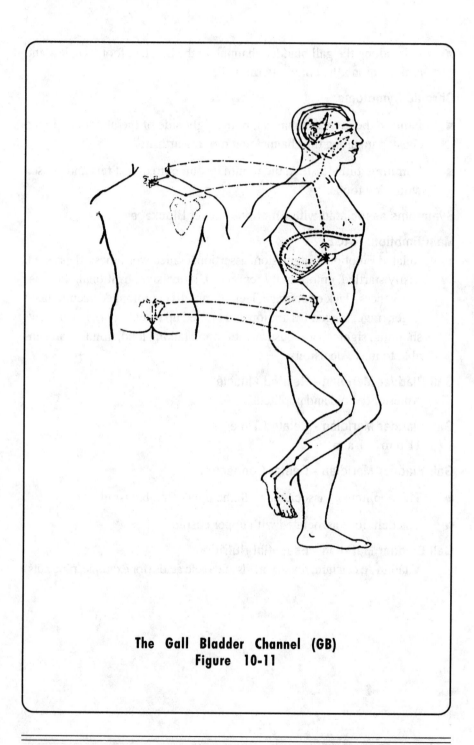

The Gall Bladder Channel (GB)
Figure 10-11

THE LIVER CHANNEL (MERIDIAN)

The liver channel begins on the dorsum of the big toe, continues across the foot to a point one unit in front of the medial malleolus and proceeds upward to spleen channel acupuncture point Sp 6 where it intersects the spleen channel. From here, it continues to the medial aspect of the lower leg, recrossing the spleen channel eight units above the medial malleolus, and thereafter, running posterior to that channel over the knee and thigh. Winding around the genitals, the channel enters the lower abdomen where it meets the conception vessel channel at points CV 2, CV 3 and CV 4 before skirting the stomach and joining with its associated organ, the liver and connecting with the gall bladder. Then the channel continues upward, across the diaphragm and costal region, traverses the nasopharynx, connecting with the tissue surrounding the eye. Finally, the channel ascends across the forehead and meets the governing vessel channel at the vertex.

A branch separates below the eye and encircles the inside of the lips. Another branch separates in the liver, crosses the diaphragm and reaches the lung. This channel is associated with the liver and connects with the gall bladder. It is also joined directly with the lungs, stomach, kidneys, brain and other organs.

Symptoms Associated with the Physical level

Headaches, vertigo, blurred vision, tinnitus, fever, spasms in the extremities and pain along the channel.

Symptoms Associated with the physiological level

- Pain in the costal region or chest, hard lumps in the upper abdomen, abdominal pain, vomiting, jaundice, loose stool, pain in the lower abdomen and hernia

- Enuresis, retention of the urine and dark urine.

- Dizziness, stroke-like conditions, irregular menses, premenstrual syndrome, reproductive organ disturbances and excessive bright-colored bleeding during menses.

Symptoms Associated with an Overactive Meridian

Excitable, cries easily, starts on several different projects at once, goes in different directions at one time, and may manifest an obsession to keep going until everything is completed.

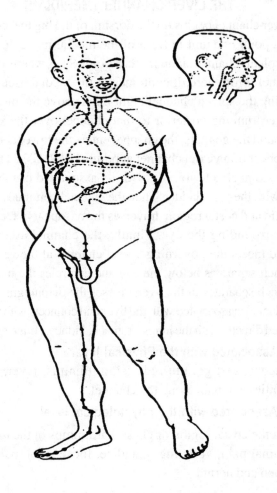

The Liver Channel (Liv)
Figure 10-12

Symptoms Associated with an Underactive Meridian

Sensation of internal cold, internal tremors, dizzy spells, lightheadedness, depression, frustration, highly irritable, mood swings and lack of interest to start a job due to lack of energy.

Acute Allergic Symptoms

- Headache at the top of the head, vertigo and blurred vision.

- Feeling of some obstruction in the throat, tinnitus and fever.

- Spasms in the extremities and pain along the channel.

Chronic Allergic Symptoms

- Abdominal pain and hard lumps in the upper abdomen.

- Pain in the intercostal region, hernia, PMS, pain in the breasts, vomiting, jaundice, loose stools and pain in the lower abdomen.

- Irregular menses, reproductive organ disturbances and excessive bright colored bleeding during menses.

- Enuresis, retention of urine and dark urine.

- Dizziness and stroke-like condition.

Symptoms Associated with Emotional Level Blockage

Main Emotion: ANGER

Related Emotions: aggression, anger with oneself, anger with others, complaining all the time, deficient liver causes fear, depression, disconnected- easily uprooted, dream disturbed sleep, easily confused, feeling wound up, finding faults with others, fluctuating mental state, frustration, inability to express anger, indifferent, irrationality, Irritability, moodiness, primed for fight, repressed anger, resentment, troubled emotions, trapped, and unhappiness.

Liver Meridian - Related Time

1 - 3:00 a.m.

Liver Meridian - Related Muscles

Pectoralis major sternal and rhomboideus.

Liver Meridian - Dental Connection
The pectoralis major sternal muscle is associated with the lower second bicuspid.

Liver Meridian - Essential Nutrition
Beets, green vegetables, vitamin A, trace minerals and unsaturated fatty acids.

THE GOVERNING VESSEL CHANNEL (MERIDIAN)

The governing vessel channel is the confluence of all the Yang channels over which it is said to "govern." There are four paths followed by the channel. The first path originates in the perineum and ascends along the middle of the spine until it reaches point GV 16 at the nape of the neck. Here, it enters the brain, ascends to the vertex, and follows the midline of the forehead across the bridge of the nose, terminating at the upper lip.

The second path begins in the pelvic region, descends to the genitals and perineum, and then passes through the tip of the coccyx. Here, it diverts into the gluteal region where it intersects the kidney and bladder channels before returning to the spinal column and then joining with the kidneys.

The origin of the third path is in common with that of the bladder channel at the inner canthus of the eye. The two (bilateral) branches from each of the inner canthii, ascend across the forehead and converge at the vertex where the channel enters the brain. Emerging at the lower end of the nape of the neck, the channel again divides into two branches that descend along the opposite sidesThe fourth path of the governing vessel channel begins in the lower abdomen and rises directly across the navel, passes through the heart and enters the trachea. Continuing its upward course, the channel crosses the cheek and encircles the mouth, before terminating at a point below the middle of the eye. This channel intersects the bladder channel at point B 12, and the conception vessel channel at point CV 1.

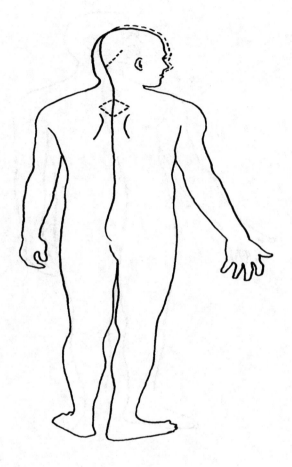

The Governing Vessel Channel (GV, Du)
Figure 10-13

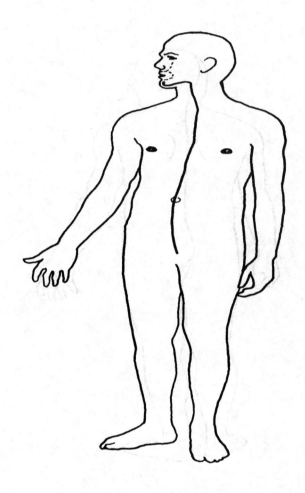

The Conception Vessel Channel (CV, Ren)
Figure 10-14

Pathological Symptoms

This channel supplies the brain and spinal region and intersects the liver channel at the vertex. Obstruction of its Chi may result in symptoms such as stiffness and pain along the spinal column. Deficient Chi in the channel may produce a heavy sensation in the head, vertigo and shaking. Energy blockages in this meridian (which passes through the brain) may be responsible for certain mental disorders. Febrile diseases are commonly associated with the governing vessel channel, and, because one branch of the channel ascends through the abdomen, when the channel is unbalanced, its Chi rushes upward toward the heart. Symptoms such as colic, constipation, enuresis, hemorrhoids and functional infertility may result.

THE CONCEPTION VESSEL CHANNEL (CV, REN)

The conception vessel channel has two routes. The first arises in the lower abdomen below conception vessel acupuncture point CV 3, ascends along the midline of the abdomen and chest, across the throat and jaw and finally winds around the mouth terminating in the region of the eye. The second course arises in the pelvic cavity, enters the spine and ascends along the back.

This channel intersects the stomach channel at acupuncture point St 1 and the governing vessel at the acupuncture point GV 28.

Pathological Symptoms

The conception vessel channel is the confluence of the Yin channels. Therefore, abnormality along the conception vessel channel will appear principally in pathological symptoms of the Yin channels, especially symptoms associated with the liver and kidneys. Its function is closely related with pregnancy and, therefore, has intimate links with the kidneys and uterus. If its Chi is deficient, infertility or other disorders of the urogenital system may result. Leukorrhea, irregular menstruation, colic, etc., are all symptoms associated with the conception vessel channel.

Any possible allergen can cause blockage in one meridian or more than one meridian at the same time. If it is blocking only one meridian, the patient may demonstrate symptoms related to that particular blocked meridian. The intensity of the symptoms will depend on the severity of the blockage. Again, the patient may suffer from one symptom, many symptoms or all the symptoms of the said blocked meridian. Sometimes, a patient can have many meridians blocked at the same time. In such cases, the patient may demonstrate a variety of symptoms, one from each meridian or many from some meridians and one or two from others. Some patients with just one meridian block can demonstrate one symptom only, but with great intensity. In some people, even though all the meridians are blocked, they may not show much reaction at all. Variations with all these possibilities make diagnosis difficult in some cases.

CHAPTER 11

SAY GOOD-BYE TO ILLNESS

Most of the acupuncture points used in eliminating energy blockages lie near vital organs. The information about the treatment points and the techniques for needling the specific points and the specific allergy elimination techniques are not described in this book. Teaching the techniques is beyond the scope of this book and has been intentionally excluded. At the present time, there are over 5,500 licensed medical practitioners trained in NAET treatment methods all over the country and outside the United States. Please visit our website "naet.com" to find a practitioner near you.

Information regarding a few important acupuncture points are discussed in this chapter. They can be used to help control any mild to moderate allergic reactions. Severely allergic patients should consult a licensed NAET practitioner for treatments. Stimulation of these points will not remove the allergies permanently, but will help temporarily to remove the energy blockages and help you to feel better.

So far, you have seen the common routes of the meridians, their internal and external courses of travel pathways (diagrams 10-1 to 10-14). You have also seen how these meridians get blocked from simple allergies, giving rise to specific pathological symptoms (physical, physiological and emotional) in the body. In Chapter 7, "Muscle-Response Testing for Allergy," you learned to test for allergies. Allergies may be the causative agents for energy blockages in particular meridians. You have learned to test and find allergens in general. You are urged to practice these testing techniques and make a habit of testing everything before exposing yourself further to food, clothing, makeup products, household chemicals, environmental agents, etc., that you know or suspect you are allergic to.

ISOLATING THE BLOCKAGES

Testing and isolating the particular blockages can be done in many ways. One method is fairly easy to understand and, with some practice, can be mastered by anyone.

Patient and tester should wash hands with soap and water before beginning the test to remove any adverse energy from the fingertips.

Step 1: Balance the patient and find an indicator muscle. Refer to Chapter 7 to learn more about balancing and MRT to test your allergies.

Step 2: Patient lies down on his/her back with the allergen (e.g., an apple) in his/her resting palm. When it is needed (to test an infant, small child, too weak or strong, old, debilitated, sick or unresponsive persons and animals), surrogate testing can also be used.

Step 3: Tester touches the points in diagram 11-1 one at a time, and tests the predetermined muscle (indicator muscle) and compares the strength of the PDM in the absence and presence of the allergen. For example, touch point "1" in diagram 11-1 with the finger tips of one hand and with the other hand test the indicator muscle (while the patient is still holding the allergen in one hand). If the test muscle goes weak, it indicates the meridian, or the energy pathways connected to that particular point, has an energy blockage.

Point "1" relates to the lung meridian. Obstruction in the energy flow anywhere in the lung meridian can make this point weak. Test all other points in table 11-1 (figure 11-1) using this technique. Write down all the weak points. For point-meridian relationships, refer to table 11-1. Using this technique, you can trace all weak meridians.

Table 11-1

Point Name	Related Meridian	Related Organ
0 Pt	Brain Test Pt	Brain
Pt 1	LU test pt	Lung
Pt 2	PHT (physical heart)	Pericardium
Pt 3	LIV test pt	Liver
Pt 4	GB test pt	Gall bladder
Pt 5	Heart test pt	Heart
Pt 6	ST test pt	Stomach
Pt 7	Kid test pt	Kidney
Pt 8	Sp test pt	Spleen
Pt 9	Colon test pt	Colon
Pt 10	TW test pt	Triple warmer
Pt 11	SI test pt	Small Intestine
Pt 12	UB test pt	Bladder

FINGER PRESSURE THERAPY

Finger pressure therapy can be used to restore the energy flow in the energy meridians by removing blockages temporarily.

Step 1: The first step for finger pressure therapy is to find the organ associated point or meridian being blocked. Find the related organ point on the table and then in diagram 11-1.

Step 2: Apply slight finger pressure, with the pad of your index finger, on the point. Hold 60 seconds at each point. Follow the order of the sequence of points given on the previous page. When the blocked meridian is found, make the associated organ point with that meridian a starting point to perform the energy balancing using finger pressure therapy. For example, if the energy is blocked in the liver meridian, make the liver organ point (point-5) the first point to begin the finger pressure. If the heart is blocked, use the heart point (point-3) as the first point in the sequence of energy balancing.

Step 3: Hold 60 seconds at each point and go through all 12 points in the order given in the table or diagram 11-1 and come back to the starting point. Then, hold 60 seconds at the starting point and stop the treatment. Always end at the starting point to complete the energy cycle.

Some patients can experience physical or emotional pain or emotional release during these treatment sessions. If the patient has an emotional blockage, it needs to be isolated and treated for the best result. Some patients can get tingling pains, sharp pains, pulsation, excessive perspiration, etc., during the treatment. In such instances, please go through another cycle of treatment. This will often correct the problem. Some commonly used acupuncture points, and their uses to help in emergency situations, are given below. Massage each of these points gently with the finger pads for one minute each. Please refer to the appropriate meridians in Chapter 10 or to the text books on acupuncture in the bibliography if you would like to learn more about these points.

RESUSCITATION POINTS

1. Fainting: GV-20, GV-26, GB-12, LI-1, PC-9
2. Nausea: CV-12, PC-6
3. Backache: GV-26, UB-40
4. Fatigue: CV-6, LI-1, CV-17, Liv-3
5. Fever: LI-11, LU-10, GV-14

For more information on revival points, refer to Chapter 3, pages 570 to 573, in "Acupuncture: A Comprehensive Text," by Shanghai College of Traditional Medicine, Eastland Press, 1981, or refer to, "Living Pain Free with Acupressure," 1997, by the author. It is available at various book stores and at our website (naet.com).

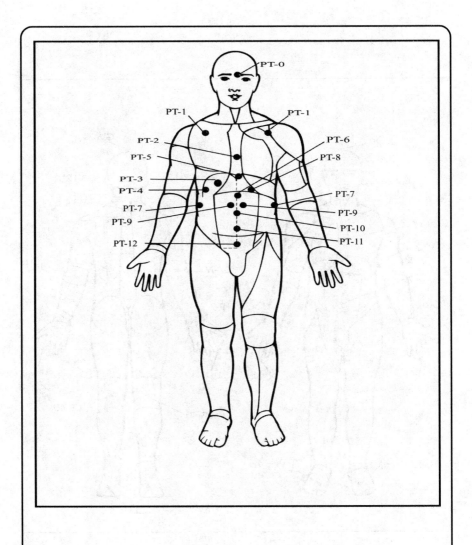

Figure 11-1
Finger Pressure Therapy Points

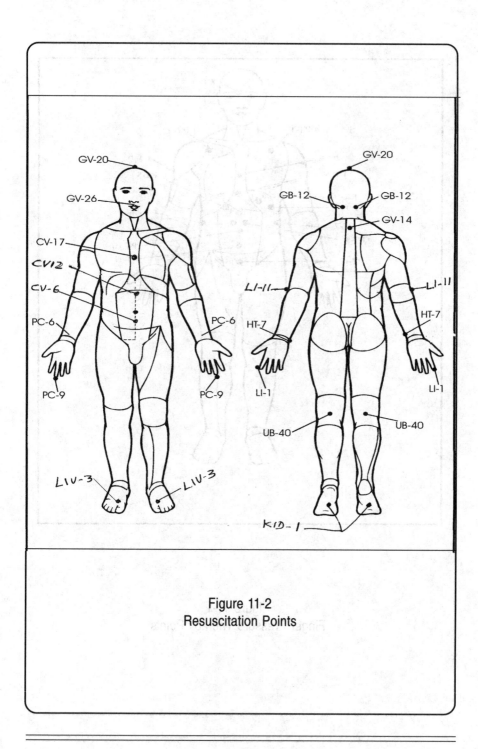

Figure 11-2
Resuscitation Points

A WORD TO THE ALLERGIC PATIENT

I have attempted to discuss most of the various types of allergic manifestations, the more common types of allergic reactions, and the prevalent Western and Oriental methods for treatment of allergies. I have presented sufficient information on NAET to free you from your immediate allergic reactions from the allergens you come in contact with in your everyday life. I have also explained in detail how to test and find your allergies on your own, the most reliable and least expensive method of allergy testing. This should help allergic patients to control allergens and prevent unexpected and unfortunate incidences by carefully preventing known allergens from affecting them. It is hoped that you will spend some time rereading every page related to testing and balancing techniques carefully and learning about this new discovery. Mild reactions can be treated using this method. This does not replace the need for visiting your doctor or an NAET practitioner. After you overcome your immediate emergency situation using this method, please make an appointment with your doctor and have him/her manage the rest of your problems. Please do not take the responsibility on yourself to continue to treat your allergies without the help of a trained practitioner. Please do not forget that these medical practitioners have sacrificed thousands of hours in their medical schools to learn how to help you and provide you with a comfortable journey towards wellness. You cannot expect to replace their knowledge with this book.

Countless examples featured on these pages have shown how many people have undergone these treatments and now enjoy good health. Allergic patients do not have to spend the rest of their lives in fear or in a bubble anymore. Instead, they can live like any normal person, provided they get treated for their allergies by doctors trained in NAET.

I hope you will take enough time to understand the material presented in this book, to learn about NTT and MRT to find allergies and to make use of the balancing techniques described herein. In addition, it is important for you to know and to understand the emergency measures that will pull you out of serious emergency situations by simply utilizing Oriental medical techniques. NAET specialists (including NAET trained acupuncturists, chiropractors, allopathic medical doctors and other medical practitioners) are available at various locations throughout the country. I cannot emphasize enough the importance of full and complete cooperation between you and your allergist. It is only by such complete cooperation that you can obtain the best results.

It is not sufficient for the patient to receive treatments regularly, although this is vitally important. He/she must also follow the other instructions if he/she hopes to attain the maximum result in a minimum time. *The NAET Guide Book*, by the author, should be read by all NAET patients. This book gives step-by-step instructions to follow during the 24 hours after NAET. Allergy treatments require repeated office visits in the beginning. Once all the known allergens are eliminated, the patient is trained to find his/her own allergens. He/she then has to see the doctor only if he/she encounters an item that bothers him which he/she can't eliminate using the above methods, or for annual follow-ups. All allergens cannot be eliminated in one or two office visits. In some severe cases, it may take as many as three visits a week for one or two years or more to achieve a condition close to normalcy. This is contingent on the patient's immune system response.

There have been a few patients with mild cases of allergies who have completed the treatments in one or two visits or in two or three months' time. These patients were either not seen again, or only on a few follow-up visits. On the average, most patients have taken anywhere from eight to twelve months to achieve satisfactory results. Some extreme cases have taken from three-and-half to four years or more to solve their problems. Allergic patients should keep this time span in mind when they approach any NAET specialists. If treatment is discontinued before completion of all the necessary basic treatments, the results will be unsatisfactory and allergic symptoms are very likely to recur. This will tend to make the patient feel that the allergy itself is to blame or that the treatment is useless. For this reason, it is better not even to start treatment than to start and discontinue too soon, or to start and then cooperate in a halfhearted manner. The allergist will discharge his/her patients with proper instructions just as soon as he/she feels it is safe to do so.

How can patients cooperate and help the doctor achieve maximum results in minimum time? After each treatment, patients are advised to stay away from the treated item for 24 hours. There are 12 energy meridians. It takes two hours for an energy molecule to pass through one meridian. To circulate through 12 meridians, it takes 24 hours. This means that the patient should not even come close to the object during that time, as its electromagnetic field can interfere with the patient's own field and negate the treatment. Patients are also advised to maintain a food diary. If the patient reacts to something violently during treatment, the offender can easily be traced and treated, preventing further pain. Patients are placed on a strict diet of non-allergic items after completion of the first three treatments. This helps the body maintain good health without having to face possible allergic items. It also speeds up the treatment process while reducing interference.

The following is a list of general directions which, it is hoped, will be of assistance to allergic patients, regardless of their symptoms.

1. The best time to begin treatments for your allergic symptoms is now. Do not wait until the next attack. It is not likely that the symptoms will decrease with the passing of time; symptoms will most likely become more severe.

2. Report regularly for treatment and as often as directed by your NAET doctor. If necessary, long breaks should only be taken after completion of the treatment for each allergen. Never take more than two days off without completing treatment for the treated allergen just in case the initial treatment failed. For example, when getting treated for a milk allergy, if you were to take five consecutive visits to clear the allergy to the sample of milk, you should take a few days or a week off from treatment soon after being cleared for the milk, and before starting treatment for another item, like beef. If you expose the brain to an allergen but you do not complete the treatment, unpleasant consequences or exaggeration of the problem can result.

A 28-year-old woman was treated for cotton. After seven consecutive treatments, she decided to go on a short vacation before being cleared of her allergy, without informing her allergist. Three months later, her husband called and asked whether NAET could help his wife's present condition. Two days into her vacation, she had slipped into a depression and refused to talk or cooperate with anyone. As a teenager, she had a nervous breakdown but recovered from the episode completely. Finally, the husband took her to a psychologist and therapist, neither of whom could help her come out of the depression. The allergist remembered that she had not completed treatment for cotton. She was brought into the office and treated for cotton and was cleared after four more treatments, a total of eleven. At the end of these treatments, she came out of her depression. This is a good example of the danger associated with letting go of treatments in midstream.

3.   Certain people may have a negative reaction to a treatment. One cannot predict reactions ahead of time. For this reason, the patient has to remain in the doctor's office anywhere from twenty minutes to an hour following the treatment. During that time, if there is an unusual reaction, the doctor will treat the patient again. If there is no reaction, the patient will be sent home with certain instructions to follow.

4.   The patient should not come close to the energy field of the allergic items after he/she leaves the doctor's office for a period of 24 hours. This is a crucial time because the brain works on a biological time clock of 24-hour cycles. During this time, the brain can reject or accept the treatment. If the brain accepts the treatment, it will generally not reject it for the rest of the patient's life.

The brain, accepting the allergen as an ally, will also make necessary changes in the chemical activity of the body and its functions. It is probable, and quite likely, that it is also capable of effecting changes in the genes, RNA, and DNA. We have not conducted experiments in the genetic field, but whenever a pregnant woman gets treated and clears an allergy, her child does not react to the mother's allergen after birth. When couples get treated for their allergies before they have children, their offspring do not react to these items at all. This tends to support the theory that the children's genes have become adjusted so as not to react.

A 22-year-old woman who had two miscarriages came to our office. We found that she was allergic to most of the foods she was eating. She was treated for most of the allergies, but then she got pregnant again and discontinued the treatments. This time she carried full term and had a normal child. She returned again, to treat for herself, as well as the child. When the child was examined, we discovered he was not allergic to the items the mother had passed before she got pregnant; however, he was allergic to the items the mother had not yet treated.

A young couple, both of whom manifested a number of allergic problems, including migraines, dizzy spells, sinusitis, joint pains etc., were treated for all their known allergies. Then they had a child. We checked the child and found that the child was absolutely healthy with no known allergies at all. Another couple, both allergic to many items, were treated for all the foods, but did not get treated for any fabrics. When their child was born, she developed severe rashes all over her body and could not wear any clothes. The parents brought the child in for evaluation, and we found she was allergic to all the fabrics, but not to the food items.

5. Soon after treatment, patients should avoid strenuous activity, exercises, heavy meals, etc., for at least three to four hours. It is possible that any of these activities can cause a sudden blockage in the energy pathway, resulting in unpleasant reactions.

6. Patients who are allergic to many items will experience various symptoms if they use the allergic items while they are undergoing treatment. In NAET treatments, the patient is asked to use or eat anything he wants except the item for which he/she is getting treated. If he/she is exposed to some other allergen, he/she can still react to that particular allergen even though this does not interfere with the current treatment; however, the patient may not feel very good. For better and faster results, the patient should avoid all other allergens. If the patient is under any other medical care for any

other symptoms, he/she is advised to continue those other treatments as before, along with the NAET treatments. This will help the patient keep his/her other health problems under control while going through the allergy treatments. This way, the body does not have to fight stress or diseases from different causes while undergoing the stress of the new treatment. Patients who have asthma, migraine headaches or other illnesses, and continue their anti-asthma medicines or pain killers, can get through these allergy treatments more easily than patients who refuse to seek Western medical supportive treatments and rely on the allergy treatments alone.

7. During treatment, patients are advised to avoid exposure to extreme weather, such as excessive heat and cold drafts. Patients with many allergies cannot tolerate extreme weather conditions because they may be allergic to the weather induced physical agents.

8. Patients are advised to practice good nutrition. They should try to eat non-allergic items, or NAET treated and cleared items, while going through this program. Patients are also advised not to over-eat or overexercise, to drink plenty of liquids, have pleasant thoughts while preparing and eating foods, and get plenty of rest. It is very important to prepare and eat foods with pleasant thoughts to avoid additional emotional blockages.

9. Remember, it usually takes several years to build up a sensitivity to the point where severe reactions occur. Do not get discouraged if relief from symptoms is delayed for some time. Just because all the symptoms do not disappear at the end of a few days' or weeks' treatment, there is no reason for discontinuing a diet or the treatments. When a few major allergies are cleared, minor allergies may be noticed more easily. Your awareness of allergies will be more pronounced after a few items have been cleared. Some patients ask, "After being cleared for some items, do I become more allergic to things I was not allergic to before?" The answer is a definite "No." The person's awareness increases and the allergic reactions stick out more noticeably after some major items have been cleared.

For example, before receiving an NAET treatment, a patient was never told that he/she had allergies. Whenever he/she had a sore throat, headache or body ache, he/she might believe that his symptoms are in fact due to a "flu" or a virus. So he/she may run to get some "Theraflu" or antibiotics. In a case of "flu," whatever he/she may take, it will normally take 7 to 21 days to get better. After treatments, if he/she gets a sore throat, he/she will begin to search for the cause, "What did I eat that was different?" And will find the answer. "Oh! It was that piece of pineapple I ate in the fruit salad that is causing these flu-like symptoms." So, actually your allergy does not increase, you just become more aware of its manifestations.

10. Avoid emotional stress and undue worry. This will bring down the immune system by increasing the energy blockages and cause more allergic reactions. If you are under a lot of stress, or sadness, you should avoid heavy meals or excessively spicy or salty meals. Try to eat simple food in liquid or pureed form to allow the food to go through the digestive tract faster without dispensing a lot of energy from the energy reservoir. You may take some digestive enzymes to help digest and assimilate the food better.

11. As you improve, your symptoms will grow less severe and less frequent, but do not stop the treatments. Try to complete treatments for all your known allergies. Otherwise, untreated allergens may build up and later cause problems.

12. Severely allergic patients should always try to carry antihistamines and oral medications or adrenaline shots with them. Severely allergic patients can get into life-threatening situations at any time with any kind of allergy. If the patient can administer the adrenaline shot or antihistamines immediately, the aftereffect will be less severe, preventing unfortunate incidents.

Additionally, specific instructions will be necessary for each patient, and these instructions vary depending on his/her sensitivities and allergic manifestations.

Statistics show that from 80 to 90 percent of allergic patients who receive proper treatments by NAET, and cooperate with the doctor, are entirely relieved of any allergy related problems or satisfactorily improved. NAET treatment can provide amazing results if done properly.

Carmel was getting treated by one of the NAET practitioners for severe pain disorders. She had constant severe pain in her liver and spleen. None of the tests showed any abnormalities, but she suffered from this excruciating pain. When she was evaluated by the doctor, she was found to be allergic to many groups except for the vitamin C group. She continued the treatments with him for 2 years. Her condition did not improve. Finally the practitioner sent her to me for evaluation. She was found to be highly allergic to vitamin C. Within 30 minutes of her treatment for vitamin C, she reported that her pain in the liver and spleen was relieved completely and had not returned in months.

A young man of 22 came in with a 2-month history of severe, acute pain in his right lateral thigh, radiating into the right knee and ankle joint. During NTT evaluation, it was discovered that he was reacting to the artichoke he ate 2 months ago. He never liked to eat artichoke, but 2 months ago he was at a party where he was served artichoke. The next morning he woke up with sciatic pain on his right thigh. He tried various treatments before he discovered NAET. His pain got worse in spite of all the pain pills he consumed. He stopped working and had to go on temporary disability. After the evaluation, I treated him for artichoke. His gallbladder and colon were blocked. Eighty percent of his sciatic pain was relieved almost instantly after the spinal treatment. After 12 minutes, he was completely free of his pain.

Artichoke seems to be a simple vegetable, but it has created many different types of pain disorders in a great number of my patients.

CHAPTER 12

THE DIGESTIVE SYSTEM

The gastrointestinal tract is made up of the organs involved with the eating and digesting of food. It includes organs from the mouth to the rectum, all of which are part of the system. Allergic reactions that affect or occur in these organs are grouped under the heading, "Allergy of the Digestive System."

Inheritance plays a large part in this type of allergy. Like asthma, migraine, headache, hay fever, and skin allergy, such allergies often appear repeatedly in families. The allergic history of a patient suffering from this type of allergy can often be traced back to the mother, father, brother, or sister. Even allergies to individual items such as milk, eggs, fish or onion may occur in two to four successive generations.

Symptoms of allergy vary between patients, depending upon many factors, such as the status of the immune system, degree of involvement of the organs and systems, age and degree of inheritance.

■ Allergy of the digestive system can manifest itself in a variety of symptoms: abdominal bloating and pain, appendicitis, burning sensation in the stomach and gastritis, belching, bleeding from any part of the digestive tract, diverticulitis, esophageal spasm, heartburn, hiatal hernia, celiac disease (Crohn's disease, irritable bowel syndrome, leaky gut syndrome), pancreatitis, peptic ulcer and ulcerative colitis.

- Anorexia, anorexia nervosa, canker sores, cold sores, fever blisters, gagging, lump in the throat, halitosis, salmonellosis, nausea and vomiting.

- Constipation, diarrhea, fecal impaction, itching of the anus and yeast infections, etc.

Although food and environmental substances are often the cause, allergic reactions to these substances are not limited to the gastrointestinal tract. Eggs, for example, may cause hives, skin rashes, asthma or headaches, rather than an allergy of the digestive system alone. Allergy of the gastrointestinal tract may cause: swelling and burning of the mouth and tongue, colitis, indigestion, colic, gall bladder symptoms, ulcer-like symptoms of the stomach and duodenum, symptoms mimicking appendicitis, or any other abdominal conditions mentioned above. The symptoms of certain allergic manifestations are so similar to cholecystitis (inflammation of the gall bladder), appendicitis, ulcers, and other abdominal diseases, that many patients have undergone needless operations, suffering and expense. Unfortunately, such treatment seldom reveals the true cause of the "symptoms." Consequently, they usually recur soon after the patient has recovered from the operation (and sometimes even sooner), leaving him/her in worse condition than before.

An example of this, as seen by an allergist, might be useful in giving the reader insight into the process. A woman suffering from an allergic condition was diagnosed as having chronic: cholecystitis, gallstones and appendicitis. She was also suffering from asthma and hay fever. The surgeon did not recognize the relationship between these conditions and her abdominal pain. She was operated on for her abdominal symptoms. Although no gallstones were found and her gall bladder was normal, it was removed. Her attacks of excruciating pain in the gall bladder region, accompanied by intense headaches and vomiting of huge quantities of mucus mixed with bile, continued to occur about once a month.

After suffering from these symptoms for nearly two more years, she underwent surgery again, only to find that no gallstones were present this time either. The symptoms grew increasingly severe, with shorter intervals of freedom from pain. For eleven years, this patient was completely disabled and confined to her bed for long periods of time, in almost constant,

MY RESPONSE TO THE FIRST NAET TREATMENT "EGG MIX"

I was treated for egg mix (egg white, egg yolk, chicken, tetra-cycline, feather mix) on my first visit with Dr. Devi Nambudripad. I followed the diet restrictions and made arrangements to sleep separate from my feather pillows and down comforter. I was distressed to learn that I had been surrounding myself each night with a source of allergic reaction. That night, I noticed my need to urinate had increased without a corresponding increase in liquid intake. The next morning I awoke free of congestion, sneezing, and foggy-headedness. I looked in the mirror and observed that my eyes were very clear and bright. I felt very energized—yet calm. I noticed that I had slept three fewer hours than I had been; my normal non-foggy-headed sleep pattern. I ate a grilled chicken pizza for dinner after the 25 hours restriction had passed. I noticed a continued increase in my need to urinate and also an increased bowel response. I felt my body detoxifying. That night I returned to my feather and down, wondering if the treatment would hold and how I would awaken. I awoke alert, again after only five hours sleep—symptom free—surrounded by my former antagonists. I retested EGG MIX four days after treatment and the results were negative—allergic response not present.

I am normally very sensitive and in tune with my body and feelings and I have a history of responding quickly to both acupuncture and homeopathic treatments when properly administered. My first exposure to N.A.E.T. is in keeping with expectations of how a successful treatment methodology is supposed to work. I will continue to maintain a record of my response to treatment for evaluation.

Sincerely,
Gui Van de Voorde, Ed.D.
culturaltransformation.Com

severe pain. During this period, she underwent five major operations to unsuccessfully cure the intense pain in the gall bladder region. Eleven years later, she required hypodermic injections of morphine two or three times weekly for her pain.

During this time, the patient had been under the care of more than a dozen different physicians who treated her for the gall bladder pain, either by surgery or with morphine injections. With the exception of the last surgeon, who referred her to an allergist, no one considered a connection between her symptoms of hay fever and asthma and her other symptoms, or saw any relation between the gall bladder pain and these allergic symptoms. The increasing doses of morphine required to relieve her pain grew to the extent that some of her physicians considered her to be a narcotics addict. Finally, an allergist was able to relieve her pain without narcotics by using adrenaline.

She requested another operation but the surgeon recognized her condition as an allergy and referred her to an allergist. Her test results indicated that she was sensitive to several foods. She was most allergic to: fish, cheese, oranges, spinach and wheat. She was also allergic to various inhalants, like pollens and dust. She was treated by desensitization treatments for the known allergens. Her symptoms began to lessen gradually and she was enjoying periods of several days that were entirely pain free.

Eventually, she was able to do her own housework again and no longer needed morphine injections. Then, a few years later, she heard about NAET. After two years of regular treatments (two-three sessions per week) she was able to resume her normal life. She secured a job in an aircraft factory and worked her regular shift of eight hours or longer. Despite the fact that several doctors had given their opinion that she would be permanently disabled, she was able to fully recover after her NAET treatments.

The type of mucus cells that occur in the nose, throat, and bronchial tubes also form the lining of the gall bladder and its ducts that open into the intestine. That is why a severe allergic reaction of the gall bladder can cause heavy production of mucus. Spasms of the gall bladder and its ducts, as well as other parts of the gastrointestinal tract, occur the same way as spasms of the bronchial tubes do.

Unfortunately, for symptoms of gastrointestinal allergy in the form of migraine headaches and for some other allergic conditions, neither skin tests nor intradermal tests are reliable in determining the patient's sensitivities. Therefore, western medical allergists are unable to determine, let alone treat, the causes of many food allergy cases. In such cases, muscle response testing is the only means of diagnosing the allergies. Neither elimination diets nor any other testing methods are helpful.

In another similar case, a woman in her thirties was seen in our office. She complained of severe pain under the gall bladder region along with numbness of the whole left side. Sometimes she also experienced pain and discomfort under the diaphragm. In addition, she suffered from severe bloating of the abdomen before her periods, indigestion, the sensations of a lump in the throat, and frequent hypoglycemic attacks. She also had repetitious Bell's palsy on the right side of the face and could not fully close her eyes or speak properly.

Two years ago, this patient had an operation to remove the gall bladder. Luckily, she had only one surgery (unlike the previous case). When she came to our clinic, we found her to be allergic to corn, wheat, eggs, meats, sugar, potassium, and milk. She was also allergic to cotton, polyester, and nylon. Her pain gradually diminished as she underwent NAET treatments. After six months of treatments, she was a new woman, without any pain, discomfort or hypoglycemic attacks. Although she still reacts to the substances as yet untreated, the reactions are less intense and of shorter duration. In addition, through our monthly patients' education seminars, she has learned to test herself for allergies and is able to detect the allergens before coming in contact with them.

PEANUT ALLERGY

A 9-year-old girl was allergic to peanuts since her early childhood. She was careful not to touch or eat them. One day, at a friend's party, she happened to take a bite of a marshmallow puff in which the hostess had added peanut butter for taste. After the first bite, she had a severe reaction. She could not breathe; her bronchioles tightened. Her mother carried Ventolin spray in her purse all the time for emergency needs, since the child was known to be asthmatic. This time the spray did not help her. Before medical help arrived, she had slipped into a coma just a few minutes after eating the peanut butter marshmallow puff. Just one bite and she was into a

EAR INFECTION

Nithya used to suffer from cold, fevers, and ear infections ever since she was born on December 20, 1997. It was a great relief to see Nithya's ear infection go away after NAET treatments. Nithya is a living proof and testimony of the effect of allergy elimination treatment by Dr. Devi Nambudripad. She was on antibiotics "Amoxicillin, Cefcil and Augmenton" for seven months continuously. On January 16, 1999, for the first time, Nithya was treated by Dr. Nambudripad for calcium mix (which included breast milk, cow's milk, and goat's milk). Twenty-five hours after the treatment, her nose stopped running, and her cold and ear infection stopped right away. Then she was treated for egg mix, vitamin C mix, vitamin B complex mix, sugar mix and iron mix from the basic NAET groups. We are extremely happy to report that for the last six months SHE IS FREE OF COLD, FEVER, RUNNY NOSE, COUGH and EAR INFECTION and she is growing healthy. She was examined by her pediatrician, Dr. Michael Cater, last week on June 21, 1999, for a wellness check up. She was perfect with a 95% score in all areas, or say 9.5 on a scale of 1 to 10. Now she is 18 months old. Our only regret is that we did not take her to Dr. Nambudripad sooner. We hope this will serve as a message to other parents with children like Nithya with various pediatric problems. Please find NAET and get them treated. Your child also can get healthy soon and you, too, can live in peace.

Sathi and Ravi Menon
Parents of Nithya.
3, De Forest, Irvine, California

life and death struggle! This shows that elimination and rotation diets do not work for highly allergic patients. Severely allergic patients can suffer from life-threatening situations by eating only a bite of an allergen once in their lifetime.

This girl was in a coma for three months. She had tried all the western medical treatments, with no positive results. Her desperate parents tried acupuncture on her. Within ten days she awoke from her coma. She was blind, her speech was slurred and her body was flaccid. She could not move or sit on her own. She received NAET treatment for peanuts and various other allergens for three to four months. At the end of that time she started walking on her own, her speech became clearer, and her eyesight started improving and returned to normal 13 months after completion of treatment.

In a similar, but unfortunately more tragic instance, peanuts were responsible for the death of an otherwise healthy 12-year-old boy in the Midwestern United States. Although he knew that he was allergic to peanuts, he accidentally ate them as an ingredient in cookies after a Little League game. He died shortly after reaching the hospital in anaphylactic shock.

Cornstarch found in many foods, sauces, etc., is a very strong allergen and can be manifested as different symptoms in different people. As a rule, few people are completely allergy-free to corn or cornstarch.

A nine-year-old boy experienced severe abdominal cramps and huge hives all over his body after eating some corn chips. A 45-year-old patient had constant breast abscesses, multiple joint pains, yeast infections, abdominal cramps and severe PMS—all from corn and cornstarch allergy. Another nine-year-old girl had severe asthma all her life and was using a breathing apparatus every two hours until she was cleared of an allergy to cornstarch. Many cases of migraine headaches improved after treatment for cornstarch. A 28-year-old nurse complained of numbness on the left side of the body, a young man of 34 had blurred vision in spite of wearing glasses, and a 14-year-old boy had frequent epileptic episodes. All of these cases recovered after treatment for cornstarch.

When infants are born, they are fed corn syrup and water from day one. It is no wonder then that they react to corn so intensely by the time they grow up. We bring about our own sickness by consuming the allergen

Peanut Anaphylaxis

Our daughter Haarnoor and son Nausher had an allergy to peanut butter and had been to the emergency room several times. Just from the smell of it, they had been in the hospital. We are not only thankful to Dr. Nambudripad, but indebted to her. Today, both our daughter and son had peanuts and had no allergic reaction. If there is any way we can be of any help or if anyone wants to call us, we will be more than happy to support and sign documents to prove it.

Sincerely,

Jumesh and Geetika Walia
Studio City, CA
jumeshwalia@hotmail.com

from a young age and thereby overloading the "toxin" in the body. Many arthritic symptoms are caused by corn and cornstarch allergy. Osteo arthritis, gouty arthritis, psoriatic arthritis, and so-called psychosomatic arthritis, all respond well to the treatment for cornstarch allergy.

CANKER SORES

Canker sores, which are classified as an allergy of the intestinal tract, are primarily due to allergies from food, drugs, and plastics, as in the case of dentures. Some people react to different salts and spices, these reactions show up as canker sores. Practically any food may be responsible for canker sores (although eggs, chocolate, corn, baking powder, baking soda, salt, nuts, and milk are very frequent offenders). Canker sores are quite often caused by one specific food item, as in the case of the man who developed blisters whenever he ate chocolate ice cream. Sometimes, people react to their own saliva, which causes canker sores and bad breath. Some people also experience a bad taste in the mouth due to an allergy to their own saliva. In some cases, an allergy to a toothbrush, mouthwash and/or toothpaste can cause canker sores, gum diseases, receding gums, cracking of the lips and corners of the mouth, and toothache.

A young man, 24-years old, suffered from severe painful canker sores from an allergy to milk and milk products. Another 15-year-old girl suffered from severely painful canker sores in addition to hives, abdominal pain and swelling of the tongue and glands in the neck. In her case, the culprits were eggs and milk.

In many cases, canker sores are associated with other, more severe allergic symptoms, as in the case of the woman with recurrent headaches, gastrointestinal disturbances, acne and almost constant canker sores for many years. Grapes and cantaloupes caused her problems. Unaware of her allergens, she had made it a practice to drink a glass of grape juice every day since childhood.

Cracking of the lips and corners of the mouth also frequently occurs in food allergy manifestations. Some cases of gingivitis (inflammation of the gums) and pyorrhea (inflammation of the gums with discharge of pus and loosening of the teeth) are results of allergy to milk, iron, and vitamin C (although they may also be caused by allergies to other substances). A

Allergy to Fish

I have had some unbelievable results from Dr. Devi's treatments. I have had all sorts of allergies all my life and have just learned to live with them, as that was my doctor's only advice. He tested me for allergies but nothing significant ever showed in the reports. I would break out in rashes on my face, my lips and eyes would swell and itch. The doctors would give me medications and ointments and gradually it would recede after weeks, only to surface again. None of my doctors knew the cause of my mysterious problem. I recently had pains in my back between my shoulders that became quite acute. It felt like I had broken a rib or something and the broken piece was piercing me on one spot. I couldn't get comfortable in any position. I was on the East Coast and went to several doctors there. After examination and X-rays, the treatment was hot and cold packs and pain medication. I didn't get any relief. I was in agony for days.

When I returned to California, one of my friends suggested that I go to see Dr. Devi. With her evaluation, in a few seconds she came up with the diagnosis: an allergy to shellfish! No X-rays, no expensive or extensive testing, no pain medication, a simple NAET treatment to my spinal area with a sample of lobster in a glass vial held in my hand! After the acupressure NAET treatment on my back (probably a minute or two) she asked me to turn over on my back. Amazing! My pain was completely gone in a couple of minutes after she treated my back! One treatment and, like a miracle, there was no more pain. I wish all medical practitioners all over the world would learn this treatment soon, so that many people can live pain free. As I said before - UNBELIEVABLE !!!

Martha Dodds
Santa Ana, CA

66-year-old patient ate some fresh avocado dip during her dinner of Mexican food. An hour later, her first upper left molar was aching. She turned out to be allergic to the lemon juice in the avocado dip.

Food allergies may cause a sore throat or secretion of tenacious, adherent mucus. Patients who suffer from this particular allergic manifestation clear their throats frequently, hacking and drawing mucus down from the posterior nasal passages in an effort to relieve the feeling of congestion. At times, this congestion is so severe that patients have the feeling that a large object is stuck in their throat, blocking the passages. Such patients often suffer from disturbed and restless sleep.

A 42-year-old female ate smoked rainbow trout at her friends' house. An hour later, she began experiencing a mild sore throat while she was driving home. In two hours, she started coughing, and she began having a tenacious secretion in her throat that was difficult to clear. She tried taking some antihistamines and decongestants at home without success. Her postnasal drip kept getting worse. She woke up around 3 a.m. having difficulty breathing. This continued until 5 a.m. when she drifted off to sleep again for a while. The 3 - 5 a.m. time relates to the lung meridian. During the daytime, she coughed and felt like she was suffering from a common cold. She suspected it was a reaction from the smoked rainbow trout, and after nine days of struggling, she asked her friends to prepare another piece of smoked rainbow trout for testing. She was treated by NAET for smoked rainbow trout and her throat cleared almost instantly. Within a couple of hours she felt normal again.

SHELLFISH ALLERGY

Many people are hospitalized from fish allergies, which can be fatal. Fish oil capsules are commonly used to reduce cholesterol and to improve circulation. Some people are extremely allergic to fish and shellfish. A 37-year-old male returned from Mexico after a two-week vacation. He woke up at 6 a.m. and rushed to the tennis court for his usual game. While he was warming up, he felt a muscle cramp, first on his right knee, and then it started moving up to his right thigh, hip joint, then to his lower back. He tumbled down on the court, unable to stand up and had to be carried to the nearest medical clinic where he received a muscle relaxant, analgesics and therapy.

a few minutes, but then the muscle spasms returned, with severe intensity. His sister, who had previously been treated by NAET, brought him to our clinic. His history revealed that he had eaten abalone shellfish three days in a row before he left Mexico. It was the first time he had ever eaten abalone. His pain, muscle spasms and discomfort were relieved completely in less than five minutes after treatment by NAET for abalone.

Sixty-five-year-old Phil suffered from pain and shingles-like lesions on the left side of his back for the last six months. He was diagnosed by his internist and was treated by medication. Phil was treated for his allergies by me about six years ago and he was doing well with his nasal and seasonal allergies. One day he accompanied his wife, who was getting treated, in my office. He came in to tell me about the new problem that he was battling for the past six months. He was in excruciating pain all the time and sleep was becoming impossible for him even with the sleeping medication.

So out of curiosity, I asked him to show me the lesion on his back. The unilateral distribution of the lesions on his back looked convincing. He was also developing another set of new lesions on his left ankle that was also very painful. I tested him using NTT and found out that these lesions were not shingles and they were due to an allergy to a supplement (salmon oil capsule) he was taking daily. He was given an expensive brand of salmon oil capsules by his nutritionist to keep his heart and circulation healthy. He was asked to bring his supplement to get treated. The next day he was treated for his supplement, "salmon oil" capsule. After the successful treatments for the supplement (three treatments), he was free of the pain and the shingles-like lesions cleared up, too.

Many cases of sea or car sickness are caused by an underlying food allergy. If you take part in any outdoor activity—playing tennis, running or boating, after eating allergic foods and happen to inhale strong gasoline or diesel fumes, cooking or frying odors, etc., you can become nauseous and even vomit or have other gastrointestinal disturbances. Some people are very allergic to car exhaust, diesel, gasoline and their smells, etc., which could contribute to their car sickness. Patients with a car exhaust allergy could collect exhaust smoke from different cars and be treated by NAET. After successful treatment for the exhaust smell, such smells should not bother them.

Allergy To Shellfish

I was diagnosed in 1975 as having gouty arthritis affecting my mid and lower back and kidney areas. My doctors told me to eliminate red meat completely from my diet. The back pain persisted for the ensuing years. My wife began treatments for asthma with Dr. Nambudripad in 1986. When she began to notice dramatic recovery from her debilitating asthma, she started insisting that I see her doctor. I did not understand anything about her treatments, but I skeptically submitted to see her more for the experience than anything else.

During diagnostic evaluation, Dr. Nambudripad performed muscle response testing for allergies. She asked if I ate much fish. I said "yes," to which she warned, "Oh, you must not; you are very allergic to any fish and it can cause you terrible backaches. But you can eliminate the allergy by treatment and you will be able to eat fish without getting backaches." Skeptically, I agreed to get treated for fish. After the treatment I was asked to wait in the post-treatment waiting room for 15 minutes, which was the usual procedure in her office. Within minutes, my back pain eased and I felt a great relief, which I hadn't felt for years. My backache has not returned in 13 years. Now I can eat fish and red meat and enjoy them without fear and without pain.

Wayne Brazil
Anaheim, CA

Allergy to Vitamin A, Fish and Shellfish

I was desperate when I came to see Dr. Devi. I was getting hives on my face and neck almost everyday for a few months. I found no relief or hope from traditional allergists. At Dr. Devi's office, I was told I was allergic to a myriad of foods. It was difficult to say which food caused my problem. I was breaking out with almost everything I ate.

Dr. Devi started me with the basic treatments. I began noticing some improvements with each treatment. Then I was treated for vitamin A mix, which included fish, shellfish, carrots and vitamin A. This treatment gave me severe reactions. During the 25-hour period, my hives and skin rashes became severe. I even had fever by the evening of the treatment. I had no energy. I visited her in the evening to check to see if I had failed the treatment. To my amazement, I was still holding the treatment. But just about 25 hours after the treatment, I felt a sudden rush of energy inside me. Then I felt a cool wave passing through me. I looked in the mirror. I couldn't believe my eyes! My neck and face looked normal ! No hives or rashes! My allergy to seafood caused my hives! I haven't had hives or rashes ever since.

Maria Meraz
Fullerton, CA

3 Year Old Constant Sciatic Pain Relieved in One Treatment !

I suffered from a right sided sciatic pain, very severe on certain days, for the past three years. It was a mystery to the medical practitioners who tried to help me with my nagging pain. While I was attending the Basic NAET training, Dr. Nambudripad selected me to demonstrate treatment for acute and/ or constant long-time pain. She found out that my pain was due to an allergy to the special brand of calcium supplement I was taking daily just over three years. I was treated for the supplement in the class and in less than 20 minutes I was 100% free from my sciatic pain and hasn't returned in two years. I still take the same supplement but no more pain!

Thank you, Dr. Devi.

Linda Cote, D.C.
Los Angeles, CA

ANGIONEUROTIC EDEMA

Angioneurotic edema, a condition characterized by patches of circum-scribed swelling of the skin, mucous membranes and viscera, is believed to be an expression of allergy. Angioneurotic edema attacks can strike at any time. The throat can swell up, making swallowing and breathing difficult or even life-threatening in certain cases. Angioneurotic edema is one of the manifes-tations of anaphylaxis. According to Oriental medical theory, energy blockage in the spleen meridian is the cause of angioneurotic edema.

A nine-year-old girl suffering from swelling all over the body was forced to stay home from school most of the time. She was found to be allergic to corn, spices, sugar, chocolate and fleece materials. After she was treated for these items, her reactions became very minimal and rare.

An 18-year-old girl with angioneurotic edema, experienced a swollen throat whenever she went jogging or walked briskly. Her test results showed her to be highly allergic to vitamin C and citrus bioflavonoid. After treat-ment for vitamin C and bioflavonoid, she did not have angioneurotic edema again. Soon after the treatment, she even started jogging every day. A year later, she ran in a marathon and completed the 26-mile race without any problem.

ANOREXIA / ANOREXIA NERVOSA / BULIMIA

Among many eating disorders, anorexia, anorexia nervosa and bulimia are getting much attention nowadays. According to Seattle's Eating Disorders Awareness and Prevention group (EDAP), an estimated 5-7 percent of America's 12 million undergraduates are afflicted with anorexia (a pathological fear of weight gain leading to extreme weight loss), bulimia ("binging" followed by purging) or binge eating (compulsive overeating). Another recent survey on the weight-obsessed, stressed-out California university coed students showed that 5-10 million females and 1 million males are suffering from eating disorders like anorexia and bulimia. The survey also showed that most of the sufferers are young (from 14 to 25), white, affluent, "perfectionistic type-A personalities." According to some of the eating disorder education and prevention groups, the major cause of the sudden rise in these disorders is because of the students' life-style. The college students are away from their families for the first time, and there is tremendous pressure to find their way in the world. Another reason among female victims is due to idolization of wispy models and skinny actresses. A recent UCLA study found that the median recovery time from anorexia is seven years.

According to NAET theory, anorexia, anorexia nervosa and bulimia are a direct result of food allergy. Anorexia is also common in young children. Nausea, vomiting, heartburn, and sour stomach are very frequent symptoms of allergy in the gastrointestinal tract and are usually accompanied by hay fever, asthma, migraine headaches, etc. Energy blockages in the stomach, spleen, liver and heart meridians are usually noted in these cases.

Anorexia nervosa and bulimia (self-induced vomiting after eating) are often also complicated with emotional blockages. In childhood or at a young age, someone may have made a negative remark about the victim's looks, which created an emotional blockage with food and caused the victim to develop bulimia. It also could be due to simple food allergy without any emotional involvement. A qualified NAET practitioner will be able to identify and treat it appropriately.

A 48-year-old female had severe heartburn, sour stomach and frequent vomiting. She happened to be allergic to her own stomach acid secretion. She was treated for her own stomach juice, and that was the end of her heartburn.

Severe intestinal flatulence could be due to poor absorption of the food in the intestinal tract. It could also be caused by the lack of intestinal enzymes, poor peristaltic movements, too much nitrogen-producing food in the diet (dried beans, etc.) or a symptom of an allergy to the basic or alkaline juice within the intestinal tract.

Regardless of what type of food he ate, a 44-year-old male would experience severe flatulence and bloating in the abdomen. He was told by a nutritionist not to mix different foods, so he tried eating only one food group at a time. He also took different kinds of enzymes before and after eating, but nothing worked. When he came to us, he was a desperate man. He was relieved of his problems when he was treated for allergy to alkaline juice and digestive enzymes from his intestinal tract.

Since the liver is the first organ that food proteins pass through after entering the blood, it is not surprising to find that allergic manifestations

ANOREXIA NERVOSA

I suffered from severe anorexia nervosa since I was 17 years old. I felt very fat and ugly, especially after I split up with Brian, my boy friend. It was a shock to me. I had no desire to eat. My weight dropped to 90 pounds and I am 5'5." Then I met Kevin and he was very different from Brian. He made me realize my problem. He found out about Dr. Devi and brought me to her for help. My parents, when they found out about my disease, forced me to go for traditional medical treatment. They did not believe in holistic treatments. With Kevin's support, I continued with NAET. I felt the difference after 5 NAET treatments. I began taking mega doses of vitamin B complex. That helped to calm my nerves. After 18 treatments, now I can say that I am quite well from my illness. I still have a few more allergies and I am taking care of them slowly. I take a treatment once every three months now. I feel very good and emotionally strong. If it was not for Kevin, Dr. Devi and NAET, I wouldn't be alive today!

Nancy S.
Fullerton, CA

affecting the liver and gall bladder occur with comparative frequency. These manifestations are not necessarily identical. For example, of the two patients having a mild allergy, one patient suffered from enlargement and swelling of the liver while the other patient suffered from intermittent low grade fever. Another patient had his gall bladder removed because of severe abdominal pain. The pain was found to be an allergic reaction to apples and beef. Another man suffered from fainting spells, frequent urination, and mild angina pectoris (heart pains due to an insufficiency of blood supply to the heart muscles), all of these symptoms were relieved by elimination of the offending foods. One patient who suffered from severe upper abdominal pains had her gall bladder removed. Subsequently, she underwent two more abdominal operations only to find out later that the pains were caused by an allergy to eggs and chicken.

PYLOROSPASM

Pylorospasm, which causes infant colic, is a spasm of the end of the stomach region called the pylorus. The contents of the stomach empty into the intestines through the pylorus. The pylorus is surrounded by folds of mucous membrane containing circular muscular fibers. When an allergy occurs, it causes them to contract spasmodically, similar to the contraction of the bronchial tubes in asthma. This very painful condition causes the child to vomit and cry almost continuously.

Such was the case of a baby boy who experienced continuous pylorospasm and vomiting after each feeding from the time he was one week old. He also had severe colicky pains, continuous skin rashes, huge hives, ulceration of the gums, heavy tongue coating, thrush, severe diaper rash, frequent colds and high fever, insomnia, and crankiness. He continued to have these symptoms until he was eight months old. His pediatrician suggested minor surgery to tighten the cardiac end or beginning of the stomach, to prevent vomiting. Before he was scheduled for surgery, he was tested by muscle response testing for allergies. The results showed him to be allergic to certain foods. He was treated by NAET soon after. He is a healthy teen-ager now. He can eat almost any food he wants without any reaction.

Another two-year-old girl with a history of vomiting after each meal was treated in our office. She also had severe colicky pains, continuous skin rashes, huge hives, ulceration of the gums, severe tongue coating, thrush, severe diaper rash, frequent colds and high fever, insomnia, and continuous crying. Her pediatrician prescribed 200 milligrams of Tagamet three times a day. The medication had no effect. She began losing weight and her growth-rate declined. Testing through NTT, she was found to be allergic to all the nutrients and food she was eating. The child was treated in our office for the basic groups (eggs and chicken, milk, vitamin C, fruits, vegetables, B complex vitamins, sugars, iron, vitamin A, salt, minerals and grains). She stopped vomiting after meals, began eating and enjoying food, gained 12 pounds in the three weeks following the treatments, and now she is a beautiful six-year-old healthy girl.

Oh Yummy Cheese!

Twelve years ago I suddenly started having "24-hour viruses" about every other day - at least that is what my internist told me each time I called to tell him how sick I was. For over a year, that was the only answer he had for the symptoms I described to him. I was trying to work as a real estate agent, but would find myself almost every other day so sick with flu-like symptoms that I could hardly get out of bed. Finally, this internist decided that it was all in my head and that I was really a manic depressive and should start taking lithium. Fortunately, before that happened, one of my customers suggested that I might have an inner ear problem, and that I should see an ear doctor. Again, fortunately, the ear doctor discovered I had a severe sinus infection. After many weeks of antibiotics and draining of the sinus, the doctor concluded that I had to be eating something I was allergic to - and so I began my trek from one allergist to another searching for help.

Thousands of dollars and several years later, I finally resorted to sinus surgery, but my constant attacks continued, as did the sinus infection. I had taken so many antibiotics that they were no longer effective. I had discovered that my worst allergy was to cheese in any form. If by accident I did eat cheese (a little in a salad dressing), I was violently ill for days.

Then, one day my whole life changed! A friend told me about Dr. Devi. I was so skeptical at first, it took me several months to agree to see her. I knew nothing of acupuncture or acupressure and could not imagine how it could help me. But in desperation I finally accepted my friend's offer to drive me there. After watching and listening to Dr. Devi's treatment of my friend, I decided I had nothing to lose...after all the time and money I had spent with no results, what was one more gamble? So began my treatments four times a week.

(continued on the next page)

Since cheese had always been my biggest problem, I decided to have her treat me for it, which would be a big test of her ability to help me.

I brought my cheese to her and, after having the treatment, I waited the required 25 hours and then went back to see if the treatment had "held." The answer was "yes," and I was told by Dr. Devi to take a bite of cheese. As much faith as I had in her at this point, I was still very frightened to take a chance, fearing it might not work and I could look forward to being so ill again for two to three days. But, at her insistence, I took a bite of the cheese and waited, convinced that it was just a delayed reaction and I would suddenly start having the usual symptoms. By bedtime, I was still feeling fine, but was sure I would awaken and find that I was right...that nothing could cure my allergy to cheese, as I had been told by several of the allergists who had tried to help me.

The next morning I was dressing for work when I suddenly remembered, "Oh, I ate cheese yesterday and I am not sick!!!" I could not believe it! I called my friend immediately and invited her to an Italian restaurant for dinner where, for the first time in twelve years, I enjoyed the largest pizza I had ever eaten! Now I knew I could finally resume the social life I had put on hold, always so afraid I would eat something unknowingly that would set off an attack. What a wonderful feeling to be able to eat again without having to "analyze" everything I put in my mouth, driving all my friends and family crazy and, I am sure, almost convincing them at times that maybe I did need that lithium!

I was cured of my allergy to cheese in 1989. This is 1999. I still enjoy my favorite cheese more than ever before. How can I ever thank you, Dr. Devi, for changing my life??!!

Dotty Johnson
New Port Beach, CA

MILK ALLERGY

Homogenized milk causes concern for many patients in the United States. Even after they are clear for the milk allergy, homogenized milk drinkers face an allergic reaction once in a while, depending mainly on what the cattle are fed. Dairies have no control over what the cows are fed every day. Most nut-oil companies, after extracting the oils, dry the leftovers into compact cakes and sell them to the dairies where they are randomly fed to the cows. When the cows secrete milk, some of the substances from the nuts are also secreted through the milk. Sometimes, if the cows are fed with hay and grasses that have been sprayed with pesticides, these substances will also be excreted in the milk.

If you have allergic tendencies, you can react at anytime when you drink milk. The particular reaction is not due to an allergy to milk, but to the pesticides or other ingredients in the milk sample. This should be kept in mind when treating for milk allergy.

In one case, the patient's abdominal distress was diagnosed as a gastric ulcer, and even the accompanying X-ray seemed to prove the diagnosis. He was under the care of the best specialists available in a large city. He was placed on what was then considered a typical ulcer diet, consisting of large quantities of milk and cream, such as custards, cream soups, and similar foods. Among other things, he drank hot chocolate made with whole milk and cream, ate chocolate pudding, and was frequently served cream of tomato soup. The few meats and vegetables he ate were ground to the consistency of baby food until they were utterly tasteless. Under this regimen, his symptoms still continued to grow worse, until he was never entirely free from pain. He carried a bottle of milk with him constantly, and he was forced to take innumerable drugs to relieve pain and sedatives to relieve insomnia.

At last, this patient was studied from the allergic standpoint, and was found to be allergic to most of the food items he was eating—especially the ones he was eating the most: milk, eggs, tomatoes and chocolate, to name a few. After the foods were eliminated from his diet, his ulcer symptoms disappeared. He had avoided milk for many years because of his ulcer. He was susceptible to attacks of abdominal pain and extreme bad breath after drinking a very small glass of milk or buttermilk. When he came to our office, he could not handle food made with even a small quantity of milk.

After being treated for food allergies by NAET, he drinks three to four glasses of milk daily without any problem.

Allergy occurs with considerable frequency in the intestines, usually causing symptoms of colic, cramping, constipation, diarrhea, soreness, and bleeding of the intestinal walls (as in irritable bowel syndrome, celiac sprue, Crohn's disease, etc.). Severe pain may result from allergies to various everyday food products such as wheat, grains, milk, corn, spices, fats, beans, proteins, meat, parasites, etc., or it could be from an obstruction in the intestines by edema (swelling) of these organs. Intestinal allergy patients frequently have a tendency to bleed in various parts of the body as in the case of a boy who had nosebleeds, bleeding from the rectum, or hemorrhaging of the conjunctiva (bloodshot eyes) whenever he drank milk.

Constipation may also be caused by an allergy of the gastrointestinal tract. The smooth muscle of the colon is a logical site for allergic spasm and could very easily cause this condition. Since the intestines are lined with mucous membrane, it is also possible for large quantities of mucus to form here, just as it does in the nasal passages. It is even possible to have a type of contact allergy in the intestines because the food is in contact with these organs for a considerable length of time. In severe allergic constipation, the muscle of the colon may contract to such a degree that very little food passes through this channel in a normal manner.

Since constipation is so frequently caused by food allergy, it is possible that many patients who load themselves with excessive amounts of bulk fruits, vegetables, bran flakes, and fibers, in an effort to keep their bowels moving, would have perfectly natural movements if their diets were allergy-free. For this reason, it is not advisable for allergic patients, or anyone else for that matter, to indiscriminately take laxatives. The very drug that is taken for this purpose may be aggravating the constipation. People who suffer from chronic constipation are often inclined to believe that there is little to be done, other than taking large amounts of laxatives regularly. Actually, in many cases the cause may be as simple as food allergies that would clear up if the offending foods were eliminated.

A 34-year-old female developed severe itching, burning and pain at the center of the tensor fascia lata muscle (a thick strip of long muscle on the outer part of the thigh). This muscle corresponds to the large intestine meridian. This lady was found to be allergic to all fibers. They made her large intestine weak. She took psyllium seed and many other fibers regularly. She was advised to cut down on her high-fiber diet for a few days. Her itching and burning diminished. Later, when she tried to put the fiber back into her diet, her itching and burning came back. At this point, she was treated for fibers and psyllium seed by NAET, and her itching never returned. She now continues to eat a high-fiber diet without any discomfort.

Diarrhea, a condition opposite of constipation, is also very frequently allergic in origin. It is often present in infancy and childhood and is frequently associated with colic, eczema, and vomiting. When the child grows up, the allergy may become manifested strongly in other symptoms, and the diarrhea may subside. However, there are cases in which diarrhea continues every day of a person's life.

A 70-year-old female suffering from moderate to severe diarrhea for 50 years was diagnosed as having pancreatitis. She moved her bowels 10-15 times per day on the average. She also suffered from hypoglycemia for years. She was found to be allergic to all grains, vegetables, fruits, fats,

Food Allergies

When I first came to Dr. Devi I couldn't eat or breathe because of a treatment I took for my allergies. I had multiple allergies to food, chemicals, air pollutants, mold – just about anything you can think of. I told her what treatment I had taken and she treated me for it and eliminated my allergy to it. I have seen Dr. Devi off and on for two years and have found a whole new world of food, fabrics and air which do not bother me now.

Betty Emms
Orange, CA

Peanut Allergy Caused hives

I am a 19-year-old college student. I was highly allergic to peanuts all my life. If I ate anything made with a trace of peanut or peanut oil, I broke out in huge hives all over, my body itched violently, and often I got severe bronchitis that did not respond to antibiotics. I became very hyper, irritable, angry and moody. I suffered from a kind of restlessness and uneasiness. I also got restless leg syndrome within minutes of ingesting peanuts. I got headaches, felt tired, depressed and unmotivated to study or do my regular chores following any exposure to peanuts.

I would sit many hours daily in the bath tub with Epsom salt to detox my body. The Epsom salt bath gave me some relief from the constant itching. Eventually, after a couple of months, I would gradually feel better. Then I was introduced to NAET. I was treated for all the basics, peanuts, peanut oil, peanut butter, smell of the peanuts and peanut mold (aspergillus). After I was cleared for peanuts and peanut products (peanut butter ice cream, cookies, peanut butter, etc.), I no longer react to them. Every now and then I eat a peanut butter sandwich, cookies or ice cream with no adverse reactions. Dr. Devi has taught and instructed my mother to check me for any allergy against each new batch of peanut products she buys and brings into the house. I have learned to check my allergies using the "O" ring test before I eat any peanut product. I was treated about four years ago. I haven't reacted ever since. Thanks to NAET.

Deepak Moosad
Phoenix, AZ

sugars, and proteins. When she was treated for all these, her diarrhea of 50 years' duration stopped, and her hypoglycemia improved. At age 75, she enjoys her life better than she ever did before.

When allergic constipation exists, it may cause the intestines to retain the fecal matter (unabsorbed residues of intestinal excretions) until it is putrefied, causing intermittent attacks of constipation and diarrhea. In some cases, milk causes such severe diarrhea that even a few drops are sufficient to bring on an attack.

Very often, both constipation and diarrhea occur in conjunction with other allergic symptoms. A 42-year-old man had bilious attacks since childhood, migraine headaches on and off, abdominal pain and discomfort, mucous colitis, irritable bowels, severe allergy to gluten, intermittent constipation and diarrhea, frequent canker sores, dry mouth, lethargy, insomnia, occasional hives, frequent urination, and periodic bloody stools. He also suffered from frequent colds and bronchitis and had a constant postnasal drip. He was treated by various medical doctors, an internist, a gastroenterologist, a urologist and a dermatologist. None of the treatments gave him any relief from his symptoms. Finally, he was seen by an allergist who could not find any allergy to food items but found him to be severely allergic to cat hair, forcing him to give his cat away.

When he was finally seen in our office and tested by muscle response testing, we discovered he was allergic to many of the food items he was eating: chicken, carrots, peas, raisins, and a popular brand of tea. These were his major diet items. He stayed away from all the offending foods. In less than two weeks, he became symptom-free. He was then treated by NAET, and freed of allergic reactions to the items. Now, he can eat almost anything and rarely reacts to any food. He was also treated for cat hair and has another cat, which he can enjoy without a problem.

IRRITABLE BOWEL SYNDROME

The root cause of most of the diseases often found in the gut, beginning with nausea, poor digestion, heartburn, reflux, bloating, cramps, diarrhea, gas, constipation, abdominal pains, nervous stomach, etc., is allergy. If not taken care of immediately, they can lead you to cough, colds and flu, fever, sinusitis, bronchitis, heart attacks, migraines, mental and emotional imbalances, irritabilities, arthritis, Crohn's disease, irritable bowel syndrome, bladder infection, menstrual disorders, skin disorders, stroke, cancer and even death.

Irritable bowel syndrome (IBS) is a disorder affecting the intestines. According to western medical researchers, no particular cause has been found; however, diet, drugs, hormones and emotional factors have been found to be major triggers for this disorder.

The commonly experienced symptom of IBS is pain in the abdomen, predominantly after meals. Other symptoms are periodic diarrhea or constipation, lower abdominal pain, pain after eating, bowel movements immediately after eating, cramps in the lower abdomen, bloating, flatulence, nausea, headache, depression, fatigue, anxiety and poor concentration.

Through NTT, our patients with IBS have been found to be highly allergic to foods. When they get treated for most of their food allergies, they become symptom-free and pain-free.

Twenty-four-year-old Sean suffered from IBS for 6 years. He suffered from severe abdominal cramps all the time and was very allergic to drugs. He could not eat anything and always had diarrhea. He lost 70 pounds in one year, could not work or study, was very depressed and began isolating himself from all his friends.

A friend referred him to NAET. He began the treatment right away. With each treatment his symptoms improved. After 30 food groups, he became absolutely asymptomatic. He found a job and decided to return to college part-time. He can eat all foods now without triggering any abdominal discomfort or pain.

Colitis is characterized by: looseness of bowels, diarrhea, colic, belching, vomiting and varying symptoms of the stomach and intestines. Very often allergic in origin, certain types of colitis are caused by amoeba (parasite) and bacteria. This type of colitis or dysentery is very common in the tropics, and parasites are frequently brought into the country by returning travelers. In these cases, most of the time the parasites are allergens. However, the parasitical type of colitis is usually quite readily diagnosed by laboratory methods. When these tests are negative, it is wise to consider the possibility of allergy. Another type of colitis, called nonspecific colitis, cannot be diagnosed by laboratory tests. This type usually occurs in nervous, excitable or unstable individuals with the nervous state being blamed for the colitis.

Extremely nervous individuals may be allergic to their own adrenaline. Extreme nervousness often accompanies and aggravates various allergic manifestations, such as colitis. These people are also very allergic to B complex vitamins.

A 38-year-old female always complained of diarrhea and severe perspiration of her palms before going to any official meeting. She was a bank manager and had several of these meetings every week. She was allergic to her own adrenaline. After she was treated for adrenaline by NAET, she never had that problem again.

Allergies to milk, wheat, grains, gluten, spices, and fruits are the most frequent causes of allergic colitis. To a lesser degree, allergies to vegetables, fish, meat, and other foods will also undoubtedly be responsible for this condition.

Mucous colitis has very similar symptoms to those of ordinary colitis, except that large quantities of mucus are formed in the intestine and passed through the bowels. At one time, this condition was known as "asthma of the bowels," which frequently occurs in people who have other allergic manifestations like asthma. The respiratory tract and the intestines are lined with the same kind of mucous membranes. Large quantities of mucus form in the respiratory tract when a person has bronchial asthma, and the same thing happens in the intestines when an allergy affects the bowels.

For several years, a 38-year-old man had suffered from profuse watery diarrhea associated with abdominal cramps and the passage of bloody mucus. He had mucous colitis. Some of his other symptoms were nausea, soreness in the upper abdomen, and a severe allergic skin condition. Careful laboratory studies and repeated examinations by various leading specialists were made in an effort to determine the cause of his symptoms. But no relief had been obtained. When he came into our office, we discovered that he had severe allergies to most common foods: beef, eggs, milk, breads, fish and fruits. He was treated for these various food allergies by NAET. He became symptom-free in a few months and was able to eat many of his favorite foods without any difficulty.

Another patient was repeatedly rushed to the hospital for operations because of suspected intestinal obstructions. Each time she reached the hospital, her symptoms improved before the operation was actually performed. Finally, it was discovered that her condition was actually angioneurotic edema (swelling) of the intestine, caused by sensitivity to wheat. After the wheat allergy was eliminated, her problems disappeared. For some reason, her brain was not releasing enough adrenaline when she ate the wheat, causing the bowels to swell. When she was taken to the operating room, fear caused more adrenaline secretion, and the additional adrenaline took care of the problem.

Although all types of gastro-intestinal (GI) tract allergies are usually caused by food, some other substances: inhalants, fabrics like nylons, flannels, wool, rubber, latex products, plastics, formaldehyde, etc., may also be responsible for this condition. Usually, milk is the greatest offender, and most of these patients are sensitive to milk products. Other foods have also been found to be frequent offenders in causing ulcerative colitis. Probably a sore-like canker occurs at the site of a small lesion in the intestines and then becomes infected. When this occurs, a very large and excruciatingly painful ulcer develops.

Irritable Bowel Syndrome

Since childhood, I had a hard time eating certain types of foods. Progressively, this became worse as I was growing up. When I was 21, I was able to eat a few grains, nonfat food and some fruits. By age 23, I could not eat anything. I would go to the kitchen hungry and eat only a slice of bread or a bowl of cereal for lunch and dinner and I would be in severe pain. I had tried all possible medicines and treatments. I tried allopathy, herbs, homeopathy and iridology (with nutrition support program). I was diagnosed with Irritable Bowel Syndrome and was told that there were no treatments for it. I had gone through all possible GI tests. I suffered extreme fatigue. My weight fluctuated between 96 pounds and 110 pounds during the two years (my height is 5'10"). My body was not absorbing the nutrients from food. I did not know that my problems were due to food allergies. I used to think that they were due to weak intestines, until one day my friend told me to contact Dr. Devi and I got hold of the book, "Say Good-bye to Illness."

I started the treatment a week after reading the book. I could see the difference in my body immediately. I started becoming more energetic and gained a few pounds in a couple of weeks. It might not be too exciting, but it was a big breakthrough for me as I was always losing weight steadily in the last 24 months. Most important of all, my abdominal pains stopped. My blood report showed that my cholesterol and protein went slightly high, which meant that my body was absorbing the nutrients.

(turn to the next page)

Right now, I am not even half way through the treatment. Still, I can see how my body is responding to the treatments. I feel good when I eat non-allergic food for which I have been treated and keep away from allergic food. As soon as I eat allergic food I get intestinal problems and I start loosing weight. Dr. Devi has been very patient in answering my questions and in consoling me during bad times.

I cannot over emphasize the need for learning self-testing as explained by Dr. Devi's books. This is because you never know what food you are allergic to. For example, you may eat a loaf of bread with wheat flour, thinking that you have been treated for wheat before. But, that wheat flour may contain some chemicals or food additives, which you may be allergic to. So after eating that bread you may become sick. This happens to me often, as I am still learning this trick of testing. This testing technique would help you to remain out of trouble and would speed up your recovery while you are getting treated. A person going through this treatment would definitely have some ups and downs.

I think the key to completing this treatment successfully is to be patient about the results, cautious about the food you eat, and learn the self-testing technique. My advice to the people with IBS: there is light at the end of the tunnel - there is hope for you through NAET. Hang in there!

Anil Shah
Los Angeles, CA

Irritable Bowel Syndrome

It has been 30 years since I was diagnosed with Irritable Bowel Syndrome. During these years, my whole life-style was affected. Going on long trips, hopping on airplanes, going on vacations, sight-seeing and staying long hours away from home was out of the question. I never knew from one moment to another when I would have to use the rest-room. Everywhere I went, I made sure a rest-room was available. I tried Allopathy and Homeopathy, but to no avail. Then I was introduced to Dr. Devi by my sister, who proved to be God sent. After the first treatment itself, I felt a change in myself. My stomach was much calmer and I no longer had to make sure a rest-room was close by.

I intend to go through the whole treatment so that all my problems will disappear. Many, many thanks to you, Dr. Devi.

Vijayan Cheriyan
Santa Monica, CA

Sugar Allergy Caused My Ovarian Pain!

For many years my physical health has slowly deteriorated and the variety of foods I have been able to eat continued to decrease to where I have been only able to eat vegetables and homemade breads. I started having pancreatic difficulties, which left me unable to digest proteins, rice, fruits, raw foods and sugars. Medical tests were done to determine if there was any physiological cause for the pancreatic problems. They found no diabetes or clinical hypoglycemia, and concluded I had a hypo-hyper-glycemic response to carbohydrates. I also had developed severe cramping in the left ovary. Ultrasound tests showed only a small uterine fibroid, and no ovarian cyst. Though there has been nothing physically causing these problems, they have persisted and continued to worsen over a period of several years.

Since I have been having NAET treatments, I have seen noticeable improvements in all areas. From the very first treatment, there was a marked improvement in how the pancreas felt and responded. After clearing the sugar allergy, I was able to eat a little fruit-juice sweetened jam for the first time in years, without having a severe reaction. I was amazed at the change. Foods have started to smell and taste good again.

Prior to the treatment for the sugar allergy, I had severe cramps in the left ovary for several days. After clearing the sugar allergy, the cramping was no longer there and continues to improve. I was surprised and happy to see such a significant change so quickly, after this persisted for many years.

Though I am still in the early stages of NAET (Basic 6 treatments so far), I am very much encouraged by the changes I have experienced. It has been great to be able to eat more foods, have food smell and taste good again, and not to be in chronic pain. I am thankful to be working with such dedicated and knowledgeable people who have, in a short time, made a remarkable difference in how I feel.

Joanne Zeppertella, Escondido, CA, 760-740-5119

Crohn's Disease

I almost lost my life. I was suffering from an extremely debilitating disease known as "Crohn's disease." I was in and out of the hospital — and as every Crohn's patient discovers — treatment (other than surgical interventions) becomes large doses of prednisone (steroids) or other immunosuppressant drugs that are very harmful to the entire system. Also, once given a high dose, patients find it extremely difficult to stop taking them. NAET saved my life. Prednisone or other immunosuppressants may save the life of a patient that is bleeding or starving to death because of the disease. However, the administration of the dangerous immunosuppressants, addressing the symptoms, is the only choice, since the real CAUSE of the disease was never addressed.

Thank you for a NEW LIFE! Dr. Devi Nambudripad's NAET treatments addressed the CAUSE of Crohn's disease. My ongoing struggle to lower the dosage of prednisone was frustrated at 35 mgs. Then, after just a few treatments of NAET, to handle the various food allergies, I was able to drop the dose from 35 mg to 5 mg with no adverse affects. There were no symptoms of bleeding or starvation or relapse of the disease.

I will not face any future surgical procedure, losing any part of my intestine.

Thank you, from the bottom of my heart, Dr. Nambudripad, for discovering the cure for such a serious illness as "Crohn's" disease.

Cathy Carlson
Buena Park, CA

My Allergy to Shellfish

I just wanted to let you know that 7 years ago I became allergic to seafood, including shellfish and fish after having a sea kelp wrap at a Spa in Florida. I grew up in Bar Harbor, Maine and ate seafood all my life!

Recently, I went to see Dr. Alexander, Alexander Chiropractic Center, in Lawrenceville, GA and was treated (it took 4 times), but I can now eat shrimp, clams, scallops, etc., and I no longer break out in hives all over my body! The hives I used to get were big welts and lasted sometimes up to 2-3 weeks before they finally cleared up. What a blessing this is. I was also allergic to vitamin C, chocolate and stomach acid. Life has certainly improved! Thank you for discovering this technology.

Martha Fleck
Suwanee, GA

My 20 year old Colitis

    I have had inhalant allergies all my life as did my father and unfortunately my sons. The NAET system of therapy found that in addition, I had many food allergies some of which were my favorite foods.

    I proceeded to follow the recommended course and treat for food allergies before the environmental ones. After approximately 12 of the food allergy treatments I volunteered the information that I have had an intermittent colitis for 20 years characterized by abdominal cramps and intermittent diarrhea. Of course I had many diagnostic tests to determine the cause of my colitis including X-ray and colonoscopy and several serological tests. No one could find a cause or any pathology. Mala, Dr. Nambudripad's associate discovered through kinesiology that the cause of my colitis occured in the year of my internship.

    I was asked to place my right fist on my forehead and think about what might have happened during that year while I was receiving the NAET treatment. My father developed Hodgkin's disease and passed away during my internship. I thought that I had resolved any emotion that was attached to his death but to my surprise the discovery of the emotional attachment to my colon caused a 10 to 15 minutes convulsive like seizure of my abdomen during the NAET treatment and my eyes became teary as I began to recall his death. Later that day and thereafter, my colitis symptoms disappeared and have not returned in two years. I am very grateful to NAET therapy for the complete elimination of my long standing "psychosomatic" illness, especially, because the cure was so easy to effect.

                             Gordon R. A. Fishman M.D.
                                  Newport Beach, CA

My Onion Allergy!

I was very allergic to onions. Whenever someone cooked onions in the kitchen, the smell made me nauseous and sick to my stomach. I got huge painful hives, and severe headache if I ingested onion in any form by mistake. After treatment for onions, I don't suffer from these problems anymore.

Mohan K.
La Mirada, CA

In addition to various allergic manifestations of the digestive tract, many people suffer from mild allergies: indigestion, dyspepsia, bloating, constipation, heartburn, flatulence, etc., which are not severe enough to seek medical help. Such people often take sodium bicarbonate, antacids, laxatives, etc., for the rest of their lives and treat themselves to relieve disturbing symptoms. Pain relievers taken for headaches, arthritis, etc., may also cause GI tract irritation sometimes doing more harm than good.

In many cases of a mild gastrointestinal allergy, the symptoms do not become acute for many years. The severity of the symptoms might eventually heighten to the point that patients undergo needless surgery. In most cases, if one learns to recognize the allergic symptoms early, the length of the treatment time can be greatly reduced. If treated before the symptoms get acute, the patient can avoid development of more severe manifestations.

CHAPTER 13

ALLERGIES AND NUTRITION

Vitamins and trace minerals are essential to life. They promote good health by regulating metabolism and assisting the biochemical processes that release energy from the foods and drinks we consume.

Vitamins and trace minerals are micronutrients, and the body needs them in small amounts. The lack of these essential elements, even though they are needed in minute amounts, can create various impairments and tissue damage in the body. Water, carbohydrates, fats, proteins and bulk minerals like calcium, magnesium, sodium, potassium and phosphorus are considered to be macronutrients, taken into the body via regular food. They are needed in larger amounts. Both macro and micronutrients are not only necessary to produce energy for our daily body functions, but also for growth and development of the body and mind.

Using macronutrients (food and drinks) and micronutrients (vitamins and trace minerals), the body creates some essential chemicals called enzymes and hormones. These are the foundations of human bodily functions. Enzymes are the catalysts, or simple activators, in the chemical reactions that are continually taking place in the body. Without the appropriate vitamins and trace minerals, the production and function of the enzymes will be incomplete. Prolonged deficiency of these vitamins and minerals can produce immature or incomplete enzyme production, protein synthesis, cell mutation, immature RNA, DNA synthesis, etc., which can mimic various organic diseases in the body.

Deficiency of the vitamins, and other essentials in the body, can be due to poor intake and absorption. Nutritional imbalances can mainly be attributed to allergies. When your energy field conflicts with nutritional elements like vitamin C, calcium, B complex, etc., you cannot absorb the essential vitamins and minerals. The body cannot function properly lacking the enzymes and mediators, etc., which were to have formed in the presence of these vitamins and minerals. When the body does not produce complete enzymes, hormones and other immune mediators, our body functions will not proceed normally. The body malfunctions and continues to malfunction for a period of time and the temporary dysfunction can lead to major illness.

Vitamin and mineral deficiency syndromes can mimic many other organic diseases in the body. When the body does not function properly, dysfunction will turn into disease, causing pain. Desperate patients will start visiting professional health practitioners seeking relief for their problem. Nutritionists also play a role in treating patients, placing them on large doses of various vitamins and minerals along with certain health foods.

NUTRITIONAL DISORDERS

Helen, a 68-year-old, was diagnosed as having Lupus Erythematosus and arthritis. Her white blood cell count dropped as low as 2,000/cubic millimeters. She was advised to get a blood transfusion. During her initial visit to our office, she said that she had been taking 6 to 8 grams of vitamin C daily for the past six months. Questioning her further, it was discovered that her joint pains had begun six months ago and that the blood count drop was discovered only two months ago. She was found to be highly allergic to vitamin C, which she was treated for. Ten days after she finished the treatment for vitamin C, her white blood cell count had gone up to 7,000/cm, which is normal.

John, a 38-year-old man, had depression for most of his life. He had tried various treatments, including psychotherapy. He was found to be allergic to iron. He had wrought-iron ornamental works all over his house. When he was treated for the metal iron, his depression cleared.

Michael, age 32, who frequently had skin cancer on his face, was evaluated and found to be highly allergic to the stainless steel blade of the razor he used. The use of a popular skin cream was the cause of the beginning of skin cancer in one patient. She was allergic to vitamin A and to the skin cream. After she was treated for these substances, her lesions cleared up.

Many patients have nutritional deficiencies due to poor eating habits and will benefit from nutritional supplements and megavitamin therapy. Others may have nutritional deficiencies due to food allergies and will not show any improvements on vitamin therapy. In fact, most of them will get worse. People who get well on vitamin therapy will consider it a miracle cure because once they fill up the deficiencies, their body functions will become normal. People who are allergic to vitamins and minerals cannot absorb them because their energy fields repel the energy fields of the vitamins and minerals. When the regular food is eaten, a minute amount of vitamins and minerals are circulated through the body, creating minute fields and weak repulsion. But when a vitamin or mineral is taken in pill form, the concentration of the elements is greater than from food items, and so is the repulsion. This is possibly the reason that allergic patients get very sick on vitamin/mineral therapy.

All patients should be tested for possible allergies before they are placed on vitamin therapy. If they are found to be allergic, they should be treated for the allergies before they are supplemented with vitamin and mineral mega-doses.

A 34-year-old woman was diagnosed by a famous doctor as having chronic fatigue syndrome, Epstein-Barr virus, candidiasis and yeast infection. She was treated by him for two years, without any relief. Then, one of her friends who suffered from a similar complaint, was magically cured by a nutritionist. Hoping to get relief as well, she drove to the nutritionist's office. Her first visit cost her a few hundred dollars. She was sent home with mega-doses of vitamin and mineral supplements, along with advice to practice good nutrition. She thought, "This is it" and was whistling, "I am on the way to good health," as she drove to the health food store.

Her hopes came crashing down the next day when she woke up with severe body aches and an unbearable headache. She called the doctor, who told her that the toxins were getting out of her system because of the change of diet and vitamin/mineral supplements. She waited anxiously for the toxins to leave her body, but her condition got progressively worse. In one week's time, she ended up having bronchitis, a hacking cough, severe joint pains, severe fatigue, headaches, lack of energy, and finally some swelling of the ankles and knees. At this point, she stopped eating the health foods and vitamins. Her body aches got slightly better but her respiratory problem persisted. She tried some strong broad-spectrum antibiotics for a couple of weeks with no positive results.

She had been suffering from severe bronchitis for six weeks when she came to our office. Through NTT, she was found to be allergic to almost all the foods she was tested for, especially whole wheat, oat bran, bran flakes, etc. She was treated for all the known food allergies first, and placed on a diet of only non-allergic foods. In less than two weeks, her bronchitis got better, as well as the cough, and her energy level picked up. She was on disability when she came to our office. Three and a half months later she was working full-time.

Apart from allergies, it is necessary to know a few things about taking vitamins and minerals. Of the major vitamins, vitamin C and B complex are water soluble, while vitamins A, D, E, and K are fat-soluble. It is believed that water-soluble vitamins must be taken into the body daily, as they cannot be stored and are excreted within one to four days, although our clinical experience has proven otherwise.

When you are allergic to vitamin B complex, in many cases you cannot digest grains, resulting in B complex deficiencies. When you get treated for allergies via NAET, you can eat grains without any ill effect and will begin to assimilate B complex vitamins. In some cases, through NTT I have found B complex deficiency amounting to fifteen to twenty thousand times the normal daily-recommended allowances. After supplementing with large amounts of B complex for a few weeks (20 - 30 times of RDA amount per day), the deficiency was eliminated. Over and over, in hundreds of patients, after weeks of supplementation, we have been able to remove their vitamin B complex deficiency symptoms completely. We have received similar results with vitamin C, but more research is needed on a larger number of patients to verify these findings.

Fat-soluble vitamins are stored for longer periods of time in the body's fatty tissue and the liver. When you are allergic to fat soluble vitamins, you begin to store them in unwanted places of the body. Some of this abnormal vitamin storage can be seen as lipomas, warts, skin tags, benign tumors inside or on the surface of the body, etc.

Taking vitamins and minerals in their proper balance is important for the correct functioning of all vitamins. Excess consumption of an isolated vitamin or mineral can produce unpleasant symptoms of that particular nutrient. High doses of one element can also cause depletion of other nutrients in the body, leading to other problems. Most of these vitamins work synergistically, complementing and/or strengthening each other's function.

Vitamins and minerals should be taken with meals unless specified otherwise. Oil-soluble vitamins should be taken before meals, and water-soluble vitamins should be taken between or after meals; however, when one is taking mega-doses of any of these, they should always be taken with or after meals. Vitamins and minerals, as nutritional supplements taken with meals, will supply the missing nutrients in our daily diets.

Synthetic vitamins are produced in a laboratory from isolated chemicals with quality similar to natural vitamins. Although there are no major chemical differences between a vitamin found in food and one created in a laboratory, natural supplements do not contain other unnatural ingredients. Supplements not labeled "natural" may include coal tars, artificial coloring, preservatives, sugars, and starches, as well as other additives. Vitamins labeled "natural" may contain vitamins not extracted from a natural food source.

These days, there are various books available on nutrition to help you understand vitamins and their assimilative processes. If anyone wants more information about nutrition, there are titles listed in the bibliography section at the end of this book.

VITAMIN A

Clinical studies have proven vitamin A and beta-carotene to be very powerful immune-stimulants and protective agents. Vitamin A is essential for a variety of normal body functions. Its deficiency can cause disturbed lymphocyte production and function. A decreased lymphocyte production, or abnormal lymphocyte production, can cause decreased phagocyte activity, leading to lower immune function and autoimmune disorders.

Vitamin A is necessary for proper vision, preventing night blindness, skin disorders, acne, etc., and it protects the body against colds, influenza and other infections. It enhances immunity, helps heal ulcers, wounds and maintains the epithelial cell tissue. It is necessary for the growth of bones and teeth. Vitamin A is an antioxidant that helps to protect the cells against cancer and other diseases. Beta-carotene, from vegetable sources, converts into vitamin A in the liver, and is very good for cancer prevention. Vitamin A helps in protein assimilation, slowing the aging process, by building body resistance, fighting respiratory infections, promoting growth, maintaining clear, healthy skin, hair, nails, teeth and gums. This helps to build body resistance, fight respiratory infections, promote growth, and maintain clear, healthy skin, hair, nails, teeth and gums.

When you are allergic to vitamin A, or when vitamin A is not absorbed normally in the body, skin tags, warts, blemishes, etc., appear on the skin surface. It is a wonder vitamin. If there is a problem with proper absorption and utilization of vitamin A in the body, you can experience toxic symptoms, such as poor or blurry vision; repeated respiratory infections; lowered immunity; skin problems like rashes, boils, acne; unhealthy, wrinkled skin; premature aging; loss of hair and nails; unhealthy teeth and gums; headaches of various nature; infertility; irregular menses; pain in the joints; gastrointestinal disturbances like nausea, vomiting, diarrhea, indigestion, etc. If the allergy is treated, and if the diet is properly supplemented, the toxic symptoms can be completely eliminated.

Vitamin A works best with B complex, vitamin D, vitamin E, calcium, phosphorus and zinc. Zinc is needed to get vitamin A out of the liver, where it is usually stored. Large doses of vitamin A should be taken only under proper supervision, because it can accumulate in the body and become toxic.

Food sources of vitamin A are fish liver oil, milk and dairy products, butter, egg yolks, corn, green leafy or yellow vegetables, yellow fruits, liver, alfalfa, apricots, asparagus, beets, broccoli, carrots, Swiss chard, dandelion greens, garlic, kale, mustard, papayas, parsley, peaches, red peppers, sweet potatoes, spinach, spirulina, pumpkin, yellow squash, turnip greens and watercress.

A seven-year-old boy had a great many problems with vision. He was tested by two ophthalmologists, at two different locations, and given high-powered eyeglasses. Then he was treated by NAET for allergy to vitamin A and given large doses of vitamin A (100,000 units daily), as a supplement, for one month. Then his vision was tested again. His eyeglass power was down by 50 percent. After six months of supplementation, he was tested again and his prescription power was down even further to minimal numbers. He was given 50,000 units of vitamin A daily for another six months, then 25,000 units for one more year. Now, two years later, he doesn't need glasses at all.

Many teenagers with allergy to vitamin A get acne, blemishes and other skin problems. Many people with allergy to vitamin A develop skin tags, and warts, and pimples around the neck, arms, etc. It is also one of the causes of premenstrual syndrome. When they get treated and properly supplemented with vitamin A, the skin clears up and PMS problems become less severe.

Vitamin deficiencies can be one of the causes of infertility since the integrity of the endometrium depends on vitamin A assimilation. Vitamin A helps to form healthy mucous membrane. A 34-year-old female was trying to get pregnant for years, without any success. She was found to be highly allergic to vitamin A and essential fatty acids. After she was treated for these items, she was placed on Tankuei and peony formula (a Chinese herbal formula for regulating the hormonal functions in women, helping with infertility). Within four months, she became pregnant.

Vitamin A is also necessary to prevent aging. A 73-year-old woman, with a lot of wrinkles, was treated for vitamin A and supplemented with 75,000 IU of vitamin A daily for three months. Her wrinkles began to subside gradually. Whenever she went off vitamin A supplementation for a couple of weeks, her wrinkles would begin to return. When she realized this, she continued to take vitamin A, somewhere in the range of 25,000 to 50,000 IU, daily. This kept her skin younger and smoother without very many wrinkles.

A young girl used to get repeated upper respiratory infections. She was found to be highly allergic to vitamin A. Within a few months after being treated for vitamin A, she built up enough resistance through a high dose of supplementation that she rarely had upper respiratory infections any more.

A 54-year-old female, with many warts and pimples around the neck and near the hairline, was allergic to vitamin A. After she was treated with NAET for vitamin A, she was supplemented with 50,000 units for six months. Her skin cleared completely.

A 48-year-old male had a history of periodic bleeding from the rectum for six years. His everyday diet included lots of raw and cooked carrots and cantaloupes. Using NAET, he was treated for vitamin A and beta-carotene. This put an end to his six-year-old problem.

VITAMIN D

Vitamin D is often called the sunshine vitamin. It is a fat-soluble vitamin, acquired through sunlight or food sources. Ultraviolet rays act on the oils of the skin to produce the vitamin, which is then absorbed into the body. Vitamin D is absorbed from foods, through the intestinal wall, after they are ingested. Smog reduces the vitamin D-producing rays of the sun. Dark-skinned people and suntanned people do not absorb vitamin D from the sun. Vitamin D helps the utilization of calcium and phosphorus in the human body. It is important in the prevention and treatment of osteoporosis. It helps to improve the body's resistance against respiratory tract infections and helps to assimilate vitamin A. It also keeps skin and bones healthy. When there is an allergy to vitamin D, the vitamin is not absorbed into the body through foods, or from the sun. People with an allergy to vitamin D can show deficiency syndromes such as rickets, severe tooth decay, softening of teeth and bones, osteomalacia, senile osteoporosis, sores on the skin, blisters on the skin while walking in the sun, severe sunburns when exposed to the sun, etc. Sometimes allergic persons can show toxic symptoms if they take vitamin D without clearing its allergy. These symptoms include mental confusion, unusual thirst, sore eyes, itching skin, vomiting, diarrhea, urinary urgency, calcium deposits in the blood vessels and bones, restlessness in the sun, and inability to bear heat. Vitamin D works best with vitamin A, vitamin C, choline, calcium and phosphorus.

Food sources of vitamin D are fish-liver oils, dairy products fortified with vitamin D, alfalfa, butter, egg yolk, liver, sunshine, milk and milk products, meat, fish, eggs, cereal products, sweet potatoes, vegetable oils, beans, fruit and vegetables.

When an allergy to vitamin D is treated by NAET, the deficiency or toxic symptoms can be eliminated. With the proper supplementation, normal health can be gradually restored.

A 30-year-old male complained of restlessness when he was exposed to the sun. He also complained of canker sores in the mouth if he walked in the sun. He was found to be highly allergic to vitamins A, C, D and calcium. After treating for vitamins A, C and calcium, his symptoms were reduced dramatically, but not completely. Finally, when he was treated for vitamin D, he began to feel comfortable under the sun. He also stopped having canker sores in the mouth.

A teenager, who had severe acne on her face, was found to be allergic to vitamin D, but not vitamin A. Whenever she took supplemental vitamins A and D, she began having more acne. Whenever she took only vitamin A and avoided dairy products and fish, her skin became better. When she was treated for vitamin D, she could eat milk products and fish without causing any skin problems.

VITAMIN E

Vitamin E is an antioxidant that prevents cancer and cardiovascular disease. The body needs zinc in order to maintain proper levels of vitamin E in the blood. Vitamin E is a fat-soluble vitamin and is stored in the liver, fatty tissues, heart, muscles, testes, uterus, blood, adrenal glands and pituitary glands. Vitamin E is excreted in the feces if too much is taken. Even though it is fat-soluble, it is stored for only a short period of time in the body.

Among the numerous functions of vitamin E is its ability to suppress cellular aging due to oxidation. Vitamin E improves circulation, repairs tissue, treats fibrocystic breasts and premenstrual syndrome. It also promotes normal clotting and healing. It reduces scarring and blood pressure, helps prevent cataracts, leg cramps, age spots or liver spots. It is an antioxidant, and it protects the lungs against air pollution, supplying more oxygen to the body. It can help prevent or dissolve blood clots because it has an anticoagulant property. It promotes healing of minor wounds and skin irritation and can prevent scarring if applied locally. It has a big role in fertility. Vitamins E and A help the uterus prepare for pregnancy. Vitamin E aids in prevention of miscarriages, alleviates fatigue and helps to strengthen tired lower limbs after long walks or exercise. It also helps to reduce leg cramps by its vaso-dilating action and acts as a diuretic.

Deficiency syndrome includes destruction of red blood cells, muscle degeneration, some anemia, infertility, and heart and circulation problems. If you are allergic to vitamin E, you can show all the deficiency syndromes. After the proper elimination of vitamin E allergy, it can be supplemented for positive benefits.

Vitamin E is found in the following food sources: vegetable oils, whole grains, dark green leafy vegetables, nuts, seeds, legumes, dry beans, brown rice, cornmeal, eggs, desiccated liver, milk, oatmeal, organ meats, sweet potatoes, wheat germ, broccoli, Brussels sprouts, leafy greens, spinach, enriched flour and whole wheat.

A 38-year-old female had scaly, dry skin on her arms and legs. She tried many different creams, including cortisone creams. The dry skin peeled periodically and was quite rough, causing pain and a burning sensation all the time. When she came to us, she was tested on various items for aller-gies and found to be highly allergic to vitamin E. She was using many creams, soaps and shampoos containing large amounts of vitamin E. She also took 400 IU of vitamin E daily as a supplement. After she was treated for vitamin E by NAET, her skin became smoother and softer. She now uses the vitamin E cream effectively.

A woman came to our office with a swollen, infected, crusty, weeping area where she had her ear pierced. She had this problem for a few years now and had seen other doctors, including dermatologists. She had used a few creams, including cortisone. When she did not wear an earring, the prob-lem area began to heal but as soon as she started wearing any type of earring, the problem returned. When she brought all her earrings to test, she was found to be allergic to the earrings or the posts. While testing one of the earrings, it was found to be sticky and oily. We questioned her about the oil and discovered that she used a cream to lubricate the post before inserting it into her ear lobe. It was a highly concentrated vitamin E cream. She was found to be highly allergic to vitamin E. After treatment for allergy to the vitamin E cream by NAET, she hasn't had the problem.

VITAMIN K

Vitamin K is needed for blood clotting and bone formation, and is necessary to convert glucose into glycogen for storage in the liver. Vitamin K is a fat-soluble vitamin, very essential to the formation of prothrombin, a blood-clotting material. It helps in the blood-clotting mechanism, prevents hemorrhages like nosebleeds and intestinal bleeding, and helps reduce excessive menstrual flow.

An allergy to vitamin K can produce deficiency syndromes such as prolonged bleeding time, intestinal diseases like sprue, etc., and colitis.

Vitamin K is found in alfalfa, broccoli, dark green leafy vegetables, soy beans, black strap molasses, Brussels sprouts, cabbage, cauliflower, egg yolk, liver, oatmeal, oats, rye, safflower oil and wheat.

As mentioned earlier, allergy to vitamin K can cause blood-clotting disorders. A four-year-old boy was suffering from hemophilia since he was two years old. He bruised often in various joints, especially if he walked fast, ran or played with other kids in school. Whenever he received an attack, he had to stay home with ice compresses on the affected joints for several days. He was found to be allergic to cabbage, a staple diet in his house. When he was treated for cabbage and vitamin K by NAET, his hemophilia-like symptoms disappeared. His family doctor declared him to be in remission. He is an active 3rd grader now, without any trace of his previous symptoms.

A 38-year-old woman came in with a complaint of severe uterine bleeding for six weeks. She was one of our pioneer patients, who previously had received treatment for various allergies. She had consulted a gynecologist and the doctor could not find any reason for the sudden bleeding. When she came to our office, it was discovered that a nutritionist had placed her on various vitamin and mineral supplements about six weeks earlier. One of them was 15 alfalfa tablets, twice a day. She was found to be allergic to alfalfa and vitamin K. Within six to eight hours after being treated for vitamin K, her bleeding stopped.

Another 28-year-old girl complained of severe PMS and cramps during her periods. She noticed that if she ate salads, with alfalfa sprouts, her PMS symptoms were worse. She was found to be highly allergic to vitamin K, alfalfa and cabbage. Her PMS dramatically diminished after treatments for vitamin K.

A 42-year-old man had a unique problem. He passed and sprayed fresh blood whenever he defecated. He had no hemorrhoids, no cramps or pains. He felt lethargic and fatigued all the time. He had given up eating red meats for health reasons and was eating mostly vegetables, salads, fruits and whole grains. He was found to be allergic to vitamins C and K, which were in all the vegetables and fruits he ate. He hasn't had the above-mentioned problems in six years since he was treated for vitamins C and K by NAET.

VITAMIN B COMPLEX

Approximately 15 vitamins make up the B complex family. Each one of them has unique, very important functions in one's body. If the body does not absorb and utilize any or all of the B vitamins, various health problems can result. B complex vitamins are very essential for emotional, physical and physiological well-being of the human body. It is a nerve food, so it is necessary for the proper growth and maintenance of the nervous system and brain function. It also keeps the nerves well fed so that nerves are kept calm and the person maintains a good mental attitude. Certain B vitamins function as enzyme precursors and aid in digestion. The most important B vitamins and their function are:

B-1- Affects the nervous system and mental attitude, aids in digestion of sugar and carbohydrates, helps to treat alcoholics and reduces stress by calming the nerves.

B-2 - Aids in growth and reproduction. Promotes healthy skin, nails and hair, aids in digestion of carbohydrates, fats and proteins.

B-6 - Aids in digestion and assimilation of proteins and fats, prevents various nervous and skin disorders, reduces morning sickness and nausea in general, promotes synthesis of nucleic acids, reduces neuralgia and neuritis, and works as a natural diuretic.

B-12 - Prevents anemia, regenerates red blood cells, increases overall energy, maintains a healthy nervous system, aids in digestion of carbohydrates, fats and proteins, improves concentration, memory and emotional balance.

FOLIC ACID

Essential to the formation of red blood cells and prevents anemia; aids in protein metabolism and production of nucleic acids; helps in cell division, essential for utilization of sugar and amino acids; improves lactation, delays hair graying when used with PABA and pantothenic acid.

INOSITOL

Promotes healthy hair and prevents hair loss, aids in redistribution of body fat, lowers cholesterol, produces a calming effect. Inositol, choline, pantothenic acid and B-12 taken together help improve concentration and memory.

Allergic symptoms can appear in many forms if one is allergic to B vitamins. The doctor has to take special care to isolate the allergic vitamin and treat to alleviate the problem. B vitamins are seen in almost all foods we eat. Some of them are destroyed by cooking and heating, others are not destroyed by processing or preparation. People who are allergic to B vitamins can get mild to severe reactions just by eating the foods alone. If they are supplemented with vitamin B complex, without being aware of the allergies, such people can get exaggerated reactions. One has to be very cautious while taking B complex, commonly known as stress vitamins.

Food sources of B vitamins include whole grains, seeds, legumes, milk products, pork, liver, beef, green leafy vegetables, potatoes, nuts, eggs, fish, root vegetables, green vegetables, fruits, brewer's yeast, bran and wheat germ.

Dr. Carlton Frederic, in his book, *Psychonutrition*, tried to point out that nutritional deficiencies are the causes of most of the mental sicknesses in psychiatric facilities. He tried to prove his theory by giving large doses of vitamin B complex, especially B-12, to some of the psychiatric patients. Fifty percent of the patients were cured of their mental sickness and went back to live normal lives. But the other 50 percent made no progress or got worse.

VITAMIN C

Vitamin C, or ascorbic acid, is a water soluble vitamin and it plays a very important role in the metabolism of carbohydrates, proteins and lipids. Vitamin C is fairly stable in acid solution. It is very sensitive to oxygen. Its potency can be lost through exposure to light, heat and air.

Vitamin C is readily absorbed through the mucosa of the mouth, stomach and mostly through the upper part of the small intestine. From there, it passes through the portal vein to the liver and is distributed to tissues throughout the body. The transport mechanism may differ from person to person. The level of ascorbic acid in the blood reaches a maximum in two or three hours after ingestion, then decreases as it is eliminated in the urine and through perspiration. Most of the vitamin C is out of the body within three or four hours.

To maintain an adequate serum level, this vitamin should be taken in small amounts throughout the day. A human body stores a total of about 1,500 milligrams with moderate reserves in the liver and spleen, and high concentration in the adrenal glands.

Vitamin C is essential in the formation of adrenaline. During stress, the adrenal uses vitamin C rapidly. For this reason, more vitamin C is needed under stressful conditions. Vitamin C helps in preventing scurvy. Vitamin C promotes fine bone and tooth formation while protecting the dentine and pulp. It reduces the effects on the body of some allergy producing substances. In large doses, it can function as antihistamine and reduce allergic reactions. Allergic patients will benefit from taking adequate amounts of vitamin C every day to reduce the various reactions. But make sure you are not allergic to the vitamin C products you are taking.

Vitamin C is used in the prevention of the common cold. It is an important nutrient in treating wounds because it speeds up the healing process. It is very important in the formation of collagen, a major component of all connective tissue in the body: skin, bones, teeth, muscles, tendons, etc. Vitamin C is necessary to transport certain amino acids, such as proline and lysine, into hydroxy proline and hydroxy lysine. These hydroxy forms give stability to the collagen molecules.

Vitamin C prevents breakdown of connective tissue. It helps amino acids in the synthesis of neurotransmitters. It also helps with the absorption of iron and helps in various enzymatic functions in the body. It helps improve the healing of wear and tear of the tissues. It nourishes the tissues of the blood vessels and helps improve the elasticity of the blood vessels. Healthy blood vessels improve blood circulation. Efficient blood circulation helps to reduce serum cholesterol. Good circulation also gives good elimination; thus vitamin C helps with constipation.

Elimination of the toxins from the body brings about a good complexion in the body. It also helps to maintain the water balance in the body by redistributing or removing the excess amount of water from the body. So this is an essential vitamin in weight control.

RDA: 60 mg. for adults; 80-100 mg. for pregnant and lactating woman. It is an essential vitamin, a good antioxidant, seen in almost all the foods. Overcooking destroys it.

A few minerals are extremely essential for our daily functions. While some metals and trace minerals are mentioned here, please refer to the appropriate references in the bibliography for more information on other minerals.

CALCIUM

Calcium is one of the essential minerals in the body. Calcium works with phosphorus, magnesium, iron, vitamins A, C and D and it helps to maintain strong bones and healthy teeth. It regulates the heart functions and helps to relax nerves and muscles. It induces relaxation and sleep.

Deficiencies in calcium result in rickets, osteomalacia, osteoporosis, hyperactivity, restlessness, inability to relax, generalized aches and pains, joint pains, formation of bone spurs, backaches, PMS, cramps in the legs and heavy menstrual flow.

Food sources for calcium are milk products, soybean, sardine, oyster, salmon, nuts, dried beans and green leafy vegetables. If you are allergic to calcium, you can get deficiency syndromes, in exaggerated forms, whenever you eat foods containing calcium. When the allergy is eliminated by NAET, you can be supplemented appropriately to get maximum health benefits.

Many asthmatic people, with upper respiratory problems, respond well to calcium supplementation. Many people with abdominal pains, dysentery, insomnia, skin problems, nervousness, dyslexia, canker sores, postnasal drip, hyperactivity, obesity, and arthritis respond well to allergy treatments for calcium and later supplementation. Many women, who have heavy menstrual flow, respond well to allergy treatment for calcium and later supplementation. When people are on cortisone treatment, they need to take more calcium.

A 26-year-old female complained of heart palpitations whenever she consumed milk or milk products. She was found to be allergic to calcium. When she was treated by NAET for calcium, she stopped having heart palpitations when she ate milk products.

A 14-year-old boy complained of severe leg cramps and extreme tiredness after baseball practice. His parents complained that he was not growing tall enough for his age. One of the nutritionists advised him to take calcium supplements. He got very sick with severe joint pains and was found to be allergic to calcium. After he was treated for calcium by NAET, his cramps and joint pains got better. When he was supplemented with calcium, not only did he got stronger, he began to grow taller. He grew six inches in a few months.

A 53-year-old female had severe skin rashes and blisters, which eventually turned into ulcers. She bruised easily and had black and blue marks all over the body. She said that she started drinking more milk and taking calcium supplements to prevent osteoporosis. She was found to be allergic to milk products and calcium. When she was treated for them, her skin problems cleared up.

A 42-year-old female complained of severe backache. She took calcium pills, which only made it worse. She was not allergic to calcium, but she was allergic to the binders used to make the pills. When she was treated for the binders of the calcium pills, she stopped having the backaches. When she took calcium pills after treatment she felt more relaxed.

A five-year-old boy was very hyperactive, getting restless and noisy soon after drinking milk. He was allergic to milk and calmed down greatly after he was treated for milk and calcium.

A 36-year-old female complained of severe uterine bleeding, with heavy clots during her menstrual periods, which lasted for almost ten days each month. She had various treatments, including hormone shots, prior to coming to our office. She was found to be allergic to calcium. She was treated for allergy to calcium by NAET and supplemented with large quantities (4,000 to 6,000 mg) of calcium daily. Her periods became regular and flow became normal within two months.

A 52-year-old male with extreme pain in his left knee had five different surgeries. He was scheduled for the sixth surgery when he was seen in our office. He was a printer by profession and had to stand on his feet the whole day. He was found to be very deficient in calcium, but not allergic to it. He was 20 pounds overweight and was on fad diets to fight his mild obesity. This hard working man did not get enough calcium from his food intake to meet his daily needs. He was supplemented with 6,000 mg. of calcium daily for one month, after which he stopped having knee pains. Three years later, the still remains symptom free.

IRON

Iron is one of the essential minerals, necessary for the production of hemoglobin (red blood corpuscles), myoglobin (red pigment in muscles), and certain enzymes. In one month, women lose more iron than men. Iron requires copper, cobalt, manganese, and vitamin C for proper assimilation and is also necessary for proper metabolizing of B vitamins. Iron aids in growth, promotes resistance to disease, prevents fatigue, prevents and cures iron deficiency anemia.

Iron deficiency results in anemia. People with allergy to iron do not absorb iron from food. They suffer from iron deficiency anemia, even though they take iron supplements. A person with iron allergy can get various problems from iron supplementation or eating iron-containing foods.

Food sources for iron include apricots, peaches, bananas, black molasses, prunes, raisins, brewer's yeast, whole grain cereals, spinach, beets, alfalfa, sunflower seeds, walnuts, sesame seeds, dried beans, lentils, liver, egg yolk, red meats, pork, kidney, heart, clams, oysters, oatmeal and asparagus.

A 32-year-old male complained of backaches since he was a teenager. On certain days his backache was very severe, and he had to stay home in bed for three to four days at a time. He could not hold a permanent job and worked on a daily basis through a temporary agency. He had undergone various diagnostic tests for his backache, but no cause was found. In our office, this man was found to be highly allergic to all the foods containing iron. When he was treated for iron by NAET, he began to feel great relief from his chronic backache. Incidentally, he took 18 consecutive treatments to get desensitized for iron. This young man does not get severe backaches anymore. He was able to work full-time, without getting sick, for the past year and a half.

CHROMIUM

Chromium is an essential element to metabolize sugar, to treat diabetes, to treat hypoglycemia and to treat alcoholism. A deficiency results in arteriosclerosis, hypoglycemia and diabetes.

Food sources include whole grain cereals, wheat germ, corn oil, brewers' yeast, mushroom, liver, raw sugar, red meat, shellfish, chicken and clams.

COBALT

Cobalt is essential for red blood cells since it is part of vitamin B-12. Deficiency results in B-12 deficiency anemia.

Food sources are all green leafy vegetables, meat, liver, kidney, figs, buckwheat, oysters, clams and milk.

COPPER

Copper is required to convert the body's iron into hemoglobin. Combined with the amino acid thyroxin, it helps to produce the pigment factor for hair and skin. It is essential for utilization of vitamin C. Deficiency results in anemia and edema. Toxicity symptoms are insomnia, hair loss, irregular menses and depression.

Food sources of copper are almonds, beans, peas, green leafy vegetables, whole grain products, prunes, raisins, liver, dried beans, whole wheat, beef, most seafood and copper piping in water supply.

FLUORINE / FLUORIDE

Sodium fluoride is added to drinking water. Calcium fluoride is seen in natural food sources. Fluorine decreases chances of dental carries (too much can discolor teeth). It also strengthens the bones. Deficiency leads to tooth decay. Toxicity or allergy symptoms include dizziness, nausea, poor appetite, skin rashes, itching, yeast infections, mental confusion, muscle spasms, mental fogginess and arthritis. Treatment for fluoride will eliminate possible allergies. Food sources include fluoridated drinking water, seafood, gelatin, sunflower seeds, milk products, carrots, garlic, green leafy vegetable and almonds.

IODINE

Two-thirds of the body's iodine is in the body's thyroid gland. Since the thyroid gland controls metabolism, and iodine influences the thyroid, an under supply of this mineral can result in weight gain, general fatigue and slow mental reaction. Iodine helps to keep the body thin, promotes growth, gives more energy, improves mental alertness, and promotes the growth of hair, nails and teeth.

A deficiency in iodine can cause overweight, hypothyroidism, goiters and lack of energy. Among its food sources are kelp, seafood, iodized salt, vegetables grown in iodine-rich soil and onion.

MAGNESIUM

Magnesium is necessary for the metabolism of calcium, vitamin C, phosphorus, sodium, potassium and vitamin A. It is essential for the normal functioning of nerves and muscles. It also helps convert blood sugar into energy. It works as a natural tranquilizer, laxative and diuretic. Diuretics deplete magnesium. Alcoholics and asthmatics are deficient in magnesium.

Food sources of magnesium include nuts, soybeans, raw and cooked green leafy vegetables, almonds, whole grains, sunflower seeds, brown rice and sesame seeds.

MANGANESE

Manganese helps to activate digestive enzymes in the body. It is important in the formation of thyroxin, the principal hormone of the thyroid gland. It is necessary for the proper digestion and utilization of food. Manganese is important in reproduction and the normal functioning of the central nervous system. It helps to eliminate fatigue, improves memory, reduces nervous irritability and relaxes the mind. A deficiency may result in recurrent attacks of dizziness and poor memory.

Food sources include green leafy vegetables, spinach, beets, Brussels sprouts, blueberries, oranges, grapefruits, apricots, the outer coating of nuts and grains (bran), peas, kelp, egg yolks, wheat germ and nuts.

MOLYBDENUM

Molybdenum helps in carbohydrate and fat metabolism. It is a vital part of the enzyme responsible for iron utilization. Among its food sources are whole grains, brown rice, brewer's yeast, legumes, buckwheat, millet and dark green leafy vegetables.

PHOSPHORUS

Phosphorus is involved in virtually all physiological chemical reactions in the body. It is necessary for normal bone and teeth formation. It is important for heart regularity, and is essential for normal kidney function. It provides energy and vigor by helping in the fat and carbohydrate metabolism. It promotes growth and repairs in the body. It is essential for healthy gums and teeth. Vitamin D and calcium are essential for its proper functioning.

Food sources of phosphorus are whole grains, seeds, nuts, legumes, milk products, egg, fish, corn, dried fruits, poultry and meat.

POTASSIUM

Potassium works with sodium to regulate the body's water balance and to regulate the heart rhythm. It helps in clear thinking by sending oxygen to the brain. A deficiency in potassium results in edema, hypoglycemia, nervous irritability, and muscle weakness.

Among its food sources are all vegetables, especially green leafy vegetables, oranges, whole grains, sunflower seeds, nuts, bananas, potatoes, potato peelings, citrus fruits, melons, tomatoes, watercress and mint.

SELENIUM

Selenium is an antioxidant. It works with vitamin E, slowing down the aging process. It prevents hardening of tissues and helps to retain youthful appearance. Selenium is also known to alleviate hot flashes and menopausal distress. It prevents dandruff. Some researchers have found selenium to neutralize certain carcinogens and provide protection from some cancers.

Food sources include brewer's yeast, wheat germ, sea water, kelp, garlic, mushrooms, seafood, milk, eggs, whole grains, beef, fish, beans, most vegetables, bran, tuna fish, onions, tomatoes and broccoli.

SODIUM

It is essential for normal growth and normal body functioning. It works with potassium to maintain the sodium-potassium pump in the body. Potassium is found inside the cells and sodium is found outside. It is essential to maintain processed foods including most fast foods. Food sources are salt, shellfish, carrots, beets, artichokes, beef, brain, kidney and bacon.

SULFUR

Sulfur is essential for healthy hair, skin and nails. It helps maintain the oxygen balance necessary for proper brain function. It works with B complex vitamins for basic body metabolism. It is a part of tissue building amino acid. It tones up the skin and makes the hair lustrous and helps fight bacterial infection. Among its food sources are radishes, turnips, onions, celery, string beans, watercress, soybean, fish, meat, lean beef, dried beans, eggs, cabbage, grapes, raisins, dried foods, wines, alcoholic beverages, saccharin, Sweet and Low, sulfites and sulfates.

VANADIUM

Vanadium prevents heart attacks. It inhibits the formation of cholesterol in blood vessels. Its food source is fish.

ZINC

Zinc is essential to form certain enzymes and hormones in the body. It is very necessary for protein synthesis. It is important for blood stability and in maintaining the body's acid-alkaline balance. It is important in the development of reproductive organs and helps to normalize the prostate glands in males. It helps in treatment of mental disorders and speeds up healing of wounds and cuts on the body. Zinc helps with the growth of fingernails and eliminates cholesterol deposits in the blood vessels.

Food sources of zinc include wheat bran, wheat germ, pumpkin seeds, sunflower seeds, brewers' yeast, milk, eggs, onions, green leafy vegetables, oysters, herrings, peas, brown rice, fish, mushrooms, lamb, beef, pork, nonfat dry milk and mustard.

TRACE MINERALS

Even though trace minerals are needed in our body, they are seen in trace amounts only. The researchers do not know definite functions of the trace minerals, but deficiencies can definitely contribute toward health problems. Its food sources include alfalfa, kelp, seafood and seawater.

AMINO ACIDS

All proteins are made up of amino acids. They are the building blocks of protein. There are 22 different types of amino acids. Some can be made

The Good Old Soy Protein

Whenever I ate any kind of dairy and soybean products, my stomach and entire intestinal tract would start to spasm. They called it colic when I was a baby, and I have had it ever since. It usually began five to ten minutes after eating anything with milk, calcium, and soy. After treatment from Dr. Devi, there were no spasms when I ate the foods containing those items. My mother Cindy was the same as I, and Dr. Devi's treatment has had the same benefit for her.

Michelle Beasely
La Mirada, CA

in the body and are called nonessential amino acids. Eight are not produced in the body and are known as essential amino acids. These essential amino acids that have to be absorbed from food are lysine, methionine, leucine, threonine, valine, tryptophan, isoleucine and phenylalanine. Children also need histidine and arginine.

Food sources for essential amino acids are complete protein foods (meat, fish, poultry and dairy products). Most vegetables, grains and fruits are incomplete proteins.

LECITHIN

Lecithin is needed by every living cell in the human body. Cell membranes are largely composed of lecithin. They select and regulate which nutrients may leave or enter the cell. Cell membranes would harden without lecithin. Its structure protects the cells from damage by oxidation. The protective sheaths surrounding the brain are composed of lecithin, and the

NAET HAS IMPROVED THE QUALITY OF MY LIFE!

In April, I came to Rebecca Stearns to begin NAET. I brought test results showing I was allergic to fifty foods and suspected there were countless others. My diet had been reduced to only a handful of foods. I ate the same things day after day, month after month, and knew I would eventually become allergic to them, too. Allergies had forced me to change jobs from a management consultant travelling 80,000 miles a year to an office position in a cubicle. I could no longer enjoy my greatest passion — preparing elaborate Italian "cucina toscana" dinners for family and friends. I realized allergies had a major impact on my career and activities. But, most importantly, my health and psyche were suffering.

In just two months, NAET has improved the quality of my life. Slowly but surely, I can now eat more and more foods with no ill effects. I feast on grilled chicken. I drink my morning orange juice. I enjoy lemonade on a summer day. I measure my health by allergy clearings and create recipes to enjoy "forbidden foods." Variety is the spice of my life. Michelangelo wrote: "The idea is there, locked inside. All you have to do is remove the stone."

With each session, Rebecca Stearns' NAET touch removes allergies and unlocks the door to a healthier and better life. But, more importantly, she brings sweet hope to the allergy-weary and the prospect of a balanced and a brighter future.

I cannot recommend Rebecca Stearns and NAET more highly.

Amy Johnston
NAET Patient of Dr. Rebecca Stearn, Maryland

Lactose Intolerence

My patient Terry had been diagnosed as having "Lactose Intolerence" for many years. A touch of milk hidden in any food product gave him severe discomfort and intestinal pain instantly and lasted for days. So he took extreme precaution by reading all the labels of anything he bought at the store and very carefully avoided milk or milk product like poison. After clearing him for milk, I had to treat him for lactose separately. After clearing milk and lactose satisfactorily, I encouraged him to try a little milk and see if he was gaining on the problem. He had that scary look on his face! He left my office and by dinner time he had mustered the courage to try. Moderation was not on the agenda. He ate 1/2 a pizza with no reaction so he ate a bowl of ice cream with no reaction. So he ate another bowl of ice cream. Next morning he woke up fine. He had no usual instant intestinal pain, he had no discomfort during the night. In fact he had a better night. Terry was convinced that NAET works. On his way home he stopped at the store and bought a quart of milk and drank it on the way home. Since then he has referred in three patients and I have learned from his wife that NAET is his favorite topic of discussion.

Thank you for making that possible.
Karl Amot.

> *Karl E. Amot, D.C.*
> *233 Cajon St. #6*
> *Redlands CA 92323*

muscles and nerve cells also contain this essential fatty substance. Lecithin is composed of choline, inositol and linoleic acids. It acts as an emulsifying agent.

It helps prevent arteriosclerosis, protects against cardiovascular disease, increases brain function, and promotes energy. It promotes better digestion of fats and helps disperse cholesterol in water and removes it from the body. The vital organs and arteries are protected from fatty build-up with the inclusion of lecithin in the diet. Most lecithin is derived from soybean, eggs, brewer's yeast, grains, legumes, fish and wheat germ.

If the allergy to lecithin is eliminated and it is assimilated in the body from the daily food, the body will be able to normalize the blood serum cholesterol, which can help the overall circulation.From some of the case histories, the reader may gain an understanding of the importance of good nutrition (non-allergic nutrients) in one's life to maintain a proper balance of the body's functions. The body needs all the essential vitamins and minerals in proper proportion for its normal function. If there is any deficiency of the vitamins, minerals, trace minerals, or amino acids, it can be seen as some functional disorder or other problem. If it can be found in time and treated or supplemented with appropriate amounts, many unnecessary discomforts can be avoided.

CHAPTER 14

ALLERGY AND
THE RESPIRATORY SYSTEM

H ay fever describes the symptoms of allergic rhinitis when it occurs in the late summer due to an individual's reaction to ragweeds and sage weeds or fresh flowers and grasses. Allergic rhinitis affects an estimated 40-50 million people in the United States. Hay fever and allergic rhinitis are both characterized by symptoms of watery discharge from the nose, eyes, and throat, loss of taste and smell, and other symptoms similar to those accompanying colds. The three most common symptoms are severe sneezing, watery nasal discharge, and stuffy nose. Many patients also complain of an annoying tickle inside the nose that results in violent sneezing. Others have dry, hacking coughs, and some have a profuse watery secretion without sneezing or obstruction of the nasal passages.

Long before hay fever was recognized and diagnosed in the nineteenth century, the instances of the ailment were recorded throughout medical history. In the time of Galen, the Greek physician who lived in the second century A.D., a record was made of people who had an eccentricity to roses. According to one historian, the king of Poland during the fourteenth century had such distaste for apples that he fled even from their aroma, as if it were the most fatal poison. In 1563, Lusitanus described people who suffered attacks similar to hay fever at the mere sight of a rose. In 1693, it was said by Riedlin that the duke of Schaumburg could not bear the sight of a cat or

---

Sinus Headaches and Allergic Rhinitis

I came to Doctor Devi a year ago with sinus headaches, shortness of breath, coughing , runny nose and wheezing. Within the first two months, my sinus headaches were reduced by almost 90 percent. The coughing and wheezing are virtually all gone. Now, we are working on eliminating allergy symptoms. I have been very pleased with her treatment and I have recommended her to many others.

Jim Ashley
Anaheim, CA

---

even the odor of a hidden one without experiencing dizziness and difficulty breathing. John Bostock, an English physician, did the foundation work for our modern knowledge of hay fever.

In 1819, Dr. Bostock presented a paper before the medical society describing his own ailment that he had suffered from seasonally since childhood. Nine years later, he published a paper covering further studies of this subject calling the condition "summer catarrh." It came to be known as hay fever because, initially, many believed the reactions were caused by hay.

By 1831, another English doctor, John Elliotson, stated that hay was definitely not the culprit; pollen from fresh flowers and grasses was to blame. The term "hay fever" is actually a misnomer and incorrectly describes this condition, as it is seldom caused by hay and only occasionally produces a fever. It may be defined as an allergic manifestation that occurs seasonally and is caused primarily by pollens, although other substances may aggravate it.

ALLERGIC RHINITIS

Although allergic rhinitis (inflammation of the nose and nasal passages) causes similar symptoms to hay fever, they often persist throughout the year, and are caused by other allergens, such as food, inhalants, fabrics or other substances. Many patients suffer from both conditions simultaneous-ly, with the symptoms considerably aggravated during the pollen season.

Allergic rhinitis is a very common medical problem affecting more than 15 percent of the population, both adults and children. Allergic rhinitis takes two different forms, seasonal and perennial. Symptoms of seasonal allergic rhinitis occur in spring, summer and/or early fall and are usually caused by allergic sensitivity to pollens from trees, grasses, weeds or to airborne mold spores. Other people experience symptoms year-round, a condition called perennial allergic rhinitis. It's generally caused by sensitivity to house dust, dust mites, animal dander and mold spores. Food allergies are another possible cause of perennial nasal symptoms.

The principal symptom in children is commonly blocked nasal passages. Children suffering from hay fever tend to breathe through their mouths and have a nasal twang to their voices. If the condition continues untreated, facial deformity frequently results. In addition to the above symptoms, many patients complain of intense itching of the eyes, ears, throat, soft palate and sometimes, the face. With hay fever, the symptoms may vary considerably between patients. Many hay fever patients are very sensitive to changes in temperature and weather. Their condition is usually aggravated by cool or damp air, even though the pollen count is lower under these circumstances.

Most hay fever sufferers feel better in warm, sunny weather. This condition frequently causes the patient to feel chills almost constantly. As a

---

Hay fever and Bronchitis

I suffered from hay fever and bronchitis since the age of twelve, ever since I moved to Norwalk, California. Dr. Devi treated me for my allergy to yeast, pollens, grasses, flowers, perfumes and mold. I have been totally symptom-free for the past 13 years (since 1986).

Janna Gossen
La Mirada, CA

My Son's Asthma

My four-year old son was in one of his extreme asthmatic attacks, even using his face muscles to breathe—this after just having spent two hours on a hospital inhaler. Dr. Devi had me listen to his distressed lungs through a stethoscope and it was frightening! A few moments after one NAET treatment for water chemicals, we listened to his lungs again—and they were perfectly normal!

Vone Deporter
Woodland Hills, CA

result, hay fever patients require more bedding and warmer clothing when suffering from this ailment.

Many patients with pollen allergies will also be allergic to certain foods, as well as other inhalants and contactants. Other than pollens and grasses, the most common items found to cause hay fever are: sugar, carob, corn, wheat, beans, pineapple, tomato, banana, perfume, furniture, cats, dogs, feathers, kapok, dust, plastics, rubber and leather. Often, hay fever victims also suffer from nasal polyps, which are swellings or growths of the mucus membrane that occur within the nostrils. Nasal polyps are caused by congestion and inflammation of the mucous membrane and tend to grow or shrink in accordance with the severity of the symptoms. In some instances, they become large enough to completely block the nasal passages and even extend beyond the nostrils.

A 49-year-old patient had suffered from nasal polyps (as well as other allergic manifestations, including asthma) and had them surgically removed several times. However, the operations did not correct the problem and they continued to return. She was fed up with her incessant ill health and doctor bills. She heard about the NAET program and visited our office. She was tested for various items including pollens, trees, fabrics, chemicals and foods. While she was beginning allergy treatments, the polyps had to be removed again. She continued to receive allergy elimination treatments for a year following the surgery. Her general health improved; her asthma and other allergic symptoms were under control, just by watching her diet and life-style. The nasal polyps have stayed away for four years without any sign of regrowth. Major progress was made after she was diagnosed and treated for her allergy to formaldehyde, which is found in almost all fabrics (including labels on clothing), wood works, office products, paper products, inks, white-out, carpets and many household items.

It is extremely important that hay fever sufferers consult an appropriate allergist knowledgeable in NAET when their symptoms begin. Hay fever has a tendency to become increasingly severe with each season. The possibility of serious complications increases with each severe hay fever attack. Untreated patients are also likely to accumulate new allergens, as well as encountering increased sensitivity in their reactions.

Dust Allergy

I suffered from sneezing and runny nose if I came near any dust. I had to wear a mask if I had to go out of the house. It was very embarrassing. My social life was limited. I took allergy shots since childhood. It helped me somewhat. I was referred to Dr. Devi by my chiropractor. After being treated for dust and dust mite with NAET, I do not react to dust anymore. I am able to travel all over the world now without wearing a mask. I visited India, Greece, Egypt and many other European countries in the past couple of years without any trouble. NAET is a revolutionary technique indeed!

Dr. Toby Weiss
St. Croix, VI

> *Can Vitamin C Cause or Cure a Cold?*
>
> *I was sold on Dr. Devi's treatment when I first got treated for Vitamin C. It seemed that I would get a cold once or twice a week and was still taking 2,000 or 3,000 units of vitamin C tablets a day. She found out I was allergic to vitamin C, I got treated, and now I feel better because I can absorb the vitamin C better.*
>
> *Marla S.*
> *Anaheim, CA*

Allergic rhinitis (common cold) may be caused by any substance: house dust, occupational dusts (such as flour in the bakery, industrial dust), cosmetics, foods, household pets, animal dander, animal epithelial, chalk powder, newspaper ink, paint, plastics, chemical sprays, molds, soaps, perfumes and other chemical agents. Prompt treatment of these allergies greatly decreases the likelihood that a comparatively mild allergic manifestation, such as hay fever or allergic rhinitis, will develop into a more severe allergy, such as asthma.

ASTHMA

Asthma is one of the more serious and disabling allergic conditions. The word asthma comes from Greek, meaning "I gasp for breath." It was used by Hippocrates (460-370 B.C.) to denote certain types of breathing difficulties. Asthma is an allergic state in which the bronchial tubes constrict the passage of air, resulting in severe difficulty breathing and a whistling type of exhalation (expelling the air from the lungs). Many times, the patient also has a cough, which further aggravates his misery. These attacks occur spasmodically but can be very severe at times. Often, the sensation of suffocation is so severe that the patient feels he is choking to death. In some cases

Anaphylaxis due to shellfish

I reacted severely to fish or fish products since childhood. Whenever I ate a minute portion of fish or shellfish, my throat closed up, I couldn't breathe, I would break out with huge hives all over my body and I ended up in the emergency room for hours with cortisone and other emergency drugs. On a few occasions, I had to be hospitalized for a few days. One of my friends, who was treated by Dr. Devi for his peanut allergy, suggested that I see her for my life-threatening fish allergy. I was curious about NAET. She treated me for all the basics before she treated me for fish groups.

I had a severe reaction during the first treatment for fish. As soon as she placed the clear glass vial with the energy of fish in my hand, my hand swelled up and I broke out in red hives all over my body. I got up from the treatment table to reach for my adrenaline shot which I carried all the time with me. But she stopped me. She commanded me to turn over. She looked very confident. I obeyed her and she applied firm pressure on my back, up and down along the spine for a few times. When she finished applying the acupressure along my spine, she asked me to turn on my back. She tested my arm. I was strong. She asked me how I was doing. I was breathing better than ever and my throat did not feel restricted anymore. I looked at my bare arms. Red rashes began fading away. This is magic, I thought. She was standing in front of me with that smile of confidence, waiting for my answer. "Better," I said, with a sigh of relief. I had to have three combination treatments for fish (fish group, lungs, colon, spleen and liver, fish group and base, fish group and heat, each on a separate office visit). After completion of the treatments, she told me to hold a small portion of fish in my palm and sit for 30 minutes. I felt fine. Then she asked me to eat a small portion of fish. I had my adrenaline near me when I ate a piece of fish, but nothing happened.

Ever since I was treated for fish, I eat fish at least twice a week without any problem. This is the best discovery man (woman) has ever made in medicine.

Dave Moore
Laguna Beach, California

cases an attack of asthma does prove fatal, and the patient dies from exhaustion and the inability to breathe.

Asthma affects more than 10 million Americans and is one of the leading causes of school and work absences. In 1998 alone, asthma affected 17,299,000 people in the U.S. According to a recent study, the largest number of asthmatics (2,268,300 people) were Californians. New York had 1,236,200 people and Texas had 1,175,100 people affected by this disorder.

Asthma is the 9th leading cause of hospitalization nationally. Over one billion dollars is spent each year on health care for asthma in the U.S.

Peanut Allergy

My eight year old son had severe peanut allergy ever since he was a baby. When he was three years old he had to be taken to the emergency room after he ate a touch of peanut butter. He would get asthma, break out in huge hives and his throat would swell if he smelled peanut oil or roasted peanuts. So we never used peanuts or peanut oil in the house. It was a nightmare for me to read all the labels before I buy food products or send him to school where children eat peanuts and candies and most of them included peanuts. Then I heard about NAET. Sam was treated by NAET for peanuts. After he was treated he accidently ate a cookie with peanut. He did not have a reaction. I am not planning to feed him peanuts for meals. But I am more at ease now knowing that he will not have a life-threatening reaction if he ate peanuts accidently somewhere. Thank you Dr. Devi, for your miraculous contribution to the world!

Sharon M.
Long Beach, CA

Bronchial Asthma And Body Ache

For approximately 15 years, I have suffered with frequent colds that turn into extended bouts with bronchial asthma and extreme weakness and fatigue. The doctors treated me with extensive doses of antibiotics, steroids, antihistamines, and cough medicine. I was usually depressed and so weak I could hardly move out of bed and had to get shots every day for weeks. Along with it, my stomach would gurgle and hurt for the duration of the medication. The doctors thought the stomach problems were due to steroids.

One night I had the flu and started wheezing, so I took some of the cough medicine I used to take. I had not had a cold since I moved out of Louisiana's humid climate, but I still had some of my old cough medicine. One hour later, I awoke, aching all over, with my stomach hurting and gurgling in that old familiar way. It brought back memories of the past when I had been so sick. I called Dr. Devi and she told me to bring the cough medicine. As soon as she treated me for it I got my strength back, was no longer depressed, and my stomach felt normal. I had continuous yeast infections for years. After being treated for toilet paper they disappeared.

When I started with Dr. Devi, I had severe body pain in my neck, head and shoulders. After being treated for the labels in my clothes (cotton and silk), the pain decreased dramatically.

Carole W.
Irvine, CA

From Permanent Disability to Fully Active Life!

The doctors had told me that I would be permanently disabled and that the medicine I was taking was to the absolute limit. That was when I could not walk across the floor without sitting down and resting because my breath was so short from the asthma I had suffered with for 12 years. A friend had told me about Dr. Devi, but I thought I would wait for a while because I had no experience with acupuncture. But finally, I decided that I had no choice but to go, see and find out what would happen.

My life has not been the same ever since! Previously, I had been tested for all kinds of allergies and the doctors I had gone to had told me that my asthma was from emotions, not allergies, because the testing I had done did not show anything significant. Devi tested me with the muscle weakness test and that showed I was allergic to almost everything I was coming in contact with, including my medication and my husband.

Since coming to her, I have been able to walk, bicycle, eat foods that I no longer react to because of the treatments. I am a voice teacher and had thought I would not be able to sing any longer. Now I am singing, my medicine dosage is minimal, and I am living a life that I did not think, for me, would ever again be possible.

I thought my life was, for the most part, over—as far as looking normal. That is not true, and with Dr. Devi's help, I am living a normal life now.

Margaret Brazil
Fullerton, CA

> ### *Tomato Caused Asthma!*
>
> *I used to get severe asthma and sinusitis whenever I ate tomatoes or anything made with tomatoes. After I was treated for tomatoes by Dr. Devi, I no longer get any reactions after I eat tomatoes.*
>
> *Raymond N.*
> *Orange, CA*

An allergic tendency toward asthma (although not the actual allergic disease) is inherited. It occurs much more frequently in families that have a history of various allergic conditions. However, in the case of asthma, the tendency toward this particular allergic ailment seems to be more frequently inherited than in most other allergic diseases. For instance, a woman who suffers from hay fever may have children who suffer from some other manifestations, such as dermatitis (rather than hay fever); whereas a patient who suffers from asthma is quite likely to have children who also suffer from asthma.

Allergens, like pollens, flowers, molds and dusts most often cause asthma in asthma sufferers. In addition, asthma can be caused by allergies to almost any: food (fish, shellfish, peanuts, food additives, food colors, sulfites), clothing, chemicals (fabric softeners, detergents, shampoo, body lotion), perfumes, synthetic substances (plastics, latex, rubber goods, ceramics, tiles, cookware) and natural substances (cotton, leather). Cold, heat, dampness and moisture can cause an asthmatic reaction as well as an allergy to one's spouse, children or another human associate, or even a pet.

What are the common triggers of asthma?

- Food, drinks, vitamins, food additives, and drugs.

- Environmental allergens: house dust, dust mites, industrial dust, mold, pollen, grass, weeds, animal dander, animal epithelial.

- Air pollutants: cigarette smoke, auto exhaust, smog, chemicals, infections in the respiratory tract.

> ### Bell Pepper And Asthma
>
> *I used to get asthma, indigestion and depression whenever I ate anything with bell pepper. After I was treated by Dr. Devi for the allergy to bell pepper, I was able to eat and enjoy bell peppers without getting any asthma or indigestion and depression. Since being treated for the allergy to eggs, I do not get any of the above-mentioned problems whenever I eat eggs.*
>
> *Dianne M.*
> *Los Angeles, CA*

- Weather changes: cold, heat, humidity, fog, dampness, damp heat and damp cold.

- Exercise (Yoga exercise helps with asthma if done properly).

- Emotional factors.

Sulfites are widely publicized substances that have been added as a preservative to salads and potatoes in restaurant salad bars and in the fast food industry. The intention was to maintain freshness (or at least the appearance of freshness and flavor) as these vegetables sit out in display cases for long periods of time. Unfortunately, sulfites are salt derivatives of sulfuric acid, which many asthma sufferers are highly allergic to.

Helen, a 65-year-old patient, ordered taquitos with very tart guacamole sauce at a restaurant. She took the leftovers home for dinner. A couple of hours after eating, she suffered a severe asthmatic attack. Later, it was discovered that the sulfite added to the guacamole sauce, to preserve its beautiful green color, had triggered her asthmatic attack. The use of sulfites in foods is banned in California, but it is legal to use "whiten-all," which acts just like sulfites and also causes many allergic reactions, especially in asthma sufferers.

Asthma and Sinusitis

I came to Dr. Devi through a friend in 1985. I suffered from asthma since childhood. During the last 7 years, I developed severe sinusitis. I was on antibiotics at least 20 days a month. My symptoms were sinus headaches, shortness of breath, coughing and wheezing. Within the first two months, my sinus headaches were reduced by 90 percent. By then, the coughing and wheezing were virtually gone. I was treated by NAET for 8 months and I was completely free of symptoms. Previously, I tested positive for grasses, pollens and trees. As per her advice, I waited for 10 months more after completion of NAET to do a traditional allergy testing (RAST). I tested negative for grasses, pollens and trees this time. I am free of asthma and sinusitis for the past 14 years! Thanks to Dr. Devi and NAET.

Jimmy A.
Anaheim, CA

A 44-year-old woman had a history of asthma since childhood. Finally, through NAET, she was found to be highly allergic to bamboo. The bamboo caused an energy blockage in her lung meridian. It was discovered that both her childhood home and current house were decorated with bamboo and cane furniture. Her asthma improved after her treatment for bamboo.

WHAT IS SINUSITIS?

Sinusitis is inflammation or infection of any of the four groups of sinus cavities in the skull, which open into the nasal passages. Sinusitis is not the same as rhinitis, although the two may be associated and their symptoms may be similar. The terms "sinus trouble" or "sinus congestion"

My Chronic Nasal Infection Is No More

Shortly after beginning a new career in interior design, I suddenly contacted a nasal infection due to allergies that, up until then, I did not realize I had. The infection worsened until I finally was operated on to keep it from spreading into the brain and to alleviate the worsening pressure, frequency and intensity of asthmatic attacks. During that seven-year period I had allergy shots, cortisone shots, antihistamines, and antibiotics prescribed by numerous medical doctors, none of which worked. The year the infection worsened before the operation, I began seeing Dr. Devi who pinpointed some major allergens. After treatment for many of them, I found I no longer reacted to those particular allergens and I started on the beginning of the healing process. However, the degree of infection up until then hampered the body's ability to respond quickly; so the operation was necessary to assist the process and halt the spreading of the infection. Almost two cups of infectious materials were removed from six packed sinus cavities.

After the operation, I had asthmatic attacks to a lesser degree, but still had not cleared the body of continuing infection, and was unable to work. When Dr. Devi began assisting in the total elimination of the infection, the accelerated healing process began. Through diligence and persistence, Dr. Devi uncovered allergens (unrecognized by conventional medicines) that I had been exposed to through my work, such as resins, and formaldehyde, which were major contributors to my illness. Of course, many foods, plants, and other chemicals contributed towards my ill health, too. But it seems that NAET actually cured the body from reacting to those particular allergens. I had the sinus surgery in 1988. I haven't had any recurrence of my sinus infections or asthmatic attacks for the past ten years. I did not have to give up my job as an interior decorator-designer, which I love so much. I am so fortunate to have discovered Dr. Devi and NAET.

Shirley Reason
Diamond Bar, CA.

are sometimes wrongly used to mean congestion of the nasal passages. Most cases of nasal congestion are not associated with sinusitis.

Bina, a 44-year-old female schoolteacher, suffered from a severe, hacking, dry cough for 18 months. She tried various prescription medicines to stop the cough with no success. Her cough plagued her constantly. She could hardly sleep during the night. Frustrated with this unsolved problem, Bina came to the Nambudripad clinic. She was tested by an allergist and found to be allergic to dusts, insects, grasses and pollens. She was treated for most of the foods, fabrics, dusts, grasses, pollens and chemicals in her environment without any positive results. Finally, she was found to be allergic to her acrylic nails.

Questioning her further, we discovered that 18 months ago she had started using acrylic nails to cover up her brittle nails. Bina removed the

---

My Chronic Cough Was Cured By NAET!

I suffered from severe dry cough for four years. I coughed throughout the day. It became worse at night after I would go to bed, and early in the morning when I woke up. I tried Western medicine, holistic medicine, and homeopathic remedies for four years. Nothing gave any relief. I changed my bed linen to 100% cotton, kept my home free of dust, used air and water purifiers. I tried every possible treatment known to get relief. Then I was guided to Dr. Devi by a friend. She evaluated me in her office and, on the very first visit, asked me if I was using any special mouthwash. I used this special mouthwash every night before I went to bed and every morning after I brushed my teeth. She treated me for the mouthwash. I had to avoid it for 40 hours. My cough stopped, just as if someone had turned off a switch, after the treatment for the mouthwash. Now I use it regularly without any trouble.

Marion S.
Costa Mesa

My Asthma Medicine Caused My Asthma!

I used to get severe asthmatic attacks. I was told to take asthma medicine. Whenever I took it, my asthma got worse. Dr. Devi discovered that I was allergic to it. She treated me and now I can take my medication to reduce my asthma.

Mary B.
Anaheim, CA

nails for a day to see if that made any difference in her cough. To her amazement, she stopped coughing completely as soon as she removed the nails. The next day she was treated for the nails, and her cough of 18 months was gone.

Della, a 47-year-old patient, suffered from chronic asthma and nasal polyps. She worked in an art shop and was on disability for seven years. After her evaluation in our office, we discovered that she was allergic to formaldehyde, one of the ingredients in hundreds of substances around her in: paints, picture frames, fabrics, name tags on dresses, pressed woods, leather goods, plastics, finishing materials in many items, decaffeinated coffee, embalming fluid, ice cream, etc. Her asthma became controlled after successfully being treated for formaldehyde.

Like other allergic conditions, asthma responds very well to NAET. When beginning treatment, it is always better to combine Western medical treatments with NAET for better and faster results. After you are treated for the basic items, you can evaluate your symptoms and try to gradually reduce the dosage of any medication that you may be taking.

Ron, 44, responded well to the treatment for diphtheria, clearing his chronic bronchitis. He had inherited the tendency toward allergies from his mother, who almost died from diphtheria when she was seven. The reaction to diphtheria was manifested in him as bronchitis, sinusitis and arthritis.

Kelly, an 11-year-old girl, had severe postnasal drip and sinusitis for two years. Her family also had a water filter installed two years earlier. She was treated for the water chemicals and her problem was eliminated. Now, one year after treatment, she is still using the same filter system without any adverse effect.

Marianne, a 38-year-old woman, continued to have asthmatic attacks when in bed, despite having been successfully treated for pillows, mattress, fabrics, etc. Finally, it was determined that her rosewood bedroom set and chest of drawers were the culprits. After she was treated for rosewood, she no longer had attacks of asthma in her bedroom.

Sam, age 42, had a throat irritation and cough that always started at 4 p.m. and subsided by 8 p.m. He worked as a travel agent, and his busy hours were 4 - 6 p.m. His irritating cough made him very uncomfortable. After proper evaluation, it was discovered that he ate a certain brand of chocolate candy bar every day at 2 p.m. during his break time. By 4 p.m., the allergic reaction from the candy bar showed up as coughing spells. After treatment for chocolate, he did not have the problem again.

Asthma is not only a dangerous and distressing malady, but it also interferes with a person's ability to lead a normal life. If you suffer from asthma, you should receive prompt allergy treatment. Asthmatics should always carry inhalant sprays for quick relief in emergencies because an asthmatic attack can be triggered at any time from an unexpected contact with an allergen.

I Was Allergic to My Nasal spray

Every time I used nasal spray, my face would turn red. After NAET treatment, I could use nasal spray with no ill effects. Being asthmatic, I was taking two oral medications and using three inhalers. Since my NAET treatments from Dr. Devi for my inhalers, not only has my medication been reduced by 50%, but my oral medication has also been reduced.

Joyce Bastian
Newport Beach, CA

Environmental factors like pollens, grasses, cigarette smoke, cooking gas smell, frying food smell, perfumes, flowers, spices, burning smell, food seasoning smell, chemical smells, smell from fabrics, dust, mold, smell from animals, smell of body secretions (stool, urine, sputum, sweat, bad breath), etc., can trigger respiratory discomforts like cough, asthma, postnasal drip, throat irritation, etc. If you collect the items with the smell and treat with NAET, the allergen or its smell should not bother you after successful treatment.

Many people are allergic to the medication they take for relief. When they do not receive the expected relief from their medication, they complain to their doctors. Doctors will change to a different medication and if that doesn't work, move on to another. The doctor's and the patient's frustration can be reduced by learning NAET-muscle testing techniques (NTT). Doctors can check the medication through NTT before prescribing it. Pharmacists can check the allergy before they supply the medication to the patient. It is very essential to teach NTT to all practicing medical professionals and pharmacists. You should also learn the testing techniques in order to test yourself for the medications you are taking. You can screen allergy to the medication before you take them. This way, you can get relief from your symptoms instead of being frustrated by trying to look for different doctors and different remedies.

A 46-year-old woman had complained of severe sinusitis and respiratory problems, including asthma, for her entire adult life. When she was 18 years old, she was given cortisone injections at the hospital. She almost went into shock at that time but finally recovered from the episode. Soon after she came out of the hospital, she began experiencing severe sinus and upper respiratory problems. At age 46, when she was tested for cortisone, she reacted violently. After being treated for cortisone by NAET, her 28-year-old upper respiratory problems improved.

Cooking pans, Teflon coating on the pans, cooking sprays, kitchen materials like scrubbers, dishwashing soap, smells from: cooking, frying and seasoning, burnt food, popcorn popping, coffee brewing, meat cooking, old kitchen trash, spoiled food, rancid oils, unclean garbage disposal, cleaning chemicals, etc., can produce respiratory symptoms (asthma, sinusitis, coughing spells, dusty feeling in the throat, hay fever-like symptoms and sensation of choking) in sensitive individuals.

For her whole life, a 54-year-old female could not tolerate the smell of fried oil. Whenever she smelled any deep-fried food, she ended up with severe asthma. She was treated in our office for heated oils. Now, not only can she smell the oil, but she can also cook and eat with the family without having any trace of upper respiratory problems.

Cigarette smoking smell can trigger asthma in sensitive individuals. Such people have to isolate in their own house most of the time. They cannot go in crowds, movies, shopping malls, airplanes, entertainment parks, restaurants, etc., for fear of getting asthma. Lately, smoking is restricted in many areas in this country. Even so, smokers find their ways to pollute public areas with smoke, making it hard for smoke-sensitive individuals to live a normal life. NAET can eliminate the allergy to smoke and asthmatics can survive in smoky neighborhoods with ease.

Allergy to Wool and Cigarette Smoke

I have had a lifetime of allergies, including asthma, hay fever, sinus problems and eczema. Two of my worst allergies were to wool and cigarette smoke. I had become so allergic to wool that I could not wear it or be around anyone who wore it without choking up, developing a headache, raspy throat, and often an asthmatic attack. Since Dr. Devi's treatment for wool, I am able to wear wool for the first time in many years without producing any unpleasant symptoms. Allergy to cigarette smoke was crippling me socially. The treatment for cigarette smoke has given me more comfort socially since I don't have to isolate myself from friends. I don't know how to express my gratitude to Dr. Devi for discovering this new treatment method to eliminate allergies permanently.

Gene Fowler
Fullerton, CA

If you are sensitive to smoke, you can also be sensitive to other fumes in the air. Fireplace smoke, smell from coffee brewing, popcorn popping, cooking smell, smell from gasoline, automobile exhaust, etc., can also trigger asthma in asthmatics.

It is helpful to use air purifiers in the house if you are sensitive to these smells. There are many chemical and odor free products available to help alleviate your symptoms. During the initial NAET treatments, such aids will be beneficial. After the successful completion of NAET, you will be able to live among all these smells without them affecting your health.

Fear Triggered His Asthma

Every Saturday, my seven year old son suffered from asthma. Medication or sprays did not help him at all. I had to take him to the doctor's office or emergency room. Just by sitting in the emergency room waiting area, his asthma would go away. Saturday was his father's turn to take him for the weekend. Since he was not feeling well on Saturday night, he could not go with him. When I brought him to Dr. Devi, she found that the cause of his asthma was an emotional issue.

He was afraid to go with his father because he would have to spend the night in his room with his gay roommate. So he began having asthmatic episodes, spending Saturday evening in the emergency room. Then Sunday, his father would take him out for a couple of hours. After he was treated for his allergy and fear of his father's roommate, he stopped having Saturday night asthma.

Belle Cole
Fullerton, CA

Emotional factors can also trigger cough, asthma, sinusitis, bronchitis or any other upper respiratory disorder. Even if the cause is emotional, it can produce physical and physiological symptoms.

Five-year-old Ray was addicted to bottle-feeding. He felt comfortable with bottles. He refused to eat food any other way. His mother had to puree all his food and feed him through the bottle with a large hole in the nipple. This became his routine. Mother wanted to wean him off the bottle. Every time she would take away his bottle and try to spoon-feed him, he would develop flu symptoms and fever ranging from 102-104 degree Fahrenheit. Then he would lose his appetite and refuse to eat any food. The child cried for hours if he did not get the bottle. His parents did not like to see him crying. Crying caused upper respiratory problems, so his worried mother would give him the bottle again. As soon as he had the bottle, his fever would come down to normal and he would fall asleep. When he woke up, he would be normal again.

Hay Fever

I suffered from hay fever ever since my childhood. I was told by other medical professionals that I could reduce the symptoms by drugs, but not eliminate them. Then I studied NAET and found out that I was very allergic to milk. I drank two glasses of milk daily. When I was treated for my milk allergy, my lifelong bout of hay fever left me. I am free again to enjoy milk without being bothered by my hay fever.

Dr. Tyler Anderson, IA

This went on for four months. It was very difficult to break his habit. Finally they decided to go to Hawaii for a week. After they arrived, they told him that they forgot to bring the bottle with them, but when he got back he could have the bottle again. Until then, he would have to eat like his mom and dad did. He was also bribed with a toy. He agreed to this arrangement. With different activities in Hawaii, he forgot about the bottle for a week. When they returned, Ray did not like to drink from the bottle anymore. Our brain adapts to new habits easily.

During NAET evaluation, the NAET doctor— before proceeding with the treatments—checks out all these factors. If practiced regularly, it takes only a few seconds to rule out all these unusual factors. A NAET practitioner is well trained to test and determine the influences of emotions in the present health conditions.

If not taken care of, asthma can turn into emphysema, in which the inner lining of the lungs and the air bags (alveoli) lose their elasticity. This makes it hard for the air to go in and out of the lungs freely. Oxygen exchange between the lungs and outside air becomes difficult. In advanced cases, the expanded air bags inside the lungs give the sufferer the appearance of someone with a barrel chest. In the early stages, the patient can get prompt relief with NAET.

CHAPTER 15

ALLERGY OF THE SKIN

Skin allergy is extremely important and includes many allergic conditions, ranging from ordinary hives to severe atopic dermatitis or eczema. Skin allergies are visible to the patient, and they usually receive more attention than any other allergic problem. When they clear up and the skin returns to a normal condition, the results are so dramatic and pleasing to the patient that allergy treatment seems almost a miracle.

Symptoms of allergy vary from person to person. It depends upon many factors: the status of the immune system, degree of involvement of the organs and systems, age, and degree of inheritance. There are many types of conventional allergy tests available to detect allergies today. The most reliable, convenient, and least expensive method of allergy testing is through NTT.

Atopic dermatitis seems to be hereditary in nature. Contact dermatitis is caused, most of the time, by external contact with some allergen: wool, cotton, polyester, other fabrics, cosmetics, etc. Atopic dermatitis is an inflammation of the skin, often called eczema. It causes the skin to become patchy, with flat reddish eruptions, occurring most frequently in the folds of the neck, back of the ears, on the wrists, the arms, the groin, back of the knees, on the bend of the elbows, and in the armpits. It occurs on the surface of the flexor muscles (which serve to bend a limb or part of the body) and where irritation occurs through friction. It may occur on any part of the body, but almost invariably begins on one or more of the flexor surfaces.

My Eczema Is Gone!

Your treatments using Nambudripad's Allergy Elimination Techniques have produced quick, dynamic results for me. If I didn't understand the science behind NAET, I would truly deem it a miracle. I have suffered with eczema since I was a child. I've seen general practitioners, allergists, and dermatologists through the years, but never found much relief. The dermatologist I've been seeing over the past few years, who is also an associate professor at a local university medical school, told me there is no cure for eczema. Cream, lotions, and pills fill my briefcase. And no longer do I suffer the embarrassment of walking around with rashes on my body. The mental anguish of a lifelong problem is gone. And I don't have to poison my body with prescription drugs that do nothing but mask the symptoms.

I really do believe you will revolutionize modern medicine with your discoveries. It is time for the medical community at large to open their minds to greater understanding and begin to address allergy at its most fundamental level – energy. NAET is not hocus-pocus, it is energy medicine. I am a living testimonial to the wonder of NAET. Your treatment program has changed my life in a significant way, and for that I am grateful. Keep up the good work – your mission will no doubt change the world. When the problem recently moved to my eyelids and cortisone treatments were completely ineffective, I reached a point of desperation that ultimately led me to your clinic. In just two NAET treatments, 95% of my eczema is gone. No longer do I carry tubes of cortisone.

Kevin Glenn
Santa Margarita, CA

When atopic dermatitis occurs in infants, it is called infantile eczema, or "cradle cap" when it occurs on the scalp. As a rule, infantile eczema begins at about the age of two or three months and usually appears first in the form of a rash on the cheeks. In many infants, it is limited to the face, scalp, and neck. Frequently, however, it spreads to the arms, trunk and legs, and may become generalized over most of the body. Redness, blisters, eruptions, oozing, crusting, thickening and hardening of the skin characterize the skin lesions. It is often accompanied by intense itching, so that the baby must have his hands tied or covered with mittens to keep him from scratching. Infantile eczema is usually caused by foods. In later life, other substances (pollens, grass, fabrics, etc.) can cause eczema.

Contact dermatitis may be caused by baby oil, soaps, shampoo, clothing, diapers, laundry detergents, water, and talcum powder, etc. A six-month old baby was brought to our office with infantile eczema. Her entire body was covered with eruptions and scabs. Scaling and blisters made by scratching herself had turned the baby into a dreadful sight. She had her hands protected by cotton mittens. The mother had the baby clad in a cotton dress, cotton sheets, etc. Surrogate testing was done to determine her allergies. Since food testing by the computerized allergy tester or any other method is not reliable for infants, surrogate testing comes in very handy. Her allergies were determined and the treatments started. She was found to be very allergic to vitamin C, milk, cotton, and polyester. Within a very short time, after the causes were removed, her skin cleared up and she became a normal baby. The baby's paternal uncle had asthma, and her maternal aunt had arthritis, hay fever, and migraines, which indicated a strong allergic inheritance.

Another infant, six days old, developed rashes, huge hives, and irritability soon after coming home from the hospital. The rashes got much worse, and it was hard to put a diaper or any clothing on him. The infant was found to be allergic to mother's milk, cotton, and baby formulas. The baby's skin cleared up very nicely after being treated.

A two-year-old was brought to the office with severe itching and hives. This child was allergic only to fish. The parents were very strict and never fed fish to the child. She drank only formulas, but the parents cooked fish at home almost every day. The smell of fish caused the dermatitis.

Fourteen-year Itch!

For 14 years, I suffered from an itch around the left side of my waist line, which caused my skin to turn dark brown. I was tested for skin cancer, treated for candida, yeast, and went through cleansing programs of various kinds over the years with no results. My itching began spreading into my thighs instead of getting better. Finally, I discovered Dr. Devi. In her office she tested me for elastic and found that it was the cause of my problem. Since I was not allergic to very many foods, she treated me for the elastics on my first visit. What relief I got from that one treatment! My waistline never itched again!

Pam . B
El Segundo, CA

For seven years a ten-year-old girl had very itchy, scaly skin on the back of both palms. Her parents had tried many different doctors and different medicines to find some relief for the problem. She was found to be allergic to egg white and took seven treatments by NAET to clear it. She was not fed eggs, but eggs are in a variety of food items: mayonnaise, salad dressing, and cookies, and even in some shampoos. At the end of the session her hands cleared.

A three-month-old infant had a severe "cradle cap," itching and rashes on different areas of the body. This infant was found to be allergic to the wheat bread his mother ate every day, causing the itching and rashes throughout his body. He was allergic to wheat and was exposed to it through the mother's milk. Most of the time, infantile eczema disappears after three years of age. Allergic manifestations can occur from time to time later with exposure to various other allergens.

A female patient was allergic to the peanut butter sandwich she made for her son every day. She developed deep furrows in the palm just by handling the peanut butter. After she was treated for peanuts by NAET, her hand cleared within 24 hours. A 64-year-old woman had severe rashes and itching on her hand and had developed many open wounds that started to weep. Questioning her, it was discovered that she had bought a hose two days earlier, which was causing her dermatitis.

Alcohol is another item that has a strong tendency to cause dermatitis. A 50-year-old man suffered from contact dermatitis, rhinitis and mild dry cough for eight years. He had seen an internist, a few dermatologists and a pulmonologist in the past. He didn't receive much help from anyone. In our office, NTT revealed that his problems were related to something he was drinking everyday for eight years. His history revealed that he had a glass of wine every night with his supper. "How long have you been drinking wine with supper?"

He paused for a moment to recollect his memory and said, " Eight years to be exact. I had my first heart attack eight years ago and my cardiologist suggested that I drink a glass of wine with supper every night. I have followed his orders faithfully."

The wine was good for his heart, but not for the rest of his body. He was allergic to wine and it affected his lung and large intestine meridian, giving rise to skin and lung-related problems. After being treated for alcohol, his problem disappeared and has not returned. He still follows his cardiologist's order and drinks a glass of wine every night with his supper.

It is easy to trigger any kind of allergic reaction with any kind of substance. Therefore, it is best for you to learn to test before buying clothes, groceries or any other items. Even if you have been treated for multitudes of things, you can still react to substances you have not been treated for. If you ingest these substances by mistake and do not get treated by NAET or other means, the reaction can last, on average, three to twenty-one days. In some extreme cases, allergies from ingestion do not clear for years.

A nine-year-old girl ingested a special brand of peanut butter, and an allergic reaction manifested itself as involuntary body jerks. At the end of three years, when the exact sample of peanut butter was found and treated, her involuntary body jerks disappeared. This shows that the allergic reaction can stay within the body for an unlimited time, even though in most cases it clears up in 21 days.

A 34-year-old woman had severe allergic rashes all over her face, neck, shoulders and scalp due to her hair dye. After treatments, she could use a dye similar to the earlier one without any trouble. However, she encountered problems if she used other brands.

A seven-year-old girl developed rashes every winter. She was allergic to the sweat suit she was wearing. A 37-year-old hairdresser had to work wearing cotton gloves for four years because of her severe, weeping skin rashes on both hands. She was allergic to the water in the house she had moved to four years earlier. Another housewife used fresh lemon to clean her silverware and developed dermatitis on both hands. She was allergic to the lemon. A 46-year-old writer had eczema on his right hand. He was found to be allergic to the stainless steel pen he was using.

Another man, who had suffered the first attack of eczema at the age of five, did not consult any allergist until he was 46. By that time his entire body was covered with atopic dermatitis, which had become chronic and had so thickened and distorted the skin that the scars are likely to be permanent. During this 40-year period, the eczema had gradually spread over the entire body and was complicated by hay fever and asthma. Unlike some cases of childhood dermatitis, his symptoms did not decrease as he entered puberty. They remained present at all times and gradually increased in intensity.

When he finally consulted an allergist, he was tested and found to be sensitive to a number of foods, pollens, and other inhalants (animal epithelial, pollens, dust) as well as the medicines he was using for internal and external application. After he tried traditional allergy treatments without positive results, he came to our office. He was treated for various food allergies, fabrics, and environmental substances and showed marked improvements in his condition. However, the scars were so deep and of such long duration that his skin will probably not return to a normal state for years, even though he is absolutely asymptomatic. This is an example of neglected symptoms that are nearly impossible to correct. Had this patient consulted an allergist and received proper allergic treatment before the dermatitis became so severe, it would have cleared up entirely, without leaving any scars.

Poison ivy and poison oak are both classic examples of allergens that can cause contact dermatitis. The response to these plants is a true allergy, since not everyone reacts to them, and many times prolonged contact does not bring allergic reactions. In other individuals, one contact is sufficient to sensitize them.

A woman went on vacation at a mountain cabin and, while there, contacted poison oak, which caused a massive reaction in her. She had severe itching, blisters and hives all over her body. She went to the nearest emergency room and got cortisone shots and antihistamines, which she took for ten days.

She was still itching badly and could not obtain any relief with antihistamines when she was brought to our office. In two treatments, she was no longer itching or hurting. It took a few days for her lesions to heal. She made the mistake of breaking those blisters and draining the lymph, so the skin became infected. She had to take penicillin to prevent infection even after she cleared the allergy for poison oak. You must be careful about secondary infections because, in some cases, they can even be fatal. The primary cause may have been an allergy; but if that is not taken care of, the secondary infection takes over even if the primary cause is cleared, and can linger on until it is also handled.

There are many people allergic to their jewelry, gold, nickel, and other metals. A 39-year-old woman developed asthma from the jewelry cleaning lotion she used in her trade. A jeweler developed contact dermatitis to the sulfuric acid he used as a cleaning agent. He had to wear gloves all the time because both his hands had deep wounds.

Simon, a seven year old, suffered from a strange looking dermatological problem since he was 9 months old. His entire body itched all the time, even in his sleep. New blisters formed all over the body, mainly on his hands, legs and face every couple of days. They turned into pustules, draining pus, lymph and blood, before turning into scabs. By then another set of blisters and pustules were on their way. This poor boy was caught in the middle of an itching-blister-pustule-scab cycle. His desperate parents took him to every doctor and dermatologist in town and every specialist that they have heard of in Europe and the U.S. Simon took many kinds of antibiotics, mega-vitamins therapy, fatty acid and amino-acid therapy, went through mercury detoxification, parasite detoxification, yeast and candida program, vigorous liver and colon cleansing program and ate special sugar, spices, chemical and pesticide-free diet. In spite of all their attempts, Simon's IBPS cycle continued.

Finally, he was referred to us by one of the detox clinics. Through NTT, it was revealed that he was allergic to a fabric he was in contact with on a daily basis that was causing his skin problem. His parents brought a sample of all the different fabrics he was coming in contact with. One piece of fabric was a velvet-like material from a sofa in his grandmother's room. She moved in with the family when he was 9 months old and occupied the one bedroom house adjacent to their house on the same lot. She had moved her old sofa into the house. She took care of him when his parents went to work so he came in contact with the sofa for many hours every day. When he was treated successfully for the sofa (it took 18 days to clear the allergy), his skin cleared up. He no longer had the IBPS cycle.

Another patient, age 44, who worked as a hair dresser for twenty years, had a severe yeast problem. He was found to be allergic to human hair. Due to an allergy to fabric, a patient developed an unusual case of dermatitis that only affected his arms. After a thorough investigation, it was found that the special wool that was used to upholster his favorite chair caused his dermatitis.

Fur is often responsible for contact dermatitis, and dyed furs are especially likely to cause this type of allergic reaction. One woman developed dermatitis that first began on her face and neck, eventually spreading over her entire body surface. It was caused by the dye in her fur coat.

Stockings are sometimes finished with an alkaline substance that causes an allergic response in most allergy-sensitive people. When this is the cause of the dermatitis, washing will usually render the stockings harmless. But when it is caused by some synthetic, such as those used in the manufacture of rayon and nylon stockings, good detective work is needed to find the cause. The same type of contact dermatitis may be caused by various articles of clothing made from cotton, wool, silk, or synthetic materials.

Sometimes the cause of contact dermatitis is so unusual as to seem almost unbelievable. Such is the case of a man who developed hives on his hands when his dog licked them. He was allergic to his dog's saliva. Dog hair caused no problems for him. An executive for a big firm who spent many hours each day speaking into a dictating machine developed dermatitis around his mouth and on his right hand. He was found to be allergic to the plastic material of the mouthpiece, which he held in his right hand and pressed against his face.

A librarian who constantly handled old books developed dermatitis of her hands. It was found that she was sensitive to the glue that was made from fish products. Printers are very often sensitive to a fine lacquer-type of spray that is used for drying inks so they will not smudge. Sometimes the sensitivity is to the spray as an inhalant and, sometimes, as a contactant. A person's trade, profession, or occupation may involve contact with a wide variety of dyes, chemicals, soaps, detergents, bleaches, plants, flowers, bulbs, woods, fabrics, varnished or natural wood furniture, clothing, lacquers, rubber vulcanizers, foods, oils, greases, yeast, metals, drugs, metal polishes, celluloid, formalin, cosmetics, perfumes, and countless other substances.

Bakers are likely to become allergic to flour, sugar, and palm or cottonseed oil while barbers are very likely to contact quinine, resorcin, mercury and sulfur in hair tonics. Dentists sometimes develop a severe dermatitis due to pain deadeners. Insect exterminators are in contact with chemicals such as arsenic, formalin, sodium chloride and pyrethrum, which are used in sprays and insecticides. People in the carpet business and furriers come in contact with arsenic and paraphenyl enediamine, which are used in treating and dying the furs, as well as in the treatment of animal dander. Gardeners are in contact with various plants, arsenic, nicotine, insecticides, lime and fertilizers. Jewelers work with cyanide and sulfuric acids. Nurses are in contact with bichloride, formalin, medicated alcohol, various antiseptics and drugs. Painters use turpentine, varnish remover, varnish, lacquers, linseed oil, aniline dyes and the lead that is in the paint. Printers are in contact with arsenic, artificial coloring, and hydrocarbons in ink as well as paper, lead, and various compounds that are used to speed up the drying of the inks. Men who work in the tanning industry work with bichromate and hydrochloric acid as well as the skin of the animals. There are hundreds of others whose trades, occupations, or professions may bring them into contact with various allergens.

The acute type of urticaria (sudden skin rashes-hives) can be caused from foods like strawberries and other berries, corn, cantaloupes, peaches, fish and shellfish. The chronic type, which sometimes persists over a period of several years, is more often caused by some basic food such as eggs, wheat, milk, oranges, chocolate, onion or other vegetables. Shellfish is responsible for great many causes of hives. Such was the case of a young man who was very fond of fish, but got severe swelling of his face and throat immediately after eating it, then severe rashes all over the body within a few hours of eating. He was treated by NAET and now eats fish almost every day without any problems.

Another woman suffered from hives on her face and severe migraines after she ate. She was found to be allergic to almost all foods and fabrics. When she received treatment for most basic foods, she was cleared not only for her headaches and hives, but also from fabrics without any further treatments.

A girl who was under treatment for hay fever and asthma also had occasional attacks of angioneurotic edema. Among other foods, she was very allergic to turkey. After Thanksgiving dinner, she had the worst attack of angioneurotic edema every year. She was treated for turkey and did not get the usual attack after this year's Thanksgiving dinner.

My Cotton Bath Towel Caused My Hair Loss?

When I complained about my recent loss of hair, Dr. Devi suggested that I be tested for my cotton bath towels. I was allergic to them. After treatment, I noticed an amazing phenomenon. In the past, I had lost a lot of hair each time I washed my hair. The first morning I washed my hair following the 25-hour-treatment lay off period, I lost virtually no hair! I am sure it was the result of my treatment for cotton towel.

Medina S.

Allergy to Cosmetics

I had always been supersensitive to any cream, makeups, lotions, shampoo, conditioner, etc. My skin burned and turned blotchy red whenever I used even hypoallergenic products. The skin around my eyes became swollen and puffy and I experienced unbearable itching, especially around the sides of my nose. Sometimes I used to go around in a sneezing fit which left me all red and stuffy with frequent sore throats. I saw three different physicians and dermatologists regarding the severe itching and for these problems. All their comments were about the same, "if that is the only health problems you have, don't worry about it." A year and a half ago, Dr. Devi treated me for all the basic allergies and for lanolin and sheep wool. Lanolin, a derivative of sheep wool, is used in many cosmetics. She also had to treat me for some specific makeups. One by one, I was able to use them with no reactions whatsoever.

Elen Singer
Costa Mesa, CA

Other skin diseases that are known to have an allergic factor involved are dermographia, acne, pruritus, and psoriasis. A 27-year-old woman had severe psoriasis for the past 10 years. She worked as a hair stylist in two different locations, causing her to work seven days a week. She had no time for cooking. Being a vegetarian, a cheese sandwich was her daily lunch. She was found to be allergic to milk products. Her psoriasis cleared when she cleared the milk products.

Acne usually clears with good nutrition after treating for allergies to vitamin C, sugar, fats, starches, iron, zinc and vitamin A.

Acne Rosacea is mainly due to blockage in the spleen. B complex, grains, corn, sugar, alcohol, fats, hormones and their combinations are usual offenders.

Scabies

In March of 1997, I contracted some kind of chigger which left bite marks on the back of my calves. I believe I got these from riding horses, because it happened a second time after I was near horses.

So when in early May of 1997, I began to itch here and there on my body without a rash, I assumed somehow I had picked up body lice and was having a recurrence. I could feel what seemed like something crawling on me, but couldn't see anything. There was no rash or bite marks ever during this experience.

A medical doctor friend called me from out of state and asked how I was. I told him I was terrible and explained my running bout with mites, lice, chiggers, whatever…I just knew I had something because I could feel them crawling on me. I told him about picking something up that did leave a bite in March. The doctor said it sounds like a clear cut case of "scabies." He suggested I go buy an over-the-counter remedy called "NIX," which is designed for lice, scabies and mites.

I washed in the shampoo and sprayed my carpets and furniture in my house with the lice spray. By that time, I was having a major reaction every day. Nothing helped — not the dog shampoo for ticks and lice, or the "Nix." I thought, my gosh, these things must be deep in my carpet and bedding.

So I bought plastic covers for my mattress, sprayed my floor with an insecticide called "Repel" that I bought at the drug store, which the label says can be sprayed on the body. I also used this on carpeting and furniture. I was that desperate to get rid of the itching.

Continued next page

Then I thought of going to Dr. Nambudripad. I mentioned my continuing problem to her. I was treated for all my basic allergies earlier, including pesticides, insects mix, cosmetics, and many environmental allergens a year ago. During my evaluation, she said, "It's not scabies or ticks. It's something you're eating." But I hadn't eaten anything new or changed my eating habits ever since her treatments a year ago.

"Have you started on a new vitamin therapy ?" I said no. I have not bought any new vitamins. She asked me to wait in the "thinking room" for a few minutes and think clearly. She has this quiet dark room next to her office where she will make the patients wait for few minutes to jog their memory to recall a past event like this. I was there just a few minutes. It came to me that it was probably something in a "NutriWest" vitamin. This was the only new item I had been consuming. I had these vitamins from three years ago and decided to use them up.

I immediately went home and brought all the vitamins I take along with the NutriWest vitamin. Her testing clearly showed that I was allergic to the NutriWest vitamin. She advised me to stay away from taking it for a week and return in one week with the vitamin container itself. As soon as I stopped taking these vitamins (which have a lot of good things in them and are very expensive), my itching went away by almost 90% in a couple of days.

The following week, I went to Dr. Devi with the vitamin container. She treated me for the vitamin and I was once again my normal self. I realized that a person shouldn't take even a great vitamin like NutriWest without checking for possible sensitivity.

Lil Toth
Laguna Beach, CA

Forty-nine-year-old May was getting treated for Acne Rosacea and was showing great improvement. One day she came to the clinic with huge acne all over her body. She was reacting to the red snapper she had been eating 10-12 times a week to clean her blood, as advised by some other medical expert. She was treated for red snapper and her hives cleared.

You have to be a good detective to find the allergen causing a particular problem. Identifying the allergens is usually the hardest part. Treatment is relatively easy. Various allergic manifestations of the skin are extremely important because of their influence on patients' lives. Anyone who is afflicted with a scarred, pitted, or crusted skin is handicapped both socially and economically. To this large portion of the population, allergy elimination brings new hope and the prospect of relief from chronic allergic skin conditions once considered hopeless.

CHAPTER 16

ALLERGY AND THE JOINTS

llergy can affect the joints like any other system. Joint disorders are called arthritis. Arthritis is a hereditary disease. It is characterized by an inflammation and/or pain in the small and big joints, often accompanied by pain. The joints usually affected in the body are upper back, lower back, mid-back (all the vertebral joints), knees, shoulders, fingers, toes, ankles, wrists, elbows, hips, tempero-mandibular joints (TMJ) and neck.

Many arthritic diseases are considered to be autoimmune disorders. Most of the autoimmune disorders are allergy-based. When you are allergic to things within you (e.g., foods, drinks, clothes, etc.), around you (fabrics, chemicals, furniture, etc.), your body begins to demonstrate its displeasure by giving rise to various types of aches, pains, and discomforts in the body. Depending on the characteristics of these symptoms of the allergic reactions, and the tissue involvement, we call these symptoms by certain medical names like osteoarthritis, rheumatoid arthritis, psoriatic arthritis, lupus arthritis, Sjogren's syndrome, etc. If we can trace the involved allergen(s) in these conditions, allergies can be eliminated with NAET and health can be restored. There are many forms of arthritis which are differentiated by the symptomatology, the causative agents, the area of the affected tissue and the manner it is affected.

15-Year-Old Arthritis

I suffered from severe joint pains in the back and right side of the hips for the last 15 years. The pain used to get very bad on certain days and I could not do many of my chores. I had to stay in bed for a couple of days or so whenever I had an attack of arthritis. I had these severe attacks of pain at least a couple of times a month. I had constant, nagging dull pain on my back and hip all the time. It was severe only on certain days. I had tried many prescription medicines with no positive results.

After I was treated by Dr. Devi for basic allergies and gold jewelry, my arthritic pain left me. I never knew I had allergies before I came to Dr. Devi. When she told me that I was allergic to all the foods I was eating, and the anti-inflammatory drugs and pain pills I was taking, I did not believe her. Now, after having been treated for most of the food items and my medication, I believe that food allergy was the cause of my arthritis. I can take my medications now without fear, if and when I need them.

Bobby M
Rancho California

Symptoms of allergy vary from person to person, depending upon many factors, such as the status of the immune system, degree of involvement of the organs and systems, age and degree of inheritance.

OSTEOARTHRITIS (OA)

Osteoarthritis, the most common form of arthritis, occurs when a thin layer of cartilage inside the joint breaks down. The rough ends rub against each other, and rub against the nearest tissue. The result can be pain, swelling and stiffness. Over a period of time, loss of joint mobility may occur. Without treatment, osteoarthritis can totally incapacitate a joint, but there is much you can do with NAET now to alleviate the pain of arthritis, slow or stop its progression, reverse the process, and rebuild the joints, and eventually even lead a normal life at whatever age you may be. According to my findings, the primary cause of osteoarthritis is food allergy: allergy to proteins, milk products, calcium, vitamin C, citrus fruits, fruit juices, nightshade vegetables (tomato, onion, chocolate, peppers and onions), salt, cartilage, ligaments, hormones, certain fabrics, etc. You can treat all of these allergies successfully with NAET.

Osteoarthritis usually develops around age 40 or over. Approximately 15.8 million Americans suffer from osteoarthritis. This debilitating illness runs in families. Almost three times as many women as men are affected.

Osteoarthritis is not simply a degenerative disorder, but rather a complex derangement of articular surfaces that involves the loss of normal collagen architecture followed by an attempt by chondrocytes to produce replacement cartilage. The replacement surface is less resistant to wear than the original. Over time, full thickness cartilage loss may develop on the articular surfaces.

The pain in osteoarthritis begins gradually: aching pain in one or more joints, stiffness, and loss of mobility. Inflammation may or may not be present. The pain may progress slowly, with bad spells followed by periods of relief. It often worsens after extensive use of the joint and is more likely to occur at night than in the morning. Stiffness tends to follow periods of inactivity, such as sleep or sitting, and can be eased by stretching and exercise. Pain seems to increase in humid weather. As the disease advances, the pain may

---

Hot Pepper Sauce

I suffered from a stiff neck for 4 weeks. I tried physical therapy, chiropractic adjustments, massages and even colonics (as suggested by a friend, to get rid of the toxins). It was difficult to drive since I couldn't turn my neck from side to side or look behind. Whenever I drove, I prayed that I would not be cited by the police for any reason. Finally, I was referred to Dr. Devi by a friend. In her office, she traced my neck pains to a Thai pepper sauce I bought a month ago. Since the sauce tasted good, I ate a few drops of it with every meal. Within two hours after receiving treatment for the sauce, my stiff neck disappeared.

Mindy C.
Los Angeles, CA

---

occur even when the joint is at rest and can keep a sufferer awake at night. If you can keep a food diary, you will be able to trace the culprits causing your osteoarthritis pains. Avoid those foods causing your pain; or find an NAET practitioner near you and get your allergy to your most favorite food treated and you may not need to live in that pain too long.

Symptoms of osteoarthritis include joint pains, typically worse with use and eased with rest, and joint stiffness after nonuse. Pain in the early morning upon awakening, and pain and stiffness while standing up from sitting in one position for a while are some of the early signs of osteoarthritis. The pain can become persistent and this is often caused by allergies, especially sensitivity to foods: wheat, nuts, spices, corn, croutons, tomato, bell pepper, potato, salt, iodine containing foods (onions, turnips, sea weeds), string beans, chocolate, fish, citrus fruits, cheese, milk, yam, peach, pear and artichoke. People with osteoarthritis are also allergic to dust, pollen, fabrics and metals. In many families, even where both husband and wife work, women often do most of the cooking. Frequent exposure to different spices and foods can make women more prone than men to osteoarthritis.

A young man of 18 was seen in our office for chronic debilitating backache. His grandfather had been crippled at age 46 due to arthritis throughout his whole body. When the grandson began to show signs of early arthritis, the grandfather forced him to get allergy treatments. The grandson was allergic to many foods and fabrics. His spine, at 18, began to show osteophytic changes. When he was treated for an allergy to milk and calcium, his backache improved. He was also treated for all known allergens and supplemented with proteins, vitamins and minerals. When new X-rays were taken three years later, his spine was cleared of osteoarthritis of the bone. This proves that bone spurs can be eliminated by allergy elimination at an early age and proper vitamin supplementation.

Jani, a 23-year-old patient, suffered from a peculiar kind of arthritis. Doctors diagnosed her condition as psychosomatic arthritis and could not prescribe any medicine to help her. She was very active and worked as a registered nurse in an intensive care unit. On certain days, she complained of severe multiple joint pains, and was absent from work several times a month. Her whole body would become stiff; at times, she could not even hold a pen without stiffness and pain in her hands. Her knuckles and wrists

Osteoarthritis

I suffered from degenerative arthritis all along my football career. I had the symptoms of arthritis before I started my football life. I played with the Green Bay Packers, Cleveland Browns, Pittsburgh Steelers and L.A. Rams for 14 years. I took pain pills, had my knees aspirated and the liquid drained off occasionally. Periodically, I took cortisone shots to reduce inflammation in my knees throughout my career. I was never free of pain, even with the number of different medications I took every day. Medication helped to assuage the pain. Sometimes, I got severe indigestion and abdominal cramps after taking medication. Then I was guided to Dr. Devi and divine NAET.

After a few basic NAET treatments, my knees stopped hurting. I was also allergic to pain medication and she treated me for my medications, too. Now I can take medication if I need it without getting any discomfort. It was a relief to find out that I didn't have to take pain pills throughout the day to get me going. I continued the NAET treatments for over a year. Now my arthritic pains and indigestion are nonexistent. No more cortisone injections, no more aspiration of the joints, no more draining the synovial sacs since 1996. I am not dependent on pain pills any more. Not only that, I am blessed to eat any type of food without having to worry about getting indigestion or pains in my knees as long as I test for allergies before I eat them. Dr. Nambudripad has taught me how to test my allergies by using muscle response testing. It is a life-saving technique. Everyone should learn it.

Occasionally I still get some allergies to the items I have not treated before. With the muscle testing knowledge in my hand, I am able to locate the offenders before they get me. I am enjoying every moment in my present pain-free world. Health is Wealth! Health is Great! I will barter anything for this health! I can't thank Dr. Devi and NAET enough for helping me find this new life!

Art Hunter, Orange, CA
Ex-Football Player / RAMS / Packers / Browns / Steelers

became swollen. She was forced to spend days in bed with aspirin and water. She suffered from this problem once a week, as sure as clockwork.

When we evaluated her, we discovered that she was making home-made bread with wheat flour for her husband once a week. She never liked wheat products, so she never ate them. She used to knead the dough with her hands. She was highly allergic to wheat, and contact with the dough was the cause of her once-a-week arthritis pain.

A 72-year-old woman came to our office complaining of generalized pain and discomfort. She was experiencing swelling and severe pains in multiple joints, especially in her hands and elbow joints, as well as in her hip and knee joints. She also had pain in her entire back. She was unable to bend over to pick up anything or get up from a seated position without help. She had been asthmatic as a child and was tested for allergies, by skin tests, but none were found. She was being treated by an arthrologist and frequently took a large number of pain pills. In our office, she was tested for food allergies by NTT and found to be allergic to almost all foods, but not to pollens or dust. She was also allergic to metals and fabrics. One by one, she was treated for the food items by NAET. At the end of two months, her health had improved by 90 percent. She was referred back to her arthrologist, who took her off all her medication. After five years, she still remains symptom-free.

A 24-year-old female nutrition student was taught about the value of millet in the diet. She was excited to share this knowledge with her family. She went to a health food store, bought the millet, cooked it and ate two meals with millet. The rest of her family ate the millet only once that day. The next morning she could not get up from bed. Her joints were swollen and hurting. Her mother brought her to our office. Millet was affecting her joints. After she was treated by NAET for millet, her joint pain improved. She was also highly allergic to grains and cleared for wheat, corn and barley. Arthritis had been one of her complaints since childhood. When she cleared the grains, she cleared the arthritis.

Another girl of 23, an assistant to a chiropractor, went to work one day and found she was unable to use her left arm. She had severe pain in her left palm and could not even hold a pen. The doctor thought she had a stress fracture and offered to take X-rays, which were negative. Within four hours her pain decreased. By the time she went home, the pain was com-

Frisbee Sports Injury

About 18 months ago, while I was playing frisbee golf, my left shoulder began to hurt. I continued playing, thinking the pain might disappear, but instead the pain grew worse. Over the next few months, I gave up playing, as the pain grew worse whether I threw the frisbee disc backhand or forehand. I hoped the rest would help my shoulder muscles recover, but the lack of activity or exercise seemed to aggravate the soreness.

For the last year, I exercised lightly in hope that the pain would go away. It didn't. It grew worse. Then about 6 months ago, I noticed that simply extending my left arm fully became painful. About 3 months ago, I visited my HMO and the doctor had X-rays taken. She prescribed physical therapy. I went for about 5 sessions over the past 4 weeks and I did the light stretching exercises recommended. The pain and stiffness were reduced only slightly. On a scale of 1-10 (ten being worst), the pain reduced from about a 6 to a 5. I continued to feel pain, stiffness and a lack of free movement even after 4 weeks of physical therapy. As I was seeing only slight improvement, I remembered my old knee injury and decided to go see Dr. Devi.

As Dr. Devi was treating me for the motion of throwing the frisbee disc, the pain began to immediately and dramatically subside. Within seconds, as Dr. Devi's treatment continued, the pain reduced from a 6 (or so) to where I felt no discomfort. And I felt as though I had no more stiffness nor constrictions of my movements. For all three previously painful motions – backhand, forehand, and reaching out as far as possible, the pain was gone! Prior to Dr. Devi's treatment, when I pressed on my left scapula area, the pain level was about 6. Now, it was only a 1 and hardly perceptible.

In October 1993, I severely strained my left knee throwing a frisbee golf disc. By June 1994, my left knee had been bothering me for about 9 months. In a few weeks, we planned to go on vacation. We had reservations for Sequoia and Kings Canyon National Parks. We hoped to do lots of hiking.

(continued on next page)

(continued from previous page)

I began seeing the HMO's (my insurance career) chiropractor. In the 5-6 months that I was under his care, he never alleviated the pain.

While under the care of the HMO chiropractor, I grew steadily worse. By June 1994, I could hardly walk, and my left knee was very weak and sore. Even putting weight on my left leg hurt. I had begun walking in ways to favor my left leg. Unfortunately, this compensation threw my hips and back out of alignment. After "one week of bed rest," the HMO chiropractor suggested that I shouldn't go on vacation because I was in such poor shape and pain. I finally realized that my health and our vacation were more important than the added cost I'd have to pay to a private doctor because the HMO denied coverage for Dr. Devi's treatments at that time.

Dr. Devi asked me what I was doing when I injured my knee. I demonstrated my throwing motion of the frisbee disc. She tested me to see if I was "allergic" to that motion. I was. As she began treating me for my "allergy" to the throwing motion, I felt my left knee relax, and the pain began to subside, and I experienced an immediate cessation of the pain and weakness. I was able, for the first time in months, to put weight on my left knee without feeling any discomfort. Over the next 10 days before our vacation, my knee's strength and comfort in walking increased dramatically. While we were in Sequoia and King's Canyon Parks, my knee never bothered me. I walked several miles every day, carried heavy (for me) 50 pound suitcases and boxes of reading materials. We had a wonderful time, thanks to Dr. Devi's perceptive diagnosis and appropriate treatment. Since that one treatment about three years ago, my left knee has felt perfectly fine!

Glen Bard
Fullerton, CA

pletely gone. At home she ate some corn bread, left over from the   previous night. Within a few minutes the pain in her arm returned, more severely than before. At that moment, she realized she was allergic to corn. Her friend brought her to our office to be treated for the corn allergy. She took three treatments with NAET, ten minutes apart. At the end of the third treatment, she no longer had pain in her hand.

Her history revealed that her grandfather died of a debilitating arthritis. Both of her parents suffered from severe arthritis. Her 62-year-old father was almost crippled with arthritis. We discovered she was allergic to most grains, spices and citrus fruits. After treatment for a variety of allergies, she was able to eat most of the food without producing arthritic symptoms. Later she said that she functioned well as long as she did not eat any allergic foods, but if she ate even one allergic item that she had not been treated for, she would immediately have joint pains and stiffness. She had no other health complaints. Osteoarthritis is mainly an allergy to calcium, grains and milk. We have had hundreds of people with osteoarthritis who eliminated their symptoms completely after they were treated for milk and calcium.

In my practice, I have noticed that certain food groups cause a particular type of pain in different joints or parts of the body.

Almost all patients with acute stiff necks are linked to string bean allergies. In most cases, potatoes affect the vertebral joints. Spices affect the interphalangeal joints and wrist joints. Peppers affect the ankles, neck, back and cause general body aches. Citrus fruits affect the knee joints. Onion and sugar affect the knees. Corn affects the feet (pin prick pain), hands, and causes general body aches. Grains (wheat, millet, barley, brown rice, oats and other grains) affect all the joints in the entire body and also cause brain fatigue and brain fog.

RHEUMATOID ARTHRITIS

Rheumatoid arthritis is a degenerative joint disease that is related to the wear and tear of aging and involves deterioration of the cartilage at the ends of the bones. Rheumatoid arthritis creates stiffness, swelling, fatigue, anemia, weight loss, fever and crippling pain. It often occurs in people under 40 years of age, including young children. Almost 2.1 million Americans suffer from this disease.

Rheumatoid arthritis begins in the synovial membrane. Many joints are affected, and rheumatoid arthritis often occurs symmetrically on both sides of the body. People generally have morning stiffness that lasts for at least an hour. X-rays shows changes in the bones that differ from those occurring in osteoarthritis. In rheumatoid arthritis, blood tests often show a specific antibody, known as the rheumatoid factor, which is not present with osteoarthritis. In another blood test, levels of a factor called erythrocyte sedimentation rate (ESR) are often elevated in rheumatoid arthritis, but they are generally normal in osteoarthritis. Rheumatoid arthritis also does not usually show up in the fingertips where osteoarthritis is common. Rheumatoid arthritis may be caused by an allergy to proteins, milk products, calcium, salt, B vitamins, synovial joint, gelatin, bacteria (streptococcus, staphylococcus, salmonella, etc.), and food chemicals.

A few cases of rheumatic arthritis were found to have their origin in allergies to foods, fabrics, the patient's own tissue from the joints (body secretions, like patient's own blood, ligament, synovial membrane) and different types of bacteria. After treatment for these items, the arthritis diminished.

A 43-year-old female was diagnosed as a rheumatoid arthritic. She was taking many pain pills to get her through the day. When she came to our office, she still had swelling, pain, and stiffness in multiple joints. She was found to be allergic to some herbal tea she had been taking for years to "cleanse her body." After she stopped taking this particular herbal tea, her pain and discomfort improved. After treating with NAET for this particular tea, she became free of her symptoms.

Another woman, age 36, visited a farm along with the school children. She ate cooked chicken there and became very sick upon returning home. The next two days she spent vomiting and purging and stayed home, drinking lemon water only. When she recovered from her illness, she began having joint pains; eventually she was diagnosed as having rheumatoid arthritis. Two years later, she was referred to our office for treatment. She suffered from joint pains when she came to us. NTT exams revealed that she was suffering from a salmonella infection. She was desensitized for salmonella. Upon passing the treatment for salmonella, she also was freed from her rheumatoid arthritis.

Rheumatoid and juvenile rheumatoid arthritis are types of inflammatory arthritis that attack the synovial membranes surrounding the lubricating fluid in the joints. The cartilage and tissues in and around the joints and often the bone surfaces themselves are destroyed. The body replaces this damaged tissue with scar tissue, causing the space between the joints to become narrow, developing folds and fusing together. As in osteoarthritis, the entire body is affected, instead of just one joint.

GOUTY ARTHRITIS

Over one million Americans suffer from the agonizing symptoms of gout, according to one of the latest CDC (Center for Disease Control) reports. Gout is a persistent metabolic disease, marked by uric acid deposits in the joints, which cause painful arthritis in many joints, especially of the feet and legs.

Gout is a type of arthritis (inflammation of the joints) that mostly affects men age 40 and older. It is nearly always associated with chronic hyperuricemia, *a long-lasting, abnormally high concentration of uric acid in the blood.*

Gouty arthritis occurs more often in overweight people and those who eat rich foods. That's why it is also called the "rich man's disease." Soft tissue swelling in one or more joints, pain, swelling and discomfort in the ankle(s) and the big toe, a high level of uric acid in the blood, and formation of uric acid crystals in the joints are classic symptoms. This illness is also closely related to other foods, mainly iron, sulfites, beef, corn, milk products, citrus fruits, fruit juices, onion, protein drinks, and tomato. A high level of uric acid in the blood test is the diagnostic tool.

In a man of 26, tomato was the culprit behind his gout. A 38-year-old woman was allergic to Mexican beans that caused her gout. Another woman, 42 years old, was allergic to her leather shoes, which caused her to suffer from gout-like pain.

PSORIATIC ARTHRITIS

Psoriatic arthritis is yet another kind of arthritis. It may affect any age, but it most commonly begins between 15 to 35 years of age. Normally, skin takes about a month for its new cells to move from the lower layers of skin up to the surface. In psoriasis, this process takes only a few days, resulting in a build-up of dead skin cells and the formation of thick scales. Psoriasis may be aggravated by cuts, burns, rash, and insect bites. Medications, viral or bacterial infections, excessive alcohol consumption, overexposure to sunlight (sunburns), general poor health, cold climate, and frequent friction on the skin are also associated with flare-ups of psoriasis. Psoriasis is not contagious.

Milk, cheese, casein, lactic acid, yogurt, whey, butter, vitamin D, chocolate, coffee, caffeine, potato, tomato, egg plant, pepper, onion, fatty acids and cucumber seem the worst culprits for this kind of arthritis. For 20 years, a 72-year-old female had psoriasis all over her body along with severe arthritis. She was found to be suffering from psoriatic arthritis.

She was eating cottage cheese every day even though she never used milk in any other form. After she was treated for milk and milk products by NAET, her psoriasis disappeared and her health greatly improved.

Within a few short weeks, a 16-year-old girl had developed psoriasis on her scalp, elbow joints, knee joints and back, suffering extensive joint pain. This girl recently had taken a special liking to avocado. She was found to be highly allergic to avocado, which can cause blockage in the spleen and kidney meridians. When she was treated for this fruit, her psoriasis and joint pains cleared up. Some shampoos and soaps also can cause similar reactions on the skin.

ANKYLOSING SPONDYLITIS

Another form of arthritis is ankylosing spondylitis. A 28-year-old chiropractor complained of stiffness of his back for years and he was diagnosed as having ankylosing spondylitis since age 17. He was found to be allergic to table salt. After he was successfully treated for salt (it took about 11 treatments on salt to desensitize him completely to salt), he was free of his symptoms. A 58-year-old woman complained of severe multiple joint pain and swelling of the joints. The pain moved from joint to joint at different times. She was allergic to salt and tap water. As soon as she was treated for these items, the wandering arthritic pain that moved from place to place improved.

PSORIASIS

I suffered from psoriasis and joint pains for seven years. My skin completely cleared up after I was treated for calcium mix, cheese mix, chocolate and vitamin F (fatty acids).

Theresa B.
Long Beach, CA

INTERMITTENT HYDRARTHROSIS

Another type of arthritis is called intermittent hydrarthrosis. This is a condition in which the symptoms are intermittent swelling and excess fluid in the joints. As we've previously discussed, the typical manifestations of allergy are edema and the production of fluids. This condition is caused mainly by foods, chemicals, and fumes.

Another interesting case is worth noting. A mother had three miscarriages, and then became pregnant again. This time, she was extra careful and took all the standard precautions to prevent another miscarriage. She had severe morning sickness throughout the nine months. Finally, she gave birth to a healthy boy. Ever since, she developed severe joint pains and gained a hefty 40 pounds. And this, even though she was a vegetarian and ate salads and low caloric food items. She came to our office about the time her child turned seven, and we discovered that she had an allergy to the child. This allergy was causing the joint pains, tiredness and obesity. The child was experiencing some minor problems as well. He was hyperactive, and usually did not perform well in school, although he somehow managed to maintain a B-grade average. He was very restless, had frequent nightmares, would grind his teeth in his sleep, and refused to make friends or take part in school activities or social functions.

The patient brought out another interesting fact. Whenever she slept with her husband and son in the same bed, she did not feel as much pain in the morning as when she slept with her son alone. She became very sick with body aches, nausea and stomach cramps. She was tested for her husband, and no allergy to him was found, nor him to her. This confirmed our diagnosis. When she was with her husband and son, the husband's strong energy neutralized the son's adverse energy and so she was not affected. When she was alone with the son, his adverse energy affected her, and in this case it showed up as joint pains. After she was treated for allergy to her son, she did not have any more arthritic pain. It also made a tremendous change in the son's personality. He became more amiable, was friendlier toward others, was able to study and his grades improved. He also stopped having nightmares and grinding his teeth. His relationships with friends improved, too.

LUPUS ARTHRITIS

Lupus erythematosus is still another kind of joint problem that is accompanied by general fatigue. Systemic Lupus Erythematosus (SLE) is a disease of unknown cause that may produce variable symptoms of fever, rash, hair loss, arthritis, pleuritis, pericarditis, nephritis, anemia, leukopenia, thrombocytopenia, and central nervous system disorders. It is an autoimmune disease that results in episodes of inflammation in joints, tendons, and other connective tissues and organs. Different tissues and organs become inflamed in different people, and the severity of the disease ranges from mild to debilitating, depending on the number and variety of antibodies that appear and the tissues and organs affected.

According to the latest statistical report by CDC, lupus can occur at any age but has its onset primarily between ages 16 and 55. It occurs more frequently in women. In children, the female-male ratio is 1.4 to 5.8:1; in adults, it ranges from 8:1 to 13:1, and in older individuals, the ratio is 2:1. The prevalence of SLE is estimated to be between 4 and 250 cases per 100,000 people. In the United States, the highest incidence is among Asians in Hawaii, blacks, and certain Native Americans. The risk of SLE developing in a black American female has been estimated to be 1:250. The prevalence is about the same worldwide. The disease appears to be common in China, in Southeast Asia, and among blacks in the Caribbean, but seen infrequently in blacks in Africa. In the United States, about 90 percent of the people who have lupus are young women in their late teens to 30's (mostly women in

Sprained Ankle

My eight year daughter sustained injury to her ankles frequently in the school while playing sports. I took her for NAET and the doctor discovered that she was highly allergic to her cotton socks and leather shoes. After she was treated for cotton and leather, she hasn't injured her ankle for two years now.

Barbara Cortez
Sun Valley, CA

their childbearing years), but children, mostly girls, and older men and women are also affected.

Symptoms include malar (facial) rash, skin rash, sensitivity to sunlight, canker sores, fluid around the lungs, heart, or other organs, arthritis, inflammation of the joints, swelling and redness of the joints, nervousness or panic attacks, butterfly sensation in the stomach, kidney dysfunction, low white blood cell count or low platelet count; nerve dysfunction, brain dysfunction, brain fog, anemia, presence of antinuclear antibodies in the blood test.

The few cases treated in our office were discovered to have allergies to fabrics and materials, rather than foods. A woman of 37 was seen in our office for the possible treatment of lupus. She attended the lupus clinic regularly. She complained of severe joint pains and extreme tiredness most of the time.

She said that, lately, painkillers failed to help. She had heard about acupuncture and herbal medicine and came to our office to find out if there was any chance of relief using these techniques. Little did she know that we had something better to offer.

As with all first-time patients and a few repeat patients manifesting new symptoms, she was evaluated and tested for every allergy. She did not have many food allergies. She showed no allergies to pollens, grasses or trees; however, she was found to be allergic to all fabrics and a few chemicals.

She was wearing all cotton materials, thinking that cotton was a good alternative to synthetics. Surprisingly, for her it turned out that she was more allergic to cotton than to anything else. She said that five years earlier, at about the time she was diagnosed with lupus, she were told that synthetic materials were harmful and that natural fibers like cotton were much safer to wear. She discarded all the synthetic materials in her household and replaced them with cotton, including sofa covers and curtains. When she was treated for cotton, polyester, wood, nylon, acetic, formic and tannic acids, she was free of her joint pains and her energy level also improved. When she visited the lupus clinic a month later, she was told she was in remission.

Within a few short weeks, a 16-year-old girl had developed psoriasis on her scalp, elbow joints, knee joints and back, suffering extensive joint pain. This girl recently had taken a special liking to avocado. She was found to be highly allergic to avocado. Allergy to avocado caused blockage in the spleen and kidney meridians. When she was treated for this fruit, her psoriasis and joint pains cleared up. Some shampoos and soaps also can cause similar reactions on the skin.

Mary, 26 years old, was under treatment for lupus at a lupus clinic. She frequently suffered severe joint pains, insomnia, mental cloudiness, poor memory, mental irritability and debilitating multiple joint pains. She was tak-

---

Lupus

For the past ten years, I suffered from severe lupus pain. My joints ached all the time. I could not sleep. My joints were swollen most of the time. When I came to Dr. Devi I was not functioning at all. I also had extreme fatigue and brain fog. Dr. Devi treated me for all the basics. By the time I finished about 12 treatments I felt much better. Now, after many treatments, I have a life. I do not hurt anymore. I go out and meet my friends. I have a social life now which once was one of my dreams. I am a self-employed accountant. I was allergic to paper and ink...the tools of my profession! I work full time. I can almost eat anything. Above all, I don't have lupus anymore.

Rosemary Depauw
Marina Del Rey, CA

Allergy To Cotton Or Lupus

I wanted to thank you, Dr. Devi, for eliminating severe joint pains associated with my Lupus Erythramatosis.

When you treated me for my cotton allergy in 1986, I noticed an immediate increase in energy. I did not have to clear my throat and the dull, low level joint pain that left me cranky and emotional vanished. While my blood panel still shows a positive ANA and other irregularities, the chief of Rheumatology at UCLA is very pleased with my progress. I have eliminated all use of anti-inflammatory and other prescribed drugs. I want to express my deepest gratitude for your most loving contribution to my health. I only hope that others are able to receive as much benefit from your treatments as I have.

Eternally Grateful,

Aviva S., O.M.D., Ph.D., L.Ac. / Los Angeles, CA

ing three different kinds of analgesics every three hours to control her pain. Extremely hot, cold or cloudy weather affected her immensely. On such days, she stayed indoors taking pain pills and warm water. When she was evaluated through NTT in our office, she was found to be allergic to all the fabrics she was wearing, but not to any food or drugs. She was treated individually for cotton, polyester, acrylic, nylon, plastics, and leather. At the end of the session, we found her symptoms of lupus had greatly diminished. Her bodily disturbances with the weather changes also disappeared. She had been visiting the lupus clinic once a month. When she visited the clinic after she cleared her allergies, she showed great improvement in her laboratory blood tests. Her doctor told her the best news — her lupus was in remission. Three years later, she remains absolutely symptom-free.

ARTHRITIS DUE TO AN ALLERGY TO FABRICS

Most of the sports injuries we see among school children happen due to some allergy to whatever they eat before the fall and/or something they wear while playing. Many children are allergic to socks, shoes, shoe inserts, shin splints, knee guards, grasses, concrete floors, etc. If you find out their allergies and treat them, you may be able to prevent many sports-related injuries.

63 year old Lorna suffered from sciatic neuralgia for 4 years. She was working in a hospital operating room supply girl. Her job was to check the inventory and fill up the supplies of caps, masks, gowns, pants, etc. When she was promoted to this job, the end of first week she took very ill with severe sciatic pain. It took two weeks before she could return to work. All laboratory and radiological tests came back negative. She was given physical therapy, rest and pain controlling pills. Doctors diagnosed her condition as psychosomatic arthritis since they couldn't find anything wrong with her. She was sad at this diagnosis because she knew she had pure pain. She was not a lazy person. She enjoyed the hospital work and took pride in it. Eventually, most of her joints began aching on certain days.

When we evaluated her, we discovered that she was allergic to the nurses' uniform, especially the while pant. She was treated immediately for the uniform, and on the following visit she reported that her sciatic pain stopped bothering her an hour after the NAET treatment.

David, a 14-year-old soccer player, frequently sprained his ankles. The cause of his frequent falls: his orlon/cotton socks and canvas shoes. After he received treatment for the socks and shoes, he never sprained his ankle again throughout high school. The chemicals used in tennis shoes, mercaptobenzothiazole (MBT) and dibenzothiazyl (DBTD) are allergens to many people, and are also known to cause cancer in rats.

A 30-year-old nurse had a similar problem. She complained of a severe tenosynovitis (pain in the thumb and metacarpal joint) of both hands, more severe on the right hand, that progressed and radiated into the elbow and shoulder joints. She had nine months of physical therapy along with many analgesics, but nothing gave her relief. Her physician referred her to our office. When we examined her, she was on disability from work because of excruciating pain and an inability to perform her nursing duties. She had severe insomnia because of the pain, and she also suffered from asthma.

She was treated for various allergens in our office with NAET. Her asthma and energy improved considerably and she slept better at night.

FIBROMYALGIA

Forty-nine-year-old Lynn suffered from fibromyalgia for eight years. She suffered from constant dull pain in her thighs, knees, legs and soles. It was very painful for her to get up from a chair after sitting for a few minutes. She noticed the pain worsened after she ate dinner at restaurants. She needed help to get up from the chair after dinner. She had restless leg syndrome that bothered her mostly at night, and with the result that she suffered from insomnia. She also suffered from frequent headaches, upper backache, mid-backache, lower backache, neck and shoulder pains and pain between the shoulders through the day. She was slightly overweight even though she ate small meals, drank plenty of water, exercised regularly and fasted with juices and water frequently. Her family doctor referred her to various specialists in the field of pain control. She also visited some special pain control clinics in this country and abroad (Canada, Mexico, Europe, China) in search of some relief from her agonizing aches and pains. She was referred to us by one of her friends, who was treated by us for her osteoarthritis in 1986 and still remains free from her arthritic pains.

In our office she was evaluated thoroughly using NTT. She was dressed in a beautiful black outfit with matching black pearls around her neck and on one wrist, a watch with black dial and black strap on the other. She also had worn a black hair band, handbag and black shoe. She was not very allergic to many foods. She tested slightly allergic to the NAET basic five groups. She was moderately allergic to salt mix and table salt. But amazingly, she was found to be highly allergic to the color black.

According to Lynn, she began gaining some extra pounds eight years ago. She began dressing in black outfits ever since to make her look thin. Her husband complemented her and others began noticing her whenever she dressed in black. She began liking black more and more. She even bought black bed linens, black night gowns and underclothing. She could easily recall the beginning of her fibromyalgia symptoms. It was just a few weeks after her conversion into black clothing.

My Arthritis Said Good-bye!
I suffered from severe arhtrittis on my right knee for over a year, and have gone through different kind of medical treatment, I have limited mobility and difficulty climbing the stairs and at night I could not cover my knee with blanket, it was very painfull even with a light cloth on top of it. I am very happy that after the NAET treatment for 6 weeks with Dr. Noratus Horas in Jakarta, my knee is pain free and now I can go to work, people and friends said that I look much fresher and younger, thank you very much.

Iswardi,
Kelapa Gading Jakarta Indonesia.
phone 62-21-4529895

She was advised to avoid wearing black for few days. She converted into other more suitable colors. Her pain was reduced by 50% just by avoiding black. Eventually, she was treated for black and she began wearing black outfits on and off. She still remains free from her unusual pains.

PAIN IN THE TEMPERO-MANDIBULAR JOINTS (TMJ PAIN)

Many people suffer from TMJ pain, and we have treated many cases. Chewing gum is one of the most common causes of TMJ disorders. Spices, salt, and sugar are a few other items that contribute to this pain.

These actual case studies show that arthritis and joint pains can be the result of any number of allergies. When examining causes of arthritis, the possibility of allergies to foods, fabrics, detergents, fabric softeners, different colored materials, environmental substances, animals and other human beings, etc., should be investigated. Today, if the root cause is traced, avoidance will give relief, and NAET treatment will eliminate the allergy-related root cause altogether. In this way, you can receive total freedom from any and all allergens without adverse reactions, and you, too, can *Say Good-bye to your pain disorders!*

CHAPTER 17

ALLERGY AND
THE GENITO-URINARY SYSTEM

As stated before, there is hardly any human disease or condition in which allergic factors are not involved. Further investigations into allergies and human ailments reveal new conditions caused by various allergic reactions. Any organ or portion of the body may be involved and the allergic responses may vary greatly. Causes of certain diseases previously unknown are now recognized to be entirely or partly allergic in origin. Bladder and kidney troubles, uterine dysfunction, ovarian cysts, hormonal dysfunction, abnormal uterine bleeding, amenorrhea, osteoporosis due to hormone deficiency, premenstrual syndrome, menopausal disorders, infertility, pelvic pain, pelvic inflammation, candidal vaginitis, other types of vaginitis, warts, endometriosis, vulvodynia, pelvic congestion syndrome, non-cyclic pelvic pain, mid-cycle pain, cyclic pain, herpes simplex, genital ulcers, cysts, tumors, infections of the reproductive organs, cancer, hypertrophy or hyperplasia of male or female reproductive organs, etc., all may be the result of certain allergies and secondary effects of allergic reactions.

Symptoms of allergy vary from person to person. It depends upon many factors such as the status of the immune system, degree of involvement of the organs and systems, age and genetic factors.

Many symptoms involving the genito-urinary tract are caused by food allergy. Food allergies should be checked first if someone comes in with a complaint of acute bladder or kidney infection. A 19-year-old female, married two months earlier, came to the office with severe pain of the lower back that had started five days earlier; by the fifth day she was also experiencing chills and fever. She had no complaints of frequent or painful urination, ruling out the possibility of a bladder infection. However, she did complain of severe frontal headaches. Her blood chemistry was normal, but the urinalysis showed possible kidney infection. She was given aspirin every four hours to relieve the fever and ampicillin (antibiotic) to bring down the infection. She drank a lot of water and rested at home for the next few days.

Her fever and infection started to come down, and she felt somewhat better. The third day she drank some herbal tea made of fenugreek. Within ten minutes she began to feel internal chills along with the onset of severe rigor that lasted almost forty minutes. At the end of the rigor, her temperature shot up to 105 degrees Fahrenheit, in spite of the aspirin and ampicillin. This time she remembered drinking the herbal tea. Her husband tested her for allergy, the result was positive. They immediately brought the offending sample to the clinic. Tests in the office confirmed the positive result that the allergy was affecting the kidney meridian and kidney organ, and she was treated for the fenugreek. Her temperature came down to normal within 35 minutes after the treatment and didn't rise again. Thinking back, she remembered that she had started using this herbal tea a day before the backache started. That confirmed our diagnosis that the herbal drink was the cause of the kidney infection, which improved when the allergic reaction was removed. Now, twelve years later, she drinks her favorite fenugreek tea without any adverse reaction.

For several years, a 49-year-old man complained of frequent urination. On certain days he had severe problems, awakening to urinate at least eight to ten times during the night. He tried various treatments for this problem, including western medical treatments with various antibiotics (none of which ever worked), homeopathic medicines, herbal medicine, even straight acupuncture. Nothing gave him relief. In our office, testing through NTT revealed he was highly allergic to most foods. He was treated for wheat, sugar, iron, vegetables, meats, milk, eggs, etc. His problem still continued, so we asked him to keep a food diary. His journal revealed that he used large quantities of artificial sweeteners. He was treated for saccharin (one of the ingredients in the artificial sweeteners) and he felt better for the first 18 hours. Then his symptoms started all over. He had lost the treatment (somehow the brain did not register the new knowledge). After ten consecutive treatments, the constant bladder irritation disappeared. He is now free from bladder irritation even though he is using artificial sweeteners again.

A 46-year-old painter complained of frequent and painful urination with fever, severe bladder pain, abdominal cramping, soreness, aching in the joints and extreme nervousness. These fever symptoms disappeared whenever he stopped painting. In his case, the paint fumes caused his problem.

In some cases, allergy of the urinary tract (to food or an inhalant) may also cause dermatitis and eczema of the genital area. The allergen is excreted in the urine and comes in contact with these organs, where it causes skin allergies. Sometimes the anal region also gets skin allergies. In such cases, the irritating allergen is excreted in the stool. This was the case of a two-year-old boy who had weeping ulcers around his anal region. He had just started eating boiled eggs for breakfast a month earlier. Initially, he had common cold-like symptoms for a week. When that stopped, he started complaining of pain while urinating and defecating. He had red rashes and itching around the anus. The family physician diagnosed the problem as a result of worm infestation. Since the family had recently visited one of the developing countries, the diagnosis was very plausible.

Lab work did not show any positive results for worms. He was treated for a month without any results. Finally, his mother brought him into our office for an evaluation. He tested highly allergic to eggs. Seventy-two hours after eggs were eliminated from his diet, his wounds healed and the itching stopped. Later he was treated for eggs by NAET. The eczema that had begun to appear on his wrist and ankle joints disappeared after the treatment for eggs.

Another condition of the urinary tract that may be caused by allergies is hematuria, or blood in the urine. A 32-year-old man endured severe headaches, nausea, vomiting, sour stomach and belching for twelve years. Later he also developed severe pain in his flanks, and for many months passed a considerable amount of blood during urination. He also had a slightly enlarged prostate. All the tests (including a CAT scan) were negative, except for blood in the urine. For two months, he was kept in the hospital for tests and observation, with no change in his condition. Finally, he was sent home. A week later he developed swelling of both feet below the ankle, making it difficult for him to wear shoes. His headaches intensified and became more frequent. He began to suffer from severe insomnia.

Can Frequent Urination Be Due To Allergies?

It was a real surprise - though a very pleasant and hopeful one in today's world of disease and tension - to observe how Dr. Devi diagnosed the allergic attributes of any substance in an individual by using a very simple and practical method. This technique can be easily learned by any average person to help him escape from many pathological and even physical reactions in his/her body to the allergic substances which, of course, vary from individual to individual.

Still more surprising is the very simple (at least as seen by a layman) technique adopted by her to develop immunity in a person to his or her allergic substances. In my personal case, I have been treated for chronic problems that have been troubling me for a long time - though I am not sure whether they would have been permanent or not. I had a very long-standing problem with my urinary system. As a result of treatment by Dr. Devi, the frequency of my urination has decreased to one-fifth or even less sometimes; it is a great relief to me. Similarly, I was sneezing and having colds, especially in the mornings, very frequently for a number of years that defied many remedies. That trouble has almost disappeared now. Even more revealing is the knowledge gained by me as to how one can be allergic to scores of substances in daily use, like fruits, vegetables, and in fact all edible items, clothes, etc., which were always considered harmless. The technique of locating the allergic substance, even if it is not treated, helps a great deal and goes a long way for an individual to lead a more comfortable and trouble-free life. It is a real ray of hope for many people in these complex times.

S. M. Singh
Anaheim, CA

At this point, he came to our office for acupuncture to relieve his headaches. Thorough evaluation found him to have allergies to wheat, cantaloupe, cucumber, and onions. Upon questioning him, the man revealed that he habitually ate one raw red onion with each meal. This practice started 12 years earlier, when he read in a health magazine that eating one onion a day could prevent heart disease through its blood cleansing properties. Ever since, he continued eating onions, and this was the major cause of his health problem of 12 years.

A 39-year-old woman had bladder trouble for 22 years, but skin tests did not reveal the sensitivities. She also experienced migraine headaches. Since childhood, she suffered from sinusitis and a runny nose. She had feelings of burning in the bladder and pain in the lower abdomen, with frequent and painful urination. Sometimes she was unable to urinate and she had to go to the emergency room or to the doctor's office to have urethral dilation. Although she always suspected some foods affected her, she did not have any positive skin test for allergies, and no one could do anything for her. Finally she came to our office. The NTT indicated that she was allergic to eggs, onions, potatoes, citrus fruits, wheat, cauliflower, cabbage, almonds, pears, cinnamon, alcoholic beverages, and fabrics like cotton, polyester and leather. After 22 years of problems, she was treated by NAET and received complete relief.

Enuresis (bed-wetting), a major affliction to the victim and to his/her family, is frequently caused by an allergy. A 13-year-old boy who had severe enuresis and sinusitis was allergic to wheat, rice, garbanzo beans, chicken, eggs, peppers, sugar and gums. He was also found to be allergic to all synthetic fabrics. When he was treated for all these items by NAET, the bed-wetting stopped.

In the case of a nine-year-old boy, oranges were found to be the culprit in causing enuresis. In another, a six-year-old was allergic to avocado, cauliflower, grapes and cantaloupe, which caused enuresis. A 12-year-old girl who had this problem was found to be allergic to feathers, her comforter, oats, rice and yogurt.

Cysts in the ovaries are one of the common problems seen in fertile women. This was the case of a 32-year-old female who had frequent ovarian pains resulting from ovarian tumors and cysts. Habitually, she had to take painkillers and antibiotics, and often had to stay home from work. This woman was found to be allergic to soy and milk products. Her painful attacks dissipated after her NAET treatments. Two years later, she continues to have no further incidence of painful cysts or tumors in the uterus or ovaries. Her severe PMS also disappeared.

A 35-year-old woman had an orange-sized tumor in her uterus. She had been living with it for eight years because she refused any surgery for fear that she would suffer the same fate as her sister, who died when she was operated on for a similar tumor in the uterus.

This woman tested positive for allergies to all green vegetables, fish, milk, beef, soy products, vegetable oils, caffeine and chocolate. After she was treated for the above items, she was placed on a special Chinese herbal formula to strengthen the uterus and remove the tumors. She woke up one morning and found herself lying in a pool of blood, and in the middle of the blood was the orange-sized mass. She had passed it in her sleep.

For the last two years, Marge, a 34-year-old, had come to our office for treatment from time to time for various health conditions. During her annual checkup at her gynecologist, she discovered that she had a 3.5 x 2cm. ovarian tumor/cyst on her left side. Her doctor suggested she have it removed. She came directly to our office in tears.

Bed Wetting!

We tried everything to help our son stop bedwetting. We tried homeopathic medication, herbal medicine, waking him every 2 hours, etc., etc. He was embarrassed about it himself. Finally, we found NAET. Dr. Devi found out that his problem was due to allergies to various foods, fabrics and detergent.After he was treated for the Basic 10 groups, his flannel pajamas and detergent, he hasn't wet his bed.

Carolyn E.
La Habra, CA

NTT evaluation revealed that her cyst was caused by a particular brand of coffee that she had switched to recently. We obtained a sample of the coffee and treated her with NAET for the next three days. A week after completion of the treatments, the ultrasound could not detect the so-called tumor. Five years after that incident, she still remains tumor-free.

Most yeast infections seen in the genital area are related to allergies. In many cases, it may not actually be a yeast infection, but some allergic reaction mimicking a yeast infection.

A 51-year-old female suffering from this complaint for the past twelve years discovered she was allergic to cotton panties. Another 44-year-old woman was allergic to toilet paper. Allergies to tampons and sanitary napkins were the cause of another woman's yeast infection. After treatment, her nagging yeast problem that had been bothering her for two years subsided. Another 41-year-old woman was found to be allergic to the decaffeinated coffee she drank every day. The reaction caused a vaginal yeast problem. A 37-year-old man had a yeast infection and sores in the genital area for seven years, which cleared after treatment for allergy to wheat and sugar.

Uterine Bleeding triggered by Almond!

Uterine bleeding began in the third month of my pregnancy. I was told by my gynecologist that I would have to terminate my pregnancy because of the severity of the bleeding. I refused to believe it, so I consulted Dr. Devi. She traced the bleeding back to the almond cookies I ate, two days in a row, just before the bleeding started. I had a craving for this kind of cookie during my pregnancy. When I was treated for the allergy to that particular almond cookie, the bleeding stopped within a few hours. I carried my pregnancy to full term without any ill-effects. My baby is now a 10 year old, very healthy and intelligent child.

Shoana S.
Santa Ana, CA

Allergy to Dairy Products

I have been coming to Dr. Devi Nambudripad for two years. Along with seeing dramatic benefits in many other patients (including close friends and my husband), I have experienced personal cures for several major problems that traditional doctors could not understand, much less cure.

1. I had suffered from ovarian cysts for 16 years - the doctors kept me on birth control pills during this entire time to control the problem, but had no idea what the cause was. Treatment alternatives included either birth control pills or a hysterectomy. Dr. Devi had seen this problem occur before and found the cause to be a severe reaction to dairy products. Her treatment cleared up the problems.

2. My skin had never really "cleared up" since adolescence, especially during the summer. We have since learned that when things irritate my stomach or intestines - my skin will break out.

3. In addition, many symptoms of common "problems" such as headaches, depression, fatigue, colds, flu, bronchitis, bladder infections, and vaginal infections have been found to be caused by allergic reactions and have been eliminated with Dr. Nambudripad's treatments.

Abbye Younghanz
Tustin, CA

In many cases, infertility is caused by allergies. A 27-year-old woman had been unsuccessfully attempting to conceive a child for eight years. Our test result showed her to be allergic to vitamin A, vitamin F, iron, B complex, and chocolate. After the treatment for the allergies, she became pregnant within four months.

A 28-year-old man with a low sperm count had been trying to have a baby with his wife for the past four years. We discovered he was allergic to milk, fruits, vegetables, wheat and vitamin A. After NAET treatment, we advised him to try "Shou Wu Pian" tablets (a Chinese herb to regain vitality and strength). Three and a half months later, he called to tell us his wife was pregnant with his child.

For twelve years, a 32-year-old female with severe endometriosis had been unsuccessfully trying to have a child. She tried various infertility treatments with no luck. Finally, she came to our office where we discovered she suffered from severe PMS due to endometriosis and sinusitis. She was allergic to many foods, grasses, pollens, cotton, polyester and even her husband's semen. After completion of the allergy treatments, she underwent surgery for the removal of scar tissue in the abdomen caused by endometriosis. We then placed her on a special Chinese herbal formula "Tankuei and Peony Formula" (available at Lotus Herbs in West Covina,

---

PMS and Abdominal Cramps

When I first brought my daughter, Crista, 15 years old, to see Dr. Devi, she had just been through $1,000 worth of medical testing to find the reason for agonizing abdominal cramps and pain. She craved sugar and she consumed a lot of sugar every day in different forms. She felt slightly relieved when she ate sugar. So I couldn't keep her off the sugar products. After five NAET treatments she never experienced the pain or cramps again. She doesn't crave sugar any more. She hasn't had PMS for the past six years.

Wendy B.
Palm Springs, CA

---

and Brion Herbs in Irvine, CA.) to regulate her hormonal functions. Within five months she became pregnant, and now they have a healthy, beautiful girl.

Vaginal warts are linked to allergies. In the case of a 42-year-old woman, cotton underwear was the culprit. A 22-year-old woman with a history of vaginal warts for four years was allergic to soy products. In many people, products containing elastics can cause warts or skin tags on any part of the body on contact.

A 62-year-old man had complained of severe and constant pain across the lower abdomen, above the symphysis pubis, for four months. The author linked the problem to a reaction from the expensive leather belt he received for his birthday four months earlier. His pain subsided after he was treated by NAET.

Many women suffer from premenstrual syndrome (PMS). In some women, the problems start one week before the period and continue up to four or five days afterwards. A series of health problems can be seen in PMS sufferers. Some of the commonly seen health problems correlated with premenstrual syndrome include: weight gain, craving sweets, salt and hot spices, bloating, tiredness, cramps in the lower abdomen, nausea, mood swings, and more.

The sugar cravings are related to the spleen and stomach meridian blockages. These sufferers can also experience bloating, nausea, dull cramps

---

PMS and Sinus Headaches

Prior to NAET treatment, I had sinus headaches every month just before my periods that lasted four-five days after my periods started. I also suffered from frequent bouts of bronchitis and chronic low backache during those days.   After treating for vitamin C mix, sugar mix, salt mix and spice mix, I do not have PMS anymore.

Colleen M.
Tustin, CA

---

after the period starts, pimples on the face and neck, and light, prolonged bleeding (8-10 days).

Cravings for pungent foods such as onions, garlic, etc., are related to blockages in the lung and large intestine meridians. Before or during periods, these people can suffer from mild to severe respiratory distress, colds, sinus problems. Constipation can occur before periods and diarrhea after periods.

Salt cravings are due to blockage of the kidney meridians. One can experience thirst, water retention, frequent urination and headaches around the nape of the neck before or during the periods.

Cravings for sour things are due to liver and gall bladder meridian blockages. Pain and swelling in the breasts, severe abdominal cramps, heavy bleeding, severe mood swings, aggressive behavior, anger, and complaining are related to the liver meridian blockages.

Cravings for hot and spicy foods are connected to heart and small intestine meridian blockages. Heart palpitations, cardiac arrhythmia, insomnia, dry mouth, heavy sensations on the chest, night sweats, fatigue, overexcitement, insecurity, etc., can be caused from blockages of these meridians before and during periods.

Craving certain foods signifies that there is blockage in some meridians. If consumed in moderation, these craved foods could help to open up or strengthen the blocked meridians. However, excessive consumption will cause an imbalance of other elements within the body. This is due to depletion of other nutrients which, in turn, can increase water retention, causing even more discomfort.

A 34-year-old female would gain at least 8-10 pounds prior to her period, then lose all her water weight by the second or third day. We discovered she was allergic to sugar and salt. Her water retention stopped after she was treated for salt and sugar with NAET.

A 22-year-old female with severe abdominal cramps and indigestion throughout her periods was allergic to the sanitary napkins she used.

This may be due to a hormonal imbalance or deficiency. Certain allergies could also cause these problems. One can easily isolate the problems through kinesiological testing and provide appropriate treatments.

Female patients who complain of premenstrual syndrome may be allergic to the sanitary napkins they are using. They could easily avoid the discomfort by finding a brand that suits their bodies (tested through muscle response testing). If they still have problems after avoiding all possible allergens, they may need to see a specialist in the field to find out whether the cause lies elsewhere.

ENDOMETRIOSIS

No successful treatment has been developed in western medicine for endometriosis, a condition that affects many women. Many food allergies such as soy and milk products play a great role in this female problem.

A 28-year-old female patient had tried various treatments for endometriosis, including laparoscopy, a surgical procedure to clean the ectopic endometrial tissue. She suffered from severe premenstrual disorders and dysmenorrhea (pain during periods) as well as extreme tiredness. NTT testing revealed she was allergic to a lot of food items, including milk, soy products and poultry. After her successful treatment, her PMS and dysmenorrhea disappeared.

Another 25-year-old female was infertile due to endometriosis. She discovered she was allergic to many food items, fabrics and chemicals. Three months after she completed the treatments, she finally became pregnant. Even after the delivery, her endometriosis did not return.

Joan, a 38-year-old, had a history of repeated ovarian cysts and uterine fibroids. As a vegetarian, her diet consisted of all types of dried beans. Unfortunately, she was extremely allergic to beans and vegetable proteins. Six months after the completion of the NAET treatments, a gynecological exam and an ultrasound treatment showed no trace of fibroids or cysts. Four years after the treatments, she can still enjoy all her bean dishes while remaining cyst and tumor-free.

Potato is one of the staple foods of many people. It contains a special toxic substance called "solanin" that is a poison for many people.

In these people, the memory to produce the enzyme to digest this toxin remains dormant. Solanin causes blockages in many energy meridians and various health problems. Lumps in the breast, sudden fever, sore throat, sinusitis, uterine fibroids, acne, fatty tumors under the skin (lipoma), back aches, mid-back ache, sciatic neuralgia, joint pains and stiffness, headaches, abdominal bloating, flatulence, skin blemishes, freckles, skin rashes, skin discolorations, constipation or diarrhea, itching, dermatological problems, hives, lack of motivation, depression, vaginal yeast, etc., are some of the symptoms I have seen in people with an allergy to potato. Other root vegetables also cause problems. Since potato is used more frequently, health problems arising from potatoes are more commonly seen among consumers.

Janet, a 24-year-old, came in complaining of bilateral breast abscesses. She suffered from this problem off and on for six years, even though the recent one began four days ago. She could not even wear normal clothes due to the swelling and pain. She had eaten a large amount of potatoes four days in a row before she developed the pain and swelling of the breast. She was treated for potato immediately by NAET. Within 45 minutes, her pain reduced by 50 percent. After successful completion of the NAET treatment, her pain and swelling disappeared. Amazingly, the body healed itself by disposing the abscess filled boils naturally.

UTERINE FIBROIDS AND PARASITES

One group of health practitioners believes that parasites and flukes cause various health problems, especially fibroids, tumors, cysts, etc. There are various types of detoxification programs being used all over the country. In our time, when natural health awareness is getting much attention, every holistic doctor or clinic you contact can give you an extensive plan of their

---

No More Endometriosis or P MS

I have been receiving treatments from Dr. Devi for seven months and have noticed many improvements in my general health. Specifically, I now have no pelvic pain, which was attributed to endometriosis or PMS symptoms. Also, my allergy to caffeine, which caused heart palpitations, is now gone.

Ann M. Pagliaro
Anaheim, CA

> ### *Hormones*
>
> *Immediately after menopause and going on hormone replacement therapy, I developed a large, double-headed cyst on my left ovary. After treating my body's own hormones, plus the hormones I was taking orally, the cyst disappeared — never to return again.*
>
> *Elena Oumano, Ph.D.*
> *Author of The Handbook of Natural Folk Remedies & Natural Sex*

detoxification program. Some of them work while others don't. You can try them out to see which one would work for you. If you are not allergic to the products you are using, any detoxification program should work for you.

A 36-year old female came to our office with complaints of pain all over the body, especially in the lower abdomen (fibromyalgia), depression, general fatigue through day and night without any relief, (chronic fatigue syndrome), hypothyroidism, brain fog, weight gain, ovarian cysts, uterine fibroids, pedal edema, frequent headaches, nausea, severe PMS, insomnia, for over 10 years. She had seen many medical specialists through the years for the above health problems. She did not receive much help from any of those treatments. She continued to take all the prescription drugs, hoping to get some relief. She also visited many holistic professionals and went through many cleansing programs. Finally she read about NAET in the "Alternative Medicine Digest" and came to see us. After all the basic treatments, she was treated for baking soda and baking powder, which were strong allergens for her. After completion of that treatment she reported that she started her periods on the following day. And she also noticed that she passed 3 - 4 inch long worms and flukes from her uterus. She had no PMS with her period and her uterine fibroid was reduced in size.

MORNING SICKNESS

Morning sickness during pregnancy is linked with some kinds of allergies. The mother may be allergic to foods, vitamins (calcium, zinc, vitamin C, etc.), or even to the embryo or fetus in some cases.

A 28-year-old woman came to our office when she was three months pregnant. She constantly felt nauseated and she vomited frequently. The only way she could keep anything in her stomach was if she was fed intravenously. She was allergic to sugar, salt, zinc, vitamin C and vitamin B complex. She became well again after successful NAET treatment.

A 27-year-old woman was four months pregnant with her third child. She complained of continuous cramps in the lower abdomen since the time of conception. The pain and discomfort disturbed her eating and sleeping patterns, and she lost a lot of weight. She was examined by her gynecologist every week and placed on complete bed rest, making her cramps even worse. Her blood test revealed that she was producing antibodies against the baby. Her doctor advised her to have an abortion because of the severe health risks involved. NTT at our clinic revealed that she was allergic to the fetus. She was treated for the allergy to the fetus with NAET. In less than four hours the painful cramping was reduced. She had a good night's sleep for the first time in four months. She woke up the next day with no abdominal cramps and there was no recurrence for the remainder of her pregnancy. A blood analysis after a week showed no further antibody production.

Many pregnant women suffer from pre-eclampsia and eclampsia. Some women get high blood pressure and their feet and body swell. Other symptoms are excessive weight gain, restlessness, sleeplessness, shortness of breath, skin rashes, itching, nausea, light-headedness and an inability to urinate freely. Pregnant mothers may be allergic to the prenatal vitamins they faithfully take. Kinesiological allergy testing for prenatal vitamins at prenatal clinics could prevent many of these symptoms.

A 39-year-old pregnant woman felt sciatic pain during her eighth month of pregnancy. In spite of all the physical therapy she was receiving, her pain was so severe she had to be confined to bed 24 hours a day. Her physician husband brought her to our office where NTT revealed that she was highly allergic to the prenatal vitamin she was taking every day. Her sciatic pain was immediately relieved after one NAET treatment.

Around certain times of the month some men become irritable or emotional and suffer from insomnia. They should be checked for hormone imbalance and if allergy is found they should be treated.

Emotions play a great part in female and male disorders. Often if the problem is emotional in origin, NAET gives lasting, permanent relief of the symptoms. Please read Chapter 20 for more on emotional blockages.

CHAPTER 18

ALLERGY AND
THE BODY, MIND AND SPIRIT

aximize your emotional health by balancing your body, mind and spirit. It's easier said than done. Can we really do it? If so, how do we do it? Is it possible to have an allergy to your own feelings? Is it possible to have an allergy to your own thoughts? Is it possible to have an allergy between two humans? Why not?

Why are some people always happy while others are never happy?

Why do some people have good health while others haven't even heard the word?

Why do some people make a lot of money while others work so hard day and night and don't even make enough to make ends meet?

Why do some people have loving and caring parents, siblings, husband/wife, children and friends while others have just the opposite?

Why do some people find the right job, meet the right people to work with, get appreciation in whatever they do and reach ultimate success and maintain it while others are unhappy at work, change jobs many times, never get recognition for the hard work they do, and embrace failure in everything they do?.

Some people might say, "It's your karma."

In my opinion, fate, destiny and karma are all words used in describing uncertainty. These are compromising and soothing words that the conscious mind uses to comfort the inner child when something didn't quite work out the way you wanted it to happen.

When you break down the purpose of life, three simple elements stand out as basic needs:

• To be healthy
• To have enough money
• To share it with someone who cares about you

The familiar expression, "May you be blessed with HEALTH, WEALTH AND HAPPINESS!" probably arose to stress the importance of these basic needs.

If you have these three basic needs in good standing, you have a satisfactory life. To achieve this, people do different things: eating, buying new clothes, using cosmetics, schooling, finding a good job, working, resting, watching television and movies; reading books, interacting with people, dating, marrying, traveling, vacationing, producing children and helping them grow up; taking care of animals, plants, flowers, etc. If you look at the various actions, you realize that all of them fall under the three basic needs. If you look around, you will see that everyone is competing to acquire health, wealth and happiness. Some succeed, some fail, and others stay in the middle. It is difficult to find people who are well balanced in all three categories. If you are well balanced, you would be the most satisfied person in the world. How can you achieve this? Is it possible?

If you want to see definite results, you need to work on the real problems. First, you need to find the problem. If you look for a problem, you will find it. If you can find it, you can fix it through NAET. If you follow the right method, it is easy to find the problem.

The Method for Finding an Emotional Blockage is: Asking Questions

Who do you ask? Who has all the answers about you? Who has a genuine interest in you? Who is interested in maintaining your good health, good fortune and happiness?

"YOUR BRAIN," of course, has all the answers about you.

The brain and nervous system work around the clock to take care of the body's needs, watching and protecting it from any physical, physiological and/or emotional harm. The electromagnetically sensitive nervous

Bipolar Disorder

Our daughter was diagnosed with Bipolar disease in 1981. She became ill while in her first year of college out-of-state, and at the end of the year we took her home in a suicidal depression. After seeing psychologists and getting no help, we finally had to have her hospitalized, as she seemed to be intent on killing herself. In the state hospital, she was diagnosed with manic depression with schizo-affective disorder. She was in the hospital for four months, came home heavily drugged, and was again hospitalized seven months later for another three months.

Since that time, she has been hospitalized every ten or eleven months for anywhere from seven to eleven weeks at a time. In between episodes, her dosages would be lowered and she would become somewhat functional. But nothing prevented her from being hospitalized a few months later.

After a couple of years on this merry-go-round, we began to look into alternative therapies, since the orthodox medical route was helping only minimally. We realized that not only was a cure impossible, but that the medications weren't even able to keep her out of the hospital. Of course, through all this she had psychiatrists who were unable to help with her illness, which involved depression, hallucinations, and bizarre and sometimes violent behavior.

Our daughter has had at least a dozen alternative therapies, including acupuncture treatments with various fine acupuncturists. Some of these treatments helped to get her past most of the side effects of her medications – but nothing prevented her from re-entering a hospital some months later.

(Continued on next page)

In February, 1997, she again began acupuncture treatments. She asked to do this because she remembered feeling somewhat better after her past treatments. She began treatment with a young woman named Rebecca, whom we had met many years before. After four sessions, Rebecca said that our daughter was ready for NAET. My response was, "But she is not allergic to anything." You see, she had never exhibited any of the usual signs of allergic reaction. Rebecca said, "She is a highly allergic person." I didn't really believe her, but we decided to give it a try since we felt that we had nothing to lose. So she began NAET treatments.

She has, through the past 16 years, been on numerous antipsychotic, anti-manic, and anti-convulsive medications, and on extremely high doses each time she was hospitalized, as her manic and schizoid episodes were so profound. Now, 18 months after beginning the NAET treatments, our daughter is off all but a very small amount of her last remaining medication. Each time her medicines have been lowered, thanks to NAET, she has seen a naturopathic physician who utilizes herbs and homeopathics to make sure she remains stable while her body is adjusting to the decrease.

We have a young male friend who has now begun NAET treatments, and almost immediately began to lift from his severe clinical depression. For the first time in many years, he is hopeful for his future. The mental illness from which so many suffer often begins with a very sensitive body. Ingesting foods (or taking in any substance) that the body doesn't want to accept upsets the balance of various organ systems which, over the course of years, culminates in an assault on the most vulnerable part of the body.

In many people the most vulnerable organ is the brain, and in those people, mental illness is the result. Most often, there is no warning because there are no recognizable symptoms.

(Continued on next page)

The only symptom is the mental illness itself. *The NAET treatment completely eliminated the allergies that, for our daughter, manifested as mental illness. From what we know, the treatment should work equally well for all types of "mental illness."*

At the present time, our daughter is working at a local library, and once more, is reading two or three books at a time. Until now, she has been unable to read more than a few lines at a given time because her mind was so cloudy from a combination of drugs and the illness. She takes aerobics classes and is able to interact with "normal" people once more. Recently, she fielded questions about the NAET treatment at a lecture given by my husband and myself. That was something she could not possibly have done before NAET.

Our daughter is 36 years old, and it's as if her life is just be- ginning. The prognosis is that she will be off all medication within the next three to four months. We are lowering her medications very slowly, in spite of the fact that she has exhibited barely any symp- toms of withdrawal, thanks to the alternative methods, in addition to the NAET, that are being employed.

If any therapists utilizing NAET feel that they would like for pro- spective patients to talk to my husband or myself about our experi- ence with NAET, we would be very pleased to answer any questions or reservations they may have. Our telephone number is 1-301-656- 6819. One of us is generally available after 7:30 P.M.

It is our fervent wish that, at some point in time, "mental illness" will be only a memory. We know that, thanks to the NAET treatment formulated by Dr. Nambudripad, we have found an answer.

Helene & Fred Forrest, WA

system is very efficient in communicating with each nerve cell in the body in complete coordination, and also has the ability to connect and communicate with the electromagnetic forces of other living or nonliving beings of the universe from any distance. So, you can trust your brain to find the best answers to your questions. In other words, you can ask your brain any question and it will give you the correct answer. Each cell in your brain and the nervous system is built uniquely with specialized cell materials which have the ability to measure and assess the energy difference of various things from your internal or external environments: disturbed body functions, substances from your environment, emotional disturbances, good and bad thoughts, vibrations, temperature change like heat, cold, etc., from your own body or someone else's body, from far and near. This sharing ability of each nerve cell creates the best network communication system or the best world- wide website ever possible. This specialized communication is made possible for the nerve cell by its unique ability to transfer its electromagnetic energy in and out of the cell within the body, out of the body and to a distance of infinity. You know from your experience that your thought has the ability to travel any distance and return in the fastest speed possible. Your mind is like a monkey. A unique monkey that has the ability to jump from: one town to another, a continent to other, or one planet to another in a split millisecond. It can never stay still, even in sleep. It jumps around and gathers information and stores it in the memory bank. How many distant places and people do you visit in a split second in any given day? No one has built an adequate calculator yet to keep track of your mental travel distance or activities of one day. This hypothesis is just to show you and remind you of the ability of your brain and the nervous system. Every one of you has the same ability. But, just like anything else in the universe, it requires practice. This area of cell function needs to undergo some vigorous scientific research to understand the methodology further.

But you don't have to wait to finish the scientific research to utilize the knowledge to help you get better health. How can you do it? How can you get useful information about you from your brain and the nervous system? When you get the answer, what can you do with it? Can you reprogram your brain or reboot your brain computer to input or imprint your need in the master template? Can you erase the harmful messages from the memory and rewrite with pleasant, useful messages? Can you achieve similar status and disposition by filling your life with health, wealth and happiness?

First you need a reference point to compare and verify your findings and the results. You can use the same muscle response testing technique you learned in Chapter 7 as a source of reference points to verify your answers. This time, you are replacing the food or substance with your question.

While doing MRT, ask questions silently

- If the muscle response testing makes the test muscle go weak, the answer is "yes."

- If the muscle response testing makes the test muscle strong, the answer is "no."

- Make a list of your problems and ask your brain, while doing MRT, to give you the causes of your problems.

METHODS OF ASKING QUESTIONS

Health:

Question: Do I (you) want to be healthy? If the MRT gives a weak muscle response, your brain is saying, "Yes, I (you) want to be healthy." But if the MRT gives a strong muscle response, your brain is saying, "No, I don't want to be healthy." You have a problem there. You may have to fix that right away. Otherwise you may not get healthy. If your brain thinks you don't want to be healthy, your brain will try everything in its power to keep you unhealthy.

You can ask the brain the same question differently.

Question: Do I (you) want to be sick? If the MRT gives a weak muscle response, your brain is saying, "Yes, I want to be sick." You may have to fix that right away. Otherwise you may not get healthy. If your brain thinks you want to be sick your brain will try everything in its power to keep you sick.

But if the MRT gives you a strong response here, your brain is saying "No, I don't want to be sick. "That's a good answer for you. So you don't have to do anything about it.

Are you afraid to be healthy? Do you like sickness? Do you want to get well? Are you afraid to get well? Form your line of questions and find out which of the thoughts, statements, questions or feelings is/are having a blockage. You have to ask a specific question to get a specific answer. Break down the question in its simplest form to get the best answer. Avoid confusing your brain. If you stand in front of 100 people and ask a question about the whole group, "Is anyone in the group afraid to be healthy?" "Is anyone in this group allergic to an apple?" You may not get an appropriate answer to this type of question because it does not fit with the criteria of simplicity or specificity.

You can ask any questions related to health in this fashion. If you find a negative answer, you may need to fix it. If you find a positive answer, don't do anything with it.

Wealth:

You can ask any questions related to your financial status in this fashion.

Question: Do I (you) want to make money? If the MRT gives a weak muscle response, your brain is saying, "Yes, I want to make money." There is nothing to fix there.

If the MRT gives a strong muscle response, your brain is saying, "No, I don't want to make money." You may have to fix that right away. Otherwise you may not make any money, because your brain thinks you don't want to make any money and your brain will try everything in its power to keep you from making money.

Question: Do I (you) like money? Do you like to make money? Do you want to make money? Do you want to make lots of money? Can you make money? Can you save money? Can you spend money? Do you want to find the job you like? Do you work at a job that you like?

If you find a negative answer, you need to fix it. If you find a positive answer, don't do anything about it.

Happiness:

You can ask a variety of questions pertaining to your happiness and related issues.

Question: Do you (I) like to be happy in your (my) life? Do you want to be happy? Do you enjoy happiness? Can you be happy? Do you like others to be happy around you?

Do you like friends? Do you like to love? Do you like to be loved? Do you want to love? Do you want to be loved? Do you want to meet the right person? Do you want to get married? Do you want to have a family? If you get the positive (right) response, you don't have to do anything. If you get a negative response, you will have to find an NAET practitioner and fix it right away. Otherwise, your dreams may not come true.

You can ask questions in this fashion about any matter in your life. If there is a blockage, find an NAET practitioner near you and get treated .

You can also have an allergy to another human being, an incident, and to a thought. Whatever culture you grew up in, most of you have swallowed a lot of emotions. You were told that you were supposed to pay respect to your elders (father, mother, grandfather, grandmother, older brothers, older sisters, etc.). You were not allowed to talk back, even if the elders were wrong. Whenever the elders were angry at something or somebody, the youngsters (you) got the heat from them. Whatever emotions came along, you swallowed them most of the time. These emotions then rooted themselves in the gut wall and remained there. In some cases, these corrosive emotions ate up your gut, making lots of holes which let large undigested protein molecules escape into the circulation, leading to physical, physiological or emotional symptoms in the body. The childhood emotional blockage and abuse can cause various lifetime chronic health problems, depending upon the energy meridian it blocks: asthma, emphysema (blockage in the lung meridian); chest pains, heaviness in the chest, overwhelming emotional outbursts, crying spells, etc. (heart meridian); ulcers, digestive troubles, migraines (stomach meridian); diabetes, blood disorders, yeast, candida, fungus, tumors, cysts, etc. (spleen meridian); brain fog, brain irritability, anger, unhappy disposition, solid tumors, etc. (liver meridian); uncertainty, inability to make decisions due to fear, (gallbladder meridian); joint disorders, connective tissue disorders, etc. (kidney meridian); internal fears, leaky gut syndrome, irritable bowels, inflammation of the small bowels, etc. (small intestine meridian); insecurity, loss of control of the situation, (bladder meridian); unable to let go (large intestine meridian).

CHECK SYSTEM

People throughout the world suffer from various emotional blockages due to today's life-style. People check each other in everything they do in their lives. No one is free from this check system.

Look at this simple example:

A mother sends her son to school. She pays a fee to the school to educate him. A teacher is assigned to teach the child. If the teacher did not teach the child, he will not know his test questions. If the child did not study, he will not pass the test. If he did not pass the test, he will not be promoted. If he continues to fail the test, his mother is going to take him out of the school. If the child did not attend school, the school will not get paid. The teacher will not get paid. If the teacher did not get paid, she will not work there. The school will not function without money and a teacher.

Look at any aspect of the life-style around you. You can see a similar check system everywhere. Everyone is entangled with one another by this check system. People who follow the check system closely win and live with less emotional blockages. People who do not follow the system carefully will swallow lots of emotions every day. These unresolved emotions will adhere to the gut wall and begin to eat it up, creating health disorders. Until you understand this and find a way to move it out of its location (wherever it is rooted), you may not meet your basic needs — health, wealth and happiness.

As you swallow emotions, you need to eliminate them immediately. Do not collect them. Until now, people talked about emotional issues, some people understood the importance of recognizing them; others thought these issues might lead to health disorders. But no one quite knew how to remove them exactly. Now there is an easy, self-treatment method to clear your troubled emotions in the privacy of your home through NAET. This technique has been tried out on many hundreds of patients in my office with excellent results. It is designed to help you free yourself from your entanglements and achieve your basic needs of life. Use it as freely and frequently as you need to and you will be able to attain your dreams!

METHOD

The best time to clear your day's emotions is each night before you go to sleep. However small it may be, clear the emotion on the same day it happened. This can prevent you from accumulating emotions and causing other health problems tagged on to the emotional issues in later life.

You may go to an NAET practitioner near you to remove your blockages with NAET, a slightly different procedure needing professional knowledge. You can get results with certain emotions using the following technique. You can also treat your young ones using a surrogate (read Chapter 7) with this same method.

NAET EMOTIONAL SELF-TREATMENT

Find a calm and comfortable area where you can be alone with your thoughts without anyone disturbing you. You are advised to sit or lie down with your eyes closed. Closing you eyes will help you to concentrate better. Do not do this procedure in a standing position. Some people may experience problems in maintaining a stable equilibrium in a standing position with the eyes closed.

Methodology:

Tap and clear (See Figure 18-1 for point locations).

Step-1: Place your right three fingertips on the "pt-1" (pt-1 on the diagram) and left three fingertips on the "pt-2" (pt-2 on diagram 18-1).

While maintaining the left fingertips' contact on "pt-2," and tap on "pt-1," using right fingertips, while **reliving** your trauma, or

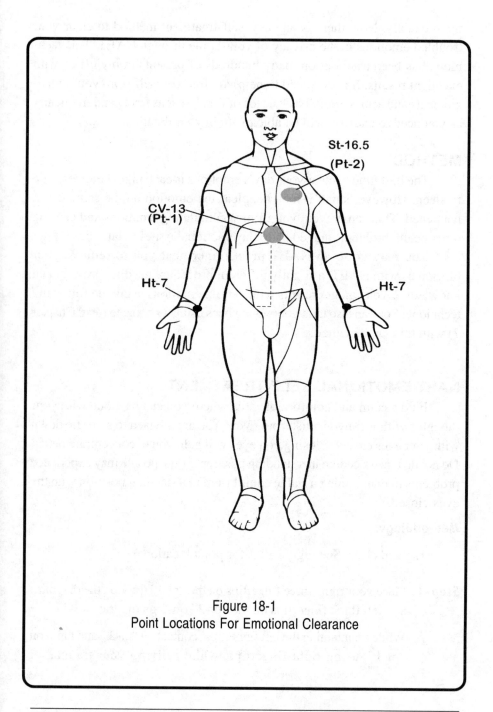

Figure 18-1
Point Locations For Emotional Clearance

incident of the day. The tapping time is 60 seconds on each point.

Step-2: Maintaining the right fingertips' contact on "pt-1," tap with the left fingertips on "pt-2," while **reliving** the memory of the incident.

Step-3: Massage clockwise on point "pt-1," then on "pt-2," one minute each, while thinking positive or pleasant thoughts about the incident.

PERSON-TO-PERSON ALLERGIES

You all know and talk about "body chemistry" and "incompatibility" in personal relationships. How did these concepts come into usage? Is there really something like body chemistry and incompatibility, or could this be an allergy between human beings?

You know that you could be allergic to different substances. You could be allergic to other living things like plants, insects and pets. Everyone accepts this as a fact. Many people sneeze, faint and get hives in the presence of a cat or a dog. Animal epithelial and dander cause a great many allergy problems among sensitive people. Saliva or other secretions of animals can cause allergic reactions in humans. If this is possible, humans could also be allergic to other humans, and their secretions, because each one of you has your own unique electromagnetic energy field that can interact positively or negatively, as it does with many substances. If these energy fields interact negatively, they can lead to allergic reactions or discomfort in one person or the other, or both.

A 42-year-old female was having problems with her marriage for the last couple of years. Joe was a devoted husband but could not make his wife happy. She nagged him and ordered him about all the time and insulted him in front of his friends. When she was alone, she loved him and regretted her behavior. They almost broke up twice during fifteen years of married life. Now, for the third time, they were getting ready for a separation. During one of her office visits, the woman poured her heart out to me. She said that she loved her husband so much that whenever she was away from him she got physical pains just thinking of him. For some reason, whenever they were together, he irritated her. The days almost always ended in fights, with the result that nights found them in separate beds. She also suffered from various allergies and manifestations like migraine headaches, gastrointestinal allergies and arthritis. She wanted to keep the marriage together, but for some reason could not express her love to her husband. They had consulted a marriage counselor a few times, but that did not help.

I advised her to try muscle response testing at home, for a possible allergy to each other. The next day these two were among the first group of patients in my office. Their tests showed that they were allergic to each other, and they both wanted to be treated. They said that they had spent fifteen precious years fighting and, if there was a way to stop that pattern, they wanted it to happen as soon as possible so they could enjoy the rest of their lives. A month later, after treatments for each other, there was a bouquet of red roses in the office and a note that said: "Thank you, doctor, for helping us. We are going on our second honeymoon to the Caribbean; things can't be better between us." Six years later they are still in love.

A 28-year-old woman had three miscarriages and finally gave birth to a baby boy. Soon after childbirth, she became very ill with aches, pains, and severe arthritis. She was very thin and tall before childbirth, but began to gain weight after the baby was born. In one month's time, she gained about forty pounds even though she had not increased or changed her intake of food and had kept up with all her usual activities. This really puzzled her, and her doctors as well. She joined an exercise program, which gave her some relief from her aches and pains, but not any weight loss. She tried all kinds of medicines and treatments, without positive results. The child refused to sleep in the crib, and slept by his mother's side every night. The mother became sicker and sicker with her migraines and joint disorders. Then one day the child fell very sick with fever and an ear infection. The woman's mother came and stayed with her to give her a helping hand with the sick child. The child started sleeping with the grandmother. When the child stopped sleeping in the mother's bed, the mother started feeling better.

The grandmother stayed for a few more weeks, until the baby's mother was well; then she left. The child started spending the nights with his mother again, and in a few days the mother was sick again. Her arthritis and joint pains returned. Her fogginess of mind returned. She was lethargic and sick, even worse than before. Her worried husband took her to different doctors and tried all possible treatments. Nothing seemed to help her. Finally, someone guided her to our office. Her history was reviewed over and over. Her son was four years old by that time and still slept in her bed. The mother was a very energetic, smart, slim woman without any health problems before the child was born. Now, all of a sudden, she was the sickest person in the world. Again, when the grandmother stayed with her and the child spent most of his time with the grandmother, the mother recovered from her illness! When the grandmother left and the child started to spend more time with his mother, she became sick again. Her history of the pattern of her illness, morning fatigue and general body aches gave us the clue.

The mother was allergic to her son, as you undoubtedly have figured out. She treated for the allergy to the son, and on completion of the treatment felt better, physically and mentally. She did not wake up hurting in the mornings. She also began losing weight soon after the treatment, and shared that she wanted to be included in this book, hoping it might help many other unsuspecting victims of allergy. Throughout her pregnancy, she suffered from severe morning sickness and headaches, vomiting, nausea and tiredness, until the day of delivery. She was living on medication, one dose every four hours, throughout her pregnancy to keep her nausea under control. From this, we can form a hypothesis that pregnant women who have severe morning sickness and other pregnancy-related sickness may be allergic to the fetus. The repulsion between the two energy fields may be the cause of miscarriages.

Many of the causes of infertility may be attributed to various allergies. If the couple are allergic to each other, or if the woman is allergic to the man's sperm, conception will not be possible. Infertile couples who do not show any other physical or physiological abnormalities should be checked for possible allergies. They may become fertile when the allergies to each other are cleared.

A 32-year-old female was trying to get pregnant for eight years. All the tests with the couple were normal. In our office they were tested for various things and found to be within normal limits. Finally, it was found that the wife was allergic to the husband's semen. After she was treated for the semen, she was pregnant within three months.

Another woman had been suffering from severe asthma for 15 years. She was on disability due to asthma when she came to our office. She was treated for various food allergies, environmental allergies, etc. Still her asthma bothered her every night. Finally, she was found to be allergic to her husband and made the connection between her 15-year marriage and the 15-year asthmatic history. She was treated by NAET for her husband, and the asthma left her.

An allergy between two people: to husband and wife, to mother and son, to daughters, to fathers, to brothers or sisters or other family members, business partners, employer and employees, co-workers, teachers and students — all these may sound unbelievable, but it is true, as we have discovered. How many of you have seen once-happy relationships end in fights and disharmony? How many of you have seen fighting between parents or simple arguments and friction between brothers and sisters and when they grow up, end in severe fights and broken relationships? Many parents grow to hate their children and vice versa. How many of the most loving couples end up in divorce, hating each other for the rest of their lives?

Two siblings in their early fifties came to our office for allergy treatments. Even though they lived miles apart, they could not stand to be around each other for even a few minutes. They had been like that all their lives, always clashing and fighting with each other whenever they met. Both had a lot of allergies to various substances and to each other. They were treated by NAET for all the known allergens, including each other. Now they are the best of friends, as siblings should be. They said that they are making up for lost time.

All of these external factors can turn into internal problems. If not taken care of right away, they can cause severe illnesses. Your electromagnetic field is unique and different from others. Therefore, it is quite possible to have a variety of results from attraction or aversion between the energy fields whenever they are in proximity.

A 46-year-old female had suffered from joint pains, extreme tiredness and asthma for the past 12 years. Before then, she was healthy and without any complaints. Her mother had suffered from asthma all her life and had died of it at the age of 44. The daughter had no sign of any allergy until she was 34 years old. She was tested and evaluated for allergies by four other allergy specialists and found to have no trace of allergies. She had to spend most of her time in and out of hospitals for joint pains and asthma. Within a day or so after checking into the hospital she was better. When she returned home, she started wheezing within a few hours. Thinking that the house was the problem, her family moved.

In our office, through NTT we found she was negative for allergies to foods, pollens, grasses, environmental items, hormones, fabrics, chemicals, etc. She had been married for 12 years and had her first attack of asthma a month after the wedding. Searching her memory, she recalled that her joint pains and tiredness started at least a week or two before her asthma. She was tested for her husband, to whom she was highly allergic. Curiously, he was not allergic to her. She was treated for the allergy to him, which took seven days to clear. After she cleared the allergy to her husband, her joint pains disappeared and her asthma also decreased. She has not had to take medicines to control her asthma ever since.

Astrologers talk about compatibility. Could it be true? You have heard of people becoming ill after they are married or after living together in close proximity. You have seen people gain good fortune or even win a lottery or a jackpot on their honeymoon trip to Las Vegas. You also have seen some partnerships do well in business, in spite of all the odds against them, while others go bankrupt, even though both partners were hard-working and honest.

Similarly, you see a lot of your friends who were in love get married and in a few months they hate each other and separate. Body chemistry and compatibility are not new to our vocabulary; however, it is difficult to explain why these happen. Various phrases such as "lack of understanding," "cheating," "mean," etc., can describe these behaviors.

You may have seen or heard events like the following before:

A father lost his job the day after the son was born; a healthy man took ill soon after getting married; a bridegroom was bitten by a snake and died on the wedding night; a previously very healthy bridegroom had a heart attack on the wedding night; a healthy bride developed severe asthma the day after the wedding night and the asthma continued for years; a healthy bride became bedridden a few months after the wedding; a new mother died after childbirth, a new mother became a lunatic after childbirth and had to be kept in restricted confinement; a father-in-law took ill and died two days after the bride's arrival into the family; the mother-in-law had a stroke and was hospitalized the day after the wedding, and some bystanders may have commented that his wife brought him bad luck.

These are nothing but the negative or positive effect of two electro-magnetic charges between bodies. Just like other external or internal factors causing energy blockages, two different charges between human bodies can also create energy blockages and imbalances or diseases in each other. If the two charges are suitable to each other, they help to keep the energy meridians free of blockages in each other.

Some children suffer from various minor illnesses like hay fever, abdominal cramps, learning disability, lack of concentration, hyperactivity, etc. It is possible that these children are allergic to their parents or some other family members in the house. Such children could turn away from home, looking for comfort elsewhere, because they were allergic to their own parents, and they were being suffocated in the house due to the adverse energy. Neither the children nor the parents understood what was happening to them. Their efforts to survive seemed to take precedence. When the parents planned to have children, they had a lot of pleasant dreams for the future. When the children were born, no one rejoiced more than the parents. If the energy between parents and children was well-matched, a lot of happiness could come to the house. The father could get a promotion soon after the child's birth. The mother could inherit a large amount of money or property from a distant uncle because she was the closest known heir alive when he suddenly died.

How many of you have heard or experienced the wild but true stories like the one seen in "Problem Child?" Of course, you might say that is just a story! But surely you have met lots of problem children. The child in the movie "Problem Child" could have been born with an adverse magnetic force around him towards his parents. If the adverse magnetic energy towards his family and friends was corrected, he or his family and friends would not have suffered such misfortunes.

You may have seen certain family misfortunes take place soon after a child is born, but never associated them with allergies. In one case the father became unemployed as soon as the child was born. Another father lost his hand and a leg in an accident. Yet another couple, while they were bringing the infant home from the hospital, met with an accident. Both parents died on the spot, but the infant survived. Another mother became disabled, due to postpartum complications. In such cases, if the child's energy is very strong or adverse for the mother, the mother's life also could be in danger. If the parents' energy (mother's and father's put together) overcame the child's adverse energy, after a while the father might find a job, the mother might come out of the acute phase of illness, or their financial status might get better, but as the child grows up, problems could be manifested all over again. The parents and the child might have small arguments in the beginning. Later on, small arguments could grow into big ones.

Finally, the child might feel uncomfortable around the parents, and he/she might begin to look for home or comfort elsewhere. If the children do not find the right guidance and support with non-allergic people, they may get into the wrong company, then perhaps into drugs and alcohol. Drugs and alcohol could give a temporary false sense of well-being. They might misunderstand and get into the addictive aspects. They could even leave the house and wander away, looking for drugs and alcohol or looking for means to acquire them. Repulsion between the parents and children could be very small in the beginning; however, if there is an energy incompatibility, small energy differences could become larger and larger as time goes by. In time, the problem would increase, causing unnecessary, unpleasant arguments and fights, which may lead the children to seek shelters, join unhealthy groups and gangs, get into drugs and alcohol or self-destructive acts.

A seven-year-old boy was brought to the office seeking help for some of his allergies. He was found to be allergic to a few food items, his mother and father, and to the grandmother who lived with his family. This child was also being treated for hyperactivity and behavioral problems. He always found some reason to argue and cry whenever he was with his parents. For example, "You don't love me, mommy, you hate me. I don't want to live in this house. I'd like to die. I wish I was never born; I wish I had another mother or father." His parents felt guilty and worried, not knowing what to do, because they loved him very much and did not know how to handle the problem. He was known as a wild child with a lot of bursting energy all through his infancy.

After he was treated for his mother, father, and grandmother, his personality changed for the better. He became quieter, felt very comfortable at home, began to express love toward everyone and even began to get good grades in school. He did not argue or fight with his parents unnecessarily after the treatments. The parents and this child were a few of the lucky ones, because they had the chance to discover his allergies on time, before they got out of hand. His parents could breathe a sigh of relief that, when he grows up, he will not get mixed up with drugs, alcohol or such unfavorable influences because he now feels secure and warm in his own home. His parents will probably never have to worry about him or his behavioral problems again.

A six-year-old male child was brought in with the complaint of hyperactivity. His mother also said that he was very destructive in the house, breaking and throwing things around, and hurting his siblings. He fought with his older siblings all the time. He hurt his younger sister and made her cry. The mother was afraid to leave him alone with his siblings, even for a few minutes.

When she brought him into our office, he appeared very restless. He paced around in the room without stopping for a moment. His mother kept telling him to calm down. He acted as if he did not hear her, but he responded fairly well to the office staff. When he was with one of the staff members, he was calm and responded to her questions. He was able to tell his name, and he helped her put a puzzle together. The moment his mother walked into the room, his behavior changed dramatically. One of his neighbors who had other children of the same age told us that this boy behaved very normally whenever he went to play with her children in her house. His mother thought that probably the cats and dogs in their house could be the culprit for this strange behavior. He was very allergic to sugar and trace minerals.

After he was treated for the food items, he still behaved the same. His older brother blamed the parents for giving him all the special attention. Once, his desperate mother said sadly that she and her husband were seriously thinking of giving him up for adoption, because he was destroying the family, and it was too much to handle him. I had an hour discussion with the parents trying to explain about person to person allergies and how it can interfere with family relationships and how we can overcome them with NAET. He was found to be allergic to his mother, father and other siblings, as well as many food items and environmental things. He was treated for all the family members. When he was treated for all the family members successfully, his behavior became normal. Two years later, he is a very happy, loving and smart boy who never gets into too much mischief. Now, the parents are glad they did not proceed with their plans to give him up for adoption.

Another young woman began to have migraines a week after her wedding. She suffered severe migraines for twenty years and was then found to be allergic to her husband. She was treated, and her migraines cleared up. Much unpleasantness might be averted if people would test themselves for possible allergies before they get into serious relationships. It is possible that in the future, when two people decide to get into a relationship or start a partnership, instead of going to an astrologer to test their compatibility, they may visit a doctor who has knowledge of NAET to find out whether they are allergic to each other.

When people get treated for each other, they no longer suffer from problems they once had. If everyone would learn this testing method and would check for allergies, this could be a happier world. Many marriages and relationships could be saved, fewer children would runaway; there would be less drug addition and other bad habits. There would be more friendship, love and caring among people rather than enemies looking for fights.

Emotional Blockages Causing Allergy-Like Symptoms

A body should be balanced physically, nutritionally and emotionally for normal health. If you are balanced, your health can be affected tremendously. NAET doctors are taught to look at the body as a whole and to administer the necessary treatments.

Emotional blockages can cause severe problems, mimicking allergies or various other common health problems. NAET doctors are trained to isolate emotional blockages from simple allergies and eliminate them permanently, in the same manner they do simple nutritional or environmental allergies. We have treated hundreds of patients who had emotional blockages which were the primary cause of their health problems.

A 25-year-old woman was seen in our office for extreme fatigue, frequent fainting attacks, nausea, anorexia, sleeplessness, frequent vomiting and general body aches whenever she ate sweets. She said that she frequently fainted as a child and vomited any time she ate sweets. She did not remember any trauma in childhood.

She showed emotional allergies to all foods, especially to sugar and chocolate. Through neuro-emotional techniques (NET discovered by

Doctor Scott Walker, Encinitas, CA) and kinesiological testing, it was discovered that she was molested by her neighbor when she was three years old. It was assumed that she was lured toward this child molester by chocolate candies, and that she was molested while she was eating these candies. She may have responded to this unexpected attack with fear. She may have also fainted when he attacked her. She may have vomited with fear, like many children do when they are frightened.

Her brain was confused because she was happy when she got the candy and ate it. But when she was attacked, she became fearful and unhappy while the candy was still in her mouth. So her brain probably received a confusing message from the messenger nerves that eating sweets (candy) was the cause of her fear and unhappiness. The brain took note of this dangerous signal, and in any future contact with anything sweet, it began giving signals about the possible danger to her health. This was the cause of her allergic reactions to all foods. She was treated for this emotional blockage with NAET. After the treatment for this trauma, she stopped reacting to food in general, and her fainting spells were gone. Three years after the treatment, while this book was being written, we contacted her and found out that she was a happy woman at that time.

A 50-year-old female complained of hypoglycemia since childhood. She was found to be very allergic to sugar. When she was treated for sugar with NAET, she cleared the physical and chemical allergy. But the emotional allergy remained the same, and her hypoglycemic reaction became exaggerated. When more investigations were done on the subject, it was revealed that when she was five years old, her parents restricted her sugar consumption, saying that sugar was bad for health. One day, one of their family friends came to visit and gave her a box full of chocolate bars as a gesture of love. But as soon as the friend left the house, her mother snatched the chocolate box from her and flushed the chocolates down the toilet   before she had a chance to eat one. The child felt very bad and she cried for a long time. The mother did not take time to explain to the child the reason for her insensitive behavior. This puzzled the child and left an unhealed wound in her heart and brain. Ever since, with each future contact with sugar or a sugar product, she experienced an unpleasant reaction that had been misdiagnosed as hypoglycemia for the past 45 years. When she was treated for this emotional blockage with NAET, she no longer suffered from hypoglycemia.

Suppose two people were fighting while eating popcorn. One got upset and walked out of the room. The second person was very angry at the person who left the room. He was thinking of a way to solve the problem or to get back at him, but kept eating the popcorn without paying any attention. In fact, at a later point, he may not even remember that he ate all that popcorn. While he was eating popcorn, his brain was stimulated with anger and resentment. The brain was not informed about the actual eating, or the actual eating was forgotten due to the priority of the situation. The brain was aware of eating popcorn, and was forced to associate that with anger and resentment, making note of this association. In a future contact with popcorn, the brain will caution its user about the previous episode of anger and resentment while he ate the popcorn, mimicking an allergic reaction. After the successful completion of treatment of an allergy, the physical and nutritional allergy may never return. But an emotional allergy can return any number of times if you are not careful to avoid unpleasant things while eating or cooking. It is very important to respect food preparation and consumption for better assimilation of the nutrients. How can you avoid the recurrence of emotional allergies?

Good Eating Habits to Prevent Emotional Blockages

Avoid eating when you are under stress. Always have pleasant thoughts while you prepare the food and eat. You can play your favorite music while you cook or eat. When you prepare the food with lots of enthusiasm and warm feelings, you blend the food with unblocked free flowing energy. This will enhance the nutritious value of the food many fold. If you cook with negative emotion, your negative electromagnetic energy will transfer into the prepared food. When the food enters your stomach accompanied by feelings of love and happiness, your body and mind will cherish the nutrients and help the body and mind grow healthy. Many people bless their food before they eat. This ritual gives the mind a chance to clear itself of all its troubled emotions and fill up with a sense of spirituality before eating. You will avoid troubled emotions and food associations when you clear your mind. It may not hold true after the blessing, if you resume arguments and negativity. So, try to eat with people who share pleasant thoughts and make eating a pleasing event. Avoid fights, exchanging bad words, bad news, etc., while eating. It will prevent repeated emotional blockages with food.

A 46-year-old woman severely reacted to Clorox and bleach. An emotional allergy was discovered with this case, too. One morning when she was a new bride of 19, she decided to scrub and clean the kitchen sink. Her father-in-law walked in and praised her, saying what a good job she did, and that he wasn't aware a sink could shine like that since he had never seen it that clean before. Her mother-in-law stood next to her with a deep hurt in her eyes. She responded, saying that she always kept the wash basin cleaner than that but he never bothered to notice it, even once. This made the daughter-in-law very unhappy and, ever since, she has reacted to the smell or touch of any chemical. After she was treated for the incident, she was able to use chemicals and detergents without any adverse reactions.

For the past few years, a 59-year-old man had frequent severe headaches after the consumption of any grain. It was discovered through kinesiological testing that he had a financial loss when he was 41. He lost his restaurant business and was very depressed about it. He may have been eating breads and grain products while he was grieving for the financial loss, and his confused brain assumed that eating the grain and grain products made him sad. So with any future contact with grains, his brain began giving warning signals such as migraine headaches. After the treatment for the incident, he no longer had the usual headaches.

A 28-year-old girl had nightmares and always woke up frightened. Then she couldn't go back to sleep for many hours. Her dream was always about burning fire. She could not remember any childhood trauma or any event that her family talked about. She was living thousands of miles away from home now. Her parents were no longer living. Through kinesiological testing, it was discovered that when she was six months old she was frightened by a scary fire. After she was treated for the emotional blockage, she no longer had scary dreams and nightmares. She was puzzled by this childhood revelation that had ruined many good years.

Finally, she visited her old grandmother, who proceeded to tell her that they had a fire when she was about six months old, and that she was sick from smoke inhalation. Everybody thought that she was sick from smoke inhalation, but she was in fact sick due to fear. If it is taken for granted that infants and small children do not understand anything and you do not explain things to them properly when a disaster takes place, their brains remain puzzled the rest of their lives. It is important to have better communication with infants and children. They may not speak in words, but they can understand you well.

A 50-year-old woman was allergic to money. She was also allergic to many food and environmental items. She was treated for the allergy to money and that cleared all the food allergies for her.

DEPRESSION

Clinical depression is a much talked about subject nowadays. It is very hard to find a normal person anymore. At some time or other, nearly everyone around us suffers from clinical depression. The increase in chemicals in our environment and pesticides in our food is a partial cause of the increasing problems. It is a chemical world with more and more chemicals thrown in it everyday. Everything you buy—vegetables, fruits, grains, meat or clothing, is treated with chemicals. Chemicals are used to kill harmful bacteria, parasites or any other disease-producing organisms.

This is an era of science and technology. Many years ago, before the discovery of germs, germicides and antibiotics, many lives were taken by infections and infectious diseases. The discovery of various chemicals, antibacterial agents, antibiotics and medicines have helped immensely to improve the quality of life. But you can be allergic to any medicine or chemical, just as you can be allergic to a natural vitamin or food. This fact needs to be recognized so allergies to beneficial chemicals and drugs can be eliminated. Then you will be able to enjoy your life using the best 21st century scientific advancements.

A 32-year-old registered nurse who was one of our patients came to our office with complaints of depression that had originally started one week earlier. She began crying desperately. She said she didn't see the need to live any longer. She felt worthless and unloved. Kinesiological testing revealed that the home-canned apples she had been eating for the past week caused her depression. The canned apples came from her mother's house in northern California. Her mother had canned them for her. In this case, she was allergic to the apples, which affected her liver and caused a blockage in the liver meridian. After being treated for the apples, her depression was gone.

Thirty-eight-year-old John had depression for most of his life. He had tried various treatments, including psychotherapy. He was found to be allergic to iron. He had wrought-iron ornamental work all over his house. When he was treated for iron, his depression cleared.

CHAPTER 19

ENVIRONMENTAL ALLERGIES

P hysical agents greatly influence our daily lives. Sensitive individuals may have abnormal reactions when exposed to weather changes: heat, sunlight, humidity, dryness, cold, cold mist, dampness, wind, drought, electricity, radiation from different sources (sun, moon, darkness, television, computer, microwave oven), gas cooktop/oven, air pressure, burns, smog and artificial lights. This abnormal reaction to physical agents can also be called an allergy. Most of the time this type of reaction occurs in patients with other allergic manifestations.

Two types of reactions can occur:

■ Contact reactions take place at the site of contact with the allergen, such as hives or rashes that develop on the portion of the body where the cold air or heat touches directly.

■ Reflex-like reactions may be more generalized or develop in the interior part of the body, such as the effect on the bronchial tubes.

A 70-year-old woman enjoyed eating ice cream. But whenever she ate ice cream she would get paroxysms of coughing or a choking sensation in the throat. When she melted the ice cream and drank it melted and warm, she did not have the cough or the choking sensation. Ice water also had the same effect on her. She felt uncomfortable in air-conditioned rooms, with cold temperatures, and got nasal congestion and a stuffy or runny nose when she walked in cold air. She was allergic to cold. When she was tested for ice cubes, she was found to be allergic to them. She did not react to hot water or tap water. There was a tremendous change in her reaction toward cold when she was treated for ice cubes. Now she does not get throat irritation or coughs when she eats ice cream, or is in an air-conditioned atmosphere.

A 55-year-old woman had just the opposite problem. She could not bear heat. She could not even drink lukewarm liquids. They made her cough and her body turn red. When she walked in the sun, she developed hives and red rashes all over her body. When she stood near a stove and cooked anything, she ended up having a headache. She was also allergic to various foods and environmental substances. After treatment for all of the other allergens, she was treated for hot water which, in turn, helped her to handle not only heat better, but all other allergens as well.

A young man of 32 reacted to sunlight in a different way. He developed canker sores as well as skin cancers on his face, two of which had already been operated on. He also had many food allergies. When he was treated successfully for vitamin D and ultraviolet rays, his reaction to sunlight diminished. He was also allergic to the sun block he used on his body. After he was treated for the sun block, ironically his skin cancer did not return and the two existing spots disappeared.

It has been recognized for many years by various physicians that extremes of temperature, particularly of cold, may bring on attacks of asthma or hives. As long ago as 1860, a physician described attacks of asthma produced in a man by applying cold water to his instep. In 1866, another physician reported that cold water invariably produced intense hives on his skin. In 1872, a physician reported the case of a 45-year-old woman whose hand would swell when it was immersed in cold water. The swelling subsided fifteen minutes after reaching its peak. Cold air produced hives on her face and neck. Eating ice cream immediately caused her intense pain in her throat and a feeling of suffocation.

Weather changes affect allergic patients greatly. Arthritic and respiratory tract allergy patients are affected badly by high or low temperatures. When the temperature falls, the humidity increases and affects asthmatics seriously, in some cases even becoming fatal. Change in altitude also can cause difficulties for allergic patients. Some people do well in high altitudes, whereas others cannot tolerate them at all. In patients with problems in high altitude, treating with NAET for exhaled air from the same person can give relief.

Some people are so severely affected by the cold that they faint or lose consciousness. Many deaths from drowning may have been caused by an allergic reaction to cold. For example, jumping into a cold water lake can cause cramping and/or drowning. The swimmer becomes immobile and/or unconscious due to the severity of the pain. The fact that the swimmer, even an expert one, died soon after eating can also be explained. The swimmer probably had a reaction to a food he/she ate, but did not have any noticeable symptom until diving into the water. The ingested food combined with the physical reaction to the cold resulted in a severe allergic attack.

As in other types of allergic responses, physical allergy may be manifested as:

- Hives or angioneurotic edema of the hands when they wash in cold water and hives on areas of the body exposed to cold air.

- Swelling of the lips or spasms of the stomach after eating cold foods.

- Allergic rhinitis and asthma may be brought on by the inhalation of cold air (responds well to wind and dampness treatment with NAET).

- Skin turning blue in cold air and red under a warm sun.

Most of the time, low concentrations of certain nutrients throw the body into imbalance, and it faces extreme discomfort when the weather changes. Lack of iron, vitamin B 12, and folic acid may cause poor quality and inadequate circulation of blood, blocking its ability to exchange oxygen and carbon dioxide properly and causing more difficulties in extreme temperatures. Many patients who have extremely cold feet or cold hands suffer from poor circulation. After treating for iron with NAET and then taking iron supplements, their circulation improves.

There are some extreme cases of patients with physical allergies. One patient complained of pains in the mouth, esophagus (the canal connecting the throat and stomach), and the stomach after drinking cold water. Cold air caused her lips and tongue to swell, made her eyes water, caused coughing, and prolonged exposure caused asthma. She was treated for basic allergies to all the essential nutrients such as calcium, iron, vitamins C and A, trace minerals, salt, B complex vitamins, sugars, and fats. By the end of these treatments she no longer suffered from an allergy to cold air. When she cleared her allergy to ice cubes, she was even able to drink cold water and eat ice cream.

Another patient, a girl who was a victim of diabetes and kidney failure, could only suck on ice cubes to quench her thirst. (She was not allowed to drink water.) She developed chronic bronchitis and a cough that did not respond to a series of strong antibiotics. After almost eight months of chronic cough, we tried to treat her for ice cubes. She took four consecutive treatments, by NAET, to clear the allergy. To our amazement, she cleared the cough and chronic bronchitis upon passing the ice cube treatments.

Another patient suffered from hives, itching, and redness of the skin, headache, diarrhea, general weakness, and fainting spells whenever she walked in the hot sun, drank hot liquids or had a hot or warm shower. She was treated for hot water and has not reacted nearly as much to heat since then. Another woman suffered from severe asthma only in the summer, but not in winter. When she was treated for food allergies, her asthmatic reaction to heat was reduced.

Very often physical allergies may exist in patients who are also allergic to other substances. While the physical allergy in itself is not sufficient to bring on an allergic attack, contact with the offending allergen plus the physical agent may precipitate an attack. An example of this type of allergy was seen in a woman who frequently suffered asthmatic attacks produced by sudden exposure to cold wind. When she was treated for the foods she was sensitive to, exposure to cold wind also lost its affect. Sometimes people are allergic to both heat and cold, and this makes them miserable all the time. Such was the case of a man who developed hives and edema, and sometimes dizzy spells, after he played tennis. When he took cold showers, he had similar complaints. He was also found to be allergic to: tennis balls, tennis rackets, shoes, soaps, shampoos, various foods, etc. After he was treated for all the known allergens, as well as for hot water and ice cubes, he no longer reacted to heat or cold.

Christmas Tree Allergy

My wife's irritating, impossible Christmas tree allergy was eliminated by Dr. Devi Nambudripad's fantastic acupuncture discoveries. Her method will revolutionize the current medical approach to allergy treatment for all people.

Dr. Stanley Y. Inouye, D.D.S., M.S.D.
Sacramento, CA

Some people are sensitive only to the sun's heat. In this case, they may be allergic to the sun's actinic rays only. These people are also allergic to various items. In the presence of other allergies, an allergy to the sun's rays brings on worse reactions. Such was the case of a man who worked on a farm and had severe dermatitis with redness, extreme swelling and itching of the face, lips, neck and hands. He could only work during the early part of the morning hours or late in the evenings. The rest of the time he spent indoors. He was also found to have various food allergies. After treatments for all the food items, his reactions to the sun were also reduced.

When physical allergy occurs in conjunction with pollen, foods or other substances, it is possible to treat the patients successfully by treating for the other nonphysical allergens. Most of the time, patients do not continue to react to the physical agents. When people suffer from allergy to physical agents only, they must be treated for cold or heat. Such cases are very rarely seen. In these rare cases, when no other treatments work, it would be wise to avoid heat-producing foods (according to Chinese nutrition theory) in heat-sensitive patients and cold-producing foods in cold-sensitive patients. The author has not seen any cases in her practice that did not respond well to some kind of allergy treatments.

Joseph, a 67-year-old man, came to our office with complaints of excruciating pain and red rashes on the lateral parts of the thigh, leg and foot for more than a week. He had seen a few professionals for this problem without any result. His pain and immobility kept increasing. Kinesiological exams focused on an allergy to the sardines he had eaten

The Beautiful Silkworms

I was suffering from headaches, rashes on my arms, backache and sinusitis. Many chiropractic adjustments brought only temporary relief. I taught preschool and was raising silkworms as a science project on life cycles. When I was treated for mulberry leaves, the symptoms cleared up and I now have used this same project, with no ill effects, for three years.

Mary Karaba.
La Mirada, CA

a week before. He was treated for sardines by NAET, and his pain and rashes disappeared in a few hours.

Margarite, a 59-year-old woman came with a history of vitiligo (white spots all over the body, some under the chin, in front of the ears, leg, back of the neck) for almost 30 years. She was found to be allergic to wool, vitamin C, dust mites, yeast, molds, fruits, yogurt, vinegar, chlorophyll, whole grains and melanin. When she was treated for these items, her white spots were replaced by normal skin pigments.

Maxine, a 72-year-old female, had chronic weeping ulcers on the tips of the fingers of both her hands for many years and had tried all the possible medicines and ointments on the stubborn ulcers. While taking her history, it was revealed that caring for roses was her main hobby. Having taken this into consideration, she was tested for the roses by muscle response testing and was found to be highly allergic to them. When she was treated by NAET for allergies, her chronic ulcers healed nicely.

Kathy, a 23-year-old woman, suffered from a type of dermatitis that did not respond to the treatments of food products, chemicals or environmental items. Various parts of her body such as the neck, lips, face, chest, etc., showed dry, cracked furrows with clear water-filled blisters that looked like first degree burns. Often she had blood and serum oozing from weeping blisters. Her history revealed that she was all right until she moved in with her fiancé a year and a half earlier. She was allergic to her fiancé's saliva. Her mysterious problem was solved when she was treated for his saliva by NAET.

INSECT AND SPIDER BITES

Many people react to bites from insects. Spider and flea bites can be fatal in some cases. Many people react to wasp and bee stings. This case study is taken from another doctor's practice. One of his patients came in with many spider bites on her arms. She was bitten while working in her vegetable garden. The bites were very painful and her arms were swollen. The doctor asked her to bring one dead spider from her garden. She was treated by NAET for allergy to the spider. After treatment, her wounds healed, and she was no longer bothered by spider bites from her garden.

Flea bites are another commonly ignored allergic item for many allergy sufferers. A nine-year-old girl, who had had severe asthma for eight years, was treated for various allergies, bringing her asthma under control. After she was treated for animal dander, cats and dogs did not bother her any more. One day she visited some of her friends who had a dog. After a few minutes, her asthma returned. She was allergic to the fleas. When she was treated for the fleas, she stopped having breathing difficulties when near cats and dogs.

Ellen, a 59-year-old patient, came to the office with a typical case of accidental serum injection poisoning. She was vacationing in New York where she was stung by a bee while boarding a bus. Although she had known that she reacted strongly to insect bites as a child, she had no idea how much the allergic condition had increased over the years. Within minutes, she was feeling nauseous and lightheaded and was having difficulty breathing. Luckily, she was taken to a hospital emergency care unit. By the time she reached the hospital, she experienced some respiratory distress. She was treated by the doctors and hospitalized for three days.

When she returned to California ten days later she was still experiencing some cellulitis in her left arm. She was brought to our office. After she received treatments by NAET to desensitize her for bee sting, the cellulitis in the arm diminished. One year later, when she was camping, bees stung her again. She panicked and her friends drove her to the nearest hospital, about 40 miles away. They sat in the hospital parking lot and waited for two long hours to see whether she was going to have any reaction. Since she felt all

Severe Reaction to Bee Sting

In 1986, I was traveling in England when I was stung by a bee on my left arm. I was treated with an antihistamine and an antibiotic. My arm grew steadily worse, I flew home in that condition, thinking that it would heal in time. Nine days later, I was entertaining a slight fever in my arm and unusual redness. It had become more swollen than ever and more uncomfortable.

My friend insisted I visit Dr. Devi. I was afraid of acupuncture. I had little knowledge of it. Visions of needles in my body was also unpleasant. If antibiotics could not help, what could she do? In desperation, I allowed her to take me to her office. I found Dr. Devi interesting and knowledgeable and her profound confidence that she could help me right then persuaded me to let her treat me. I found the treatment relaxing and even enjoyable. I could not believe that the needles did not hurt - almost immediately I felt better. By morning, after the best night's rest I had experienced in days, I found the swelling was gone! Was this my arm? It sure was! I called her and said, "It is a miracle, I am coming back today." Since that time she has treated me for all my allergies. I feel now I am "allergy free."

Ileen Coons
Fullerton, Calif.

right, they returned without entering the hospital. The next day she came to our office. She had many bee sting marks on her arms, which looked like mild prickly heat, but never experienced any unpleasant reactions.

A 79-year-old male patient from North Carolina worked as a painter when he was young and had been stung by wasps many times while on his ladder painting houses. He developed cancer, which had metastasized, throughout his body by the time it was discovered and was given six months to live. He refused any traditional treatment for his problem but was treated for various allergies, one of which was wasp stings. Soon his condition began to change. His appetite increased, and he did not feel sleepy or fatigued any more. He increased his activities and started playing golf once again. A year later, when he went to the same clinic that had given him six months to live, his doctors were amazed at his condition. "Some miracle has happened," they said. "Somehow your cancer has gone into remission." Actually, it was the repeated injection of wasp venom into his body that created the cancer. An abnormal proliferation of the cells in his body was the reaction he experienced from the wasp stings. He did not show any external reactions such as hives or swelling, etc. When he was treated for the same toxin, his body responded well and created the antidote to destroy the wasp venom and the carcinoma that was the side effect of the wasp stings. His energy level increased. When he went for a follow-up visit at the hospital, his cancer was in remission.

Many people react to fertilizers used on the soil to cultivate their kitchen garden. When they use the vegetables grown with the fertilizers, they

---

City Water Causing Fatigue And Pain

I suffered from extreme fatigue and diffused pain all over my body. My feet remained edematous. When I began treatments with Dr. Devi, she found out that city water was causing my body aches and fatigue. I do not drink the tap water. I use it to cook, clean and bathe. She treated me for the tap water. 35 hours after the treatment, my pedal edema, body ache and fatigue diminished. Every few months I would still react to water, depending on the water chemicals the city used in the purifying process. Now I recognize the symptoms and immediately test and treat my city water. Sometimes, I react to the bottled water the same way. Thanks to NAET, I don't have to run from doctor to doctor to find out the cause of my illness!

Ileen Garcia
Long Beach

> ### *Allergy To Pesticides*
>
> *When I came to Devi I had been unable to live in my home for 6 months. Our neighbor had been spraying poison. I was also allergic to our new refrigerator. After a few basic treatments, she treated me for the refrigerator and pesticides and I was able to go home right away. Three weeks later, the neighbor sprayed pesticides again and after 3 days of staying inside with the windows closed, I was able to be outside and not get sick. I will be eternally grateful. There are some things I am still having trouble with, but I am definitely on the right track.*
>
> *Nancy Saucy,*
> *Anaheim, CA*

begin to get sick. These people need to be treated for the fertilizer used on the soil.

INSECT SPRAYS

Some people get sick on insecticides that they spray on plants, flowers or inside the house for small insects. Insect sprays paralyze the respiratory system of the insects and they die in a few seconds to a minute. These sprays contain minute amount of poisons. If a sensitive individual comes in contact with the toxin, he/she can also be affected.

In some cases, drinking water and city water cause severe health problems. Water chemicals are added to the water to kill the pathogenic bacteria. If we do not kill them in the water, they can kill us when we drink the water. But some of the chemically sensitive patients are highly reactive to the chemicals added to the water. If the patients are taught to test the city water or drinking water every day by MRT, this problem can be avoided.

Diamonds Are Forever

When I began my allergy treatments with Dr. Devi, I could not get through a meal without a dripping, full nose, sometimes with difficulty in breathing, clearing my throat, sneezing, swelling around the eyes, pains in my chest, joints, and lower back, feet, and knees. I had been diagnosed as anemic, arthritic, inclined to hypochondria. I felt extremely tense, and yet by three o'clock in the afternoon, I could not stay awake, and needed a 15-minute nap to make it through the rest of the day. I had trouble climbing stairs due to weakness in my legs. The joints in my left hand caused me pain and Dr. Devi found out that I was allergic to the diamonds in my wedding band. When I drove more than half an hour I suffered from excruciating pain in my right leg and we found an allergy to the formic acid used in hard rubber products such as the gas pedal.

These treatments have totally changed my life. I am now a functioning energy-charged, healthy being, much to my delight. Now when necessary, Dr. Devi and I are able to trace any new ache or pain to a sensitivity to a material in our atmosphere or a food item, and eliminate it. I am also treating for those dormant, but possible future problems such as different diseases. I expect to expand my life-style by these treatments as well as live each day to its fullest in the optimum of health and well being.

Helene S.
Costa Mesa, CA

ALLERGY TO JEWELRY

People can be allergic to the jewelry and clothing they are wearing and sometimes to the jewelry and clothing others are wearing. They may also be allergic to items when visiting friends, shopping, attending theaters or going anywhere people congregate. A young woman who was a patient in our office complained of getting sinus blockages, pain in the upper arms and sometimes numbness on certain parts of the body whenever she sat in our waiting room. She claimed she felt better away from the office. The office staff felt guilty about this and decided to investigate.

She was scheduled for treatment at the same time as another lady who always wore a large crystal pendant. They were both in the office at the same time waiting to see the doctor. We discovered that the first woman was allergic to the crystal the other woman was wearing. The energy field of the crystal was very strong, like diamonds, and was affecting the first patient's field from ten feet away. From that day on, these two patients were scheduled at different times until the patient with the allergy could be treated for the crystal.

For ten years, a young man had constant yeast infections, chronic fatigue syndrome, emotional fatigue, night sweats, nervousness, poor memory and various mental disturbances. He had seen a number of medical doctors, chiropractors, acupuncturists, and nutritionists to get some relief. Often suicidal, he was going for psychiatric counseling regularly. Over the next six months, he was treated in our office for various allergies and showed marked progress.

He stopped having night sweats and fatigue, his memory improved and the yeast infection cleared up for the first time in ten years. He began to live normally, until three or four months later. Then all of a sudden he returned to the office in tears. He said he was almost back to where he had started. We tested him for the various items that he was once treated for and found no allergy to anything. We noticed that he was wearing a lot of jewelry: four earrings, with four different stones in one ear, a heavy necklace with a huge gold and silver pendant, eight rings on the fingers with stones (star ruby, diamond, emerald, garnet, turquoise, sapphire, etc., and a gold watch studded with diamonds). When he was tested for the stones, he was found to be highly allergic to them. He revealed that he had taken off all the jewelry when he started the treatments with us months ago. He was fond of jewelry and for ten years had always adorned himself with these jewels. Since he was feeling better, he started wearing them again and all the previous symptoms returned. He was treated for all the jewelry and once again he became healthy and happy.

CRYSTALS AND STONES

Many times, stiffness, pain in the shoulders and upper back tension can be the result of an allergy to jewelry.

Gold has been used in treatment for arthritis for years. If you are allergic to gold you can experience the exaggerated symptom of arthritis. Whenever you are allergic to a substance, it can generate the exaggerated symptom of the disease that was supposed to have been helped by the same substance.

A 27-year-old female was a victim of an allergy to gold. She was married at age 22 and, according to her custom, a tradition in India, she wore a thick gold chain around her neck. She was not allowed to remove the chain until she or her husband died. She began to have severe neck and shoulder pains. She went from doctor to doctor for some relief. One day her pain got so severe that she had to be rushed to the emergency room. X-rays of the neck showed a clean cut of the C5 vertebra exactly beneath the chain. She was kept in the hospital, and the vertebra was fused. She was all right for two months. Then she began to have the excruciating pain, all over again. This time she came to us, and we found that she was allergic to the thick gold chain she was wearing. She was treated for gold, and her neck pains and body aches disappeared. She still wears the chain around her neck. Since her treatment for gold, she does not have to worry about the reactions any more.

HEAT / COLD / DARKNESS

Helen, a 74-year-old woman, liked to drink cold water, but always choked on icy cold water. She also developed an allergic dry cough whenever she ate ice cream. She was treated for all the ingredients in the ice cream, yet her coughing spells and choking incidents persisted. She was finally treated for actual ice cubes. Afterwards, she could enjoy ice water and ice cream without choking.

John suffered from a continuous cough all winter (from October through April). When the weather warmed up, his cough got better. Every year, he went through the same problem. He drank cough syrup by bottles without any result. His friend referred him to us. When he was evaluated through NTT, he was found to be allergic to cold. He was treated for cold (ice cubes). For the past five winters in a row he has not had a cough.

Forty-nine-year-old Smith suffered from asthma all his life. As he was getting older, his attacks intensified. Inhalers and cortisone refused to work on him as before. He was forced to increase the dosage frequently to get some results. Then he heard about NAET through one of his friends. Another NAET specialist treated him for various food and environmental substances. His energy improved and he felt better overall, but his asthma did not get better. After 84 treatments, his practitioner referred him to me for evaluation. By evaluating through NTT, I found that he was reacting to dampness. He was treated for dampness immediately. In less than ten minutes, he reported that his lungs and respiratory passages opened up. "Something lifted off my chest," he exclaimed. "I can feel the air filling up my lungs for the first time in my life!" After that treatment, he did not have asthmatic attacks.

Five-year-old Ronja suffered from asthma ever since he was an infant. He was using various medications, especially in cold weather. He was treated for cold (ice) that helped his asthma about 30 percent. When he was treated for dampness, his asthma left, never to appear again in three years.

The problem for 30-year-old Michael was different. He lived near the ocean and suffered from depression until 11 a.m. He felt better when the sun came out and the fog lifted. His depression improved after he was treated for the Basic 10 treatments and cold (ice cube), cold mist, serotonin and neurotransmitters.

Many people suffer from depression during the winter season. They seem to be reactive to the long nights (darkness). They feel better when the summer returns. This is a problem for people living in places like Alaska where they have long, dark nights during winter. Some people feel better if they sit in front of bright white lights for a few hours everyday. Many people begin to have food cravings during winter. Such people may need to get treated for vitamin D, calcium, pineal gland, sugar, serotonin, fatty acids, magnet, and salt. NAET treatments can help with this condition.

Seana, 42, suffered from winter depression and became suicidal. She was found to be allergic to vitamin D, calcium, sugar, serotonin, melatonin, magnet, pineal gland, and fatty acids. After she was successfully treated for her allergies, she no longer suffered from her usual winter depression.

Esther, a 42-year-old woman, became very disturbed mentally and physically whenever it was hot. Her whole body swelled up in the hot season and/or if she walked in the sun for a few minutes. She could never drink hot liquids or eat hot foods without getting sick. Whenever she ate hot foods, she would have a paroxysmal tachycardia (very speedy heart rate) and her whole body would become red and swollen. She was treated for very hot water. A few minutes after treatment by NAET, she had abdominal cramps and severe continuous diarrhea. After clearing her treatment for hot water, her body began to adjust to the heat in a normal way.

A week after the treatment, there was a heat wave in Southern California. The temperatures reached 104 degrees. Her car broke down

---

Water, Pure Water, Can It Cause Hair Loss?

Although I was surprised when Dr. Devi suggested that I be treated for purified and tap water, I was allergic to both. After treatment, I noticed an amazing phenomenon. In the past, I had loss of hair each time I washed my hair. Since I have thick hair it has never surprised me. The first morning I washed my hair following the 25-hour-treatment lay off period, I lost virtually no hair! I am sure it was the result of my treatment for water.

Carolyn W.
Anaheim, CA

---

mid-afternoon, and she had to walk for about 15 minutes to reach the gas station for help. Amazingly, she did not react to the heat, as she would have before the treatment. She did not even have the usual foot swelling. Now she enjoys hot herbal teas and soups, and she has lost 35 pounds. In her case, the allergy to heat was the cause of her obesity.

A 38-year-old woman had second-degree burns with huge blisters as a result of a container of boiling water falling on her. After one week of extreme pain, she was treated by NAET with very hot water in a glass jar. After 24 hours the pain was gone. Within a week, her skin was healed.

Jenny, a woman of 58 years, suffered from Raynaud's disease. The tip of her fingers remained dark blue on a cold day. She was allergic to cold, citrus fruits, and cold cut meat products. She felt better when she was cleared for those items.

Bill, a 67-year-old man, used to get severe knee pains on both knees whenever it was cold or cloudy. He was found to be allergic to sodium chloride, potassium, and cold. His sodium-potassium pump probably became less active when he was surrounded by cold. This may have caused his poor circulation and water collection in his larger joints, bringing about his pain during cold weather.

Angela, a 54-year-old female patient, had a history of catching a cold after taking a shower and walking in a cold draft from the main house to her dwelling 50 yards away. She was treated with NAET in the presence of ice cubes (cold) and table fans (the draft). Successful treatment ended her problem of catching cold after showering.

Sarah, a 64-year-old patient, visited Colorado Springs. At that altitude, she noticed a shortness of breath and began sighing deeply. A local NAET practitioner treated her for carbon dioxide blown into a paper bag, Within a few hours, her breathing difficulties ceased. She was able to stay there for another week with no further problem.

Sam, a 26-year-old patient who lived near the ocean, regularly became very depressed in the early mornings until the sun came up. He was allergic to cold humid air. Using NAET, he was treated by filling a jar with ice cubes to produce cold, humid air.

Susan, a 46-year-old patient, complained of shortness of breath and swelling of her body whenever she was in the high humidity in Hawaii. She was treated by NAET with a large jar half filled with boiling water. The hot air coming from the jar simulated the humid air that caused her reaction.

LATEX ALLERGIES

To most people, latex gloves can be a very helpful item. If the allergic person uses them, it can turn into a disaster. Many people are allergic to latex gloves, one of the most common items found in hospitals. Hardly any procedure is done in the hospitals without latex gloves. If the allergic person happens to use them, it can be life threatening.

A 48-year-old woman went to the dentist for a routine cleaning. The dental hygienist put on a pair of latex gloves and began cleaning her teeth. All of a sudden, she began feeling very hot; her body became burning hot. The patient almost went into anaphylactic shock. The doctor came in and called the paramedics who revived her with the help of drugs. She had red rashes all over her body and a mild fever when she left the dentist's office. She came to our office two days later with red rashes still on her body and a fever of 100 degrees Fahrenheit.

Testing through NTT showed she was allergic to the latex gloves the dental hygienist used. She was also allergic to the chalk powder in the gloves, which affected her large intestine, heart and gallbladder meridians. She was treated for the gloves and the powder. After she was treated for the gloves, she was also treated for local anesthetics, amalgam, cleaning agents, gauze and the cotton balls. She was advised to return to the dental office to finish up the dental work. This time, she had no adverse reaction. She even had a root canal!

Later, she revealed that the allergy elimination treatment for the latex gloves and the powder was the best thing that happened to her in 15 years. She had been afraid to have any intimate relationship with her husband for many years. She reacted to his semen and broke out in rashes and blisters all over her body whenever she had intercourse. She was allergic to the condom materials and couldn't use them or be around them. Later, she was successfully treated for her husband's semen, and it goes without saying that she is a very happy woman now.

Allergy to Perfume!

Wendy W., a 44 year old assistant superintendent of education and doctoral student, could not tolerate the scent of perfume, cologne or even certain flowers without getting migraine headaches. As this was a common exposure at work related meetings and classes, she was often forced to leave work or class due to the severity of her pain. After two treatments for perfume mix, Wendy states that while she still "feels" the perfume, she has had no migraines, and has not missed work or class since, due to migraine.

An interesting side note to Wendy's story involves an earlier treatment we did for chocolate. Neither she nor I thought anything about the results of that treatment until one of her coworkers complained that Wendy never had any chocolate in her desk any more. It seemed that this person could at any time find a large supply of chocolate in Wendy's drawer, and help herself. After her treatment, Wendy's craving for chocolate gradually subsided, her stash dwindled and eventually ran out without her taking notice. Sometimes an allergy can cause a craving. This type of craving reduction is not uncommon after eliminating the allergy.

Wendy's friend Debbie, also a school superintendent and attorney had been my patient for the last few months. She began to complain of numbness in the index finger and thumb of her right hand. Myofacial release and other treatments wasn't helping. About that time I learned NAET. I tested using my new learned skill NAET-MRT. This new test revealed that Debbie's numbness was NOT a physical problem (such as carpal tunnel syndrome), but rather a chemical/nutritional allergy. Further MRT testing showed that the allergy was to lemon Ricola cough drops she had taken 6 weeks prior. Treating twice for the cough drops (15 minutes apart) ended the numbness.

NAET is awesome! Thank you for sharing it with us! We have a 100% NAET practice now. J.and M. Chianese, (330) 743-0304.

John, an infant, was one week old when his mother found him in his crib without any signs of life. He wasn't breathing. She grabbed him and shook him. Her husband called the paramedics. Within three minutes they arrived and found his heart had stopped. They revived him by using a defibrillator. John was alive once again, his breathing and heartbeat restored.

He was taken to the hospital for monitoring for 48 hours and then sent home with a beeping monitor. Whenever he stopped breathing, the beeper went

Allergy To My Car!

I started NAET treatments with Dr. Devi to get rid of my sinus allergies. One of the main problems I always had was being allergic to my car, or any other car. She treated me for my car, exhaust and gasoline. Usually, when I would get into my car, for 45 minutes to an hour I would always sneeze, hack and clear my throat and head a number of times. After passing the treatment, I have had no problems while in my car. I have driven over 100 miles at a time and no sinus drainage occurs. I am really excited about this procedure.

Mary Jean Fincher
Glendora, CA

off. At home his beeper was going off frequently, at least five to eight times a day. His mother, grandmother and father watched closely for 24 hours. Although he was doing fine in the hospital, he was having breathing stoppages frequently at home. Later on, it was found that he was allergic to the attractive plastic crib covering and other plastic accessories. After he was treated for the plastic items by NAET, his heart and breathing were fine.

Kathy, one of the secretaries in our office, was attending a computer demonstration. Five minutes after the demonstration began, she complained of feeling hot all over her body and uncomfortable. She was working at the computer keyboard. Instantly, she began having blisters on her lips, rashes on her face and a sensation of light-headedness. The author found that the keyboard (plastic) material was causing the problem. She was treated for the special plastic keyboard and sent home. When she returned to work the next day, she felt fine. Ever since, she has worked on that computer keyboard without any further ill effects.

MULTIPLE CHEMICAL SENSITIVITIES

Bill, a 49-year-old man complained of severe pains in the right elbow, the wrist joint and the first interphalangeal joints. He was treated for carpal tunnel syndrome, tenosynovitis, and tennis elbow many times before he came to our office. When he was evaluated in our office, he was found to be highly allergic to paper, one of the tools of his trade as a writer.

Food coloring causes many allergies among people. Sally, a 42-year-old patient, suffered from severe persistent perspiration on her palms, feet, axilla and groin. After careful observation, it was found that she had perspired profusely soon after she ate some lemon colored candies. She got relief from her problem after she was treated for her allergy to yellow food coloring.

Silica or silicon dioxide is a chemical compound consisting of silicon and oxygen. Silica occurs widely in rock-forming minerals called silicates, which make up much of the earth's crust (outside and inside the earth). Some of the items derived from silicates are quartz crystals, ceramics, feldspar, glass, mica, opal, silica gel, silicon and silicone. Reactions to these materials vary from person to person. One of the forms of silica is silicone used in implants mainly for cosmetic purposes. An allergy to silicone can produce various health problems in people. Silica is used in many products around us such as glass used on windows, doors, car doors, etc. People who react to silica can get sick riding in a car or sitting near a glass window or door. Silica gel is used as a sealing agent in bathrooms and places where there is a leak. It is also used in certain glues.

A 38-year-old woman who had severe migraines for 20 years came to see me. Through NTT, it was revealed that an implant was creating toxic build up in her body, causing her headaches. At that time, she told me about her silicone breast implant. Ever since she had the implant put in 20 years ago, she suffered from migraines and digestive problems. She was treated for silicone and her 20 years of migraine headaches and digestive troubles were eliminated.

Another woman got sick whenever she traveled in her car. Blame was placed on car exhaust, fumes, smell of gasoline, movement in the car, smog, etc. But through NTT, it was discovered that she was allergic to the glass in the doors, which was traced to the silica. After she was treated for silica, her travel in the car became enjoyable.

Maria, a 49-year-old woman, had severe hot flashes for the last three years. She was on hormone supplements, but nothing gave her relief. She was found to be allergic to heat, sugar and hormones. After she was cleared for these items, her hot flashes stopped completely.

Allergy to the rowing and rocking motion in a boat could be another cause of sea sickness. Some people are sensitive to various motions on land (running, jogging, cycling, dancing, playing tennis, driving a car, exercising), and in the air (airplane, roller coaster, climbing a pole or tree). These are all considered motion sickness. Many people get sea sick due to the rowing or swaying motion of the boat disturbing the inner ear balance. Allergy to salt could be another cause of sea sickness. These people may be also allergic to other minerals, fish, iodine, or the swaying motion itself. Various motions can be treated through NAET. After successful NAET treatment for rocking, swaying, or different motions, people can go and experience the same body movements without any unpleasant reactions and enjoy trips on the ocean once again.

A 24-year-old woman was on her honeymoon in the Virgin Islands when she discovered that sea travel was not designed for her. She became very ill on her return. She not only felt nauseated and dizzy, but also experienced frequent nightmares of her trip. She tested positive for allergies to salt, iodine, fish, B complex and swaying motion. A year after her treatment, she was able to take a trip to Catalina Island without any problems. Ever since, she has taken numerous ocean cruises without any ill effects.

When people get sick in the air, treatments are slightly different. A 28-year-old female got panic attacks whenever she traveled by plane. In this case, she was allergic to plastics, formaldehydes, perfumes, polyester, pesticides, airplane pillows, blankets, ear phones, peanuts, pesticides and airplane seats. On top of all that, she also had a fear of flying. Her panic attacks during flight disappeared after her NAET treatments.

If people become sick while playing tennis, golf, etc., they may be allergic to the exact positions or motions of their games. They can be treated through a surrogate for the exact motion of playing tennis, golf or any such games. If you suffer from one of these complaints, ask your NAET practitioner for help.

If you react to any type of fumes (from your home, work, outside air, air conditioning vent, gasoline smell, perfume smell, cigarette smoke, wood burning smoke, cooking oil smell, fried food smell), you may need to collect a sample before you see your NAET practitioner. Collecting a sample is a simple procedure that can speed up your treatment. Taking some wet paper towels and wiping the inside of the exhaust pipes of cars and trucks will give a satisfactory gasoline and diesel fuel sample. Or leave a wet paper towel in an open container in the area of the smell for 8 – 10 hours. Afterwards, put the paper towel in a glass jar with a lid and take it to your NAET doctor. You should also be treated for fresh gasoline, the actual cigarette, and other materials that produce the offending smells, along with the actual smell.

A 36-year-old male suffered from asthma and a Los Angeles syndrome. Whenever he traveled away from Los Angeles, his lungs cleared and so did the effects of his asthma. The moment he landed in Los Angeles, his chest tightened and breathing problems started. He was a lawyer by profession and had to make many trips in and out of Los Angeles. After he was treated for automobile exhaust, gasoline, diesel, fireplace smoke and cigarette smoke, his asthma improved, and he started to enjoy living in Los Angeles.

A young wife moved to Los Angeles with her husband from a rural village in India. They lived in a small apartment. For the first time in her life she started using natural gas for cooking. The house was also heated by gas. In a few days' time she became very tired, depressed and slept almost the entire day. Lacking energy or enthusiasm to do anything, she was unable to handle her daily chores. Worried, her husband took her to different doctors. She was treated for psychological problems and placed on antidepressants, which gave her some relief. Then she started having severe nasal congestion, headaches and backaches. At this point, she visited our office. After elimination of a few allergies by NAET, her problems were pinpointed to natural gas. After she was treated for natural gas by NAET, she improved both mentally and physically.

CHAPTER 20

ALLERGY AND
THE CIRCULATORY SYSTEM

D iseases affecting the heart and circulatory system may be influenced by various allergies. Most chronic diseases develop as a result of some severe irritation. This chronic irritant could be an allergen. People suffering from arteriosclerosis (or plaque in the blood vessels) seem to be allergic to milk products and calcium from very early childhood. The body does not digest, absorb, or assimilate the ingested calcium products through proper channels. Instead, the particles get stuck along vessels and cause obstruction of the blood flow. Another problem seen among heart and circulatory cases is allergy to iron and iron products. Allergies to these two items, along with salt (sodium) and potassium, are most common among heart patients. A large percentage of the time, allergies are linked to cardiac arrhythmia, hypertension and hypotension (high and low blood pressure respectively), varicose veins and hemorrhoids. Some hemorrhages caused by allergies may occur in various tissues of the body such as the skin, GI tract, eyes, nose and urogenital tract. People allergic to iron usually bruise easily. People with varicose veins are usually allergic to bioflavonoids (also known as vitamin P). Their varicose veins improve significantly after only a few months of treatment.

A 38-year-old man with severe varicose veins on both legs also suffered from bleeding hemorrhoids. He was allergic to vitamin P. After NAET treatment, we placed him on vitamin P supplements. In only six months, not only did his hemorrhoids stop bleeding, but the varicose veins on his legs also started disappearing. After a year, he came in for a reevaluation, and the varicose veins on his legs were minimal.

A 60-year-old woman had an extreme case of varicose veins on both legs below the knees. Her feet were also constantly swollen due to poor circulation. Nothing gave her any relief from her pain. We discovered she was allergic to vitamin P. After treatment, she was supplemented with vitamin P and her pain and swelling decreased to a bare minimum within three weeks.

Cardiac arrhythmia is produced by various allergies and can be found in any age group. A two-week-old boy happened to be allergic to his mother's milk. He had a heartbeat of 200 to 250 a minute. He was kept in a cardiac unit for the first two weeks of his life due to his cardiac arrhythmia. His anxious parents waited two weeks for the cardiac specialists to diagnose his problem. When the doctors could find no physical or physiological reason for the problem, his 22-year-old mother brought the infant to our office. She was a previous NAET patient of ours. Sure enough, we discovered he was allergic to breast milk. His heartbeat returned to normal after his breast milk treatment.

Mother's Milk

My grandson was born with an irregular heartbeat and was back at the hospital within the first ten days of his life with a racing heartbeat. Since I had been coming to Dr. Devi for about a year, I suggested to my daughter that we take him to see her. After arriving, Dr. Devi found he was reacting to his mother's milk. After being treated he went totally limp in a spread-eagle position and slept solid for seven to eight hours. Since that time, he has had no more problems with irregular heartbeat and when he is not reacting to something he has eaten, he is a grand little boy. We continue treatment with Dr. Devi.

Meg Brazil
Fullerton

A young girl of nine complained of heart palpitations one day around 4 p.m. after returning from school. Her worried parents took her to her pediatrician, and later to a heart specialist. Even though she received a certificate of good health, she kept having fast heartbeats almost daily. We evaluated her condition at our office. The food journal we asked her to keep revealed that she ate at least six to ten chocolate bars a week. Her allergy to chocolate was affecting her heart. After treatment for chocolate, she was able to eat it without producing any discomfort.

A 72-year-old female complained of cardiac arrhythmia and dizzy spells. She also had hypertension, severe arteriosclerosis, hearing loss, migraine headaches, abdominal cramps, swelling of both feet, and she had a mild to moderate number of varicose veins. Our tests revealed she was highly allergic to cereals, milk products, chicken, turkey, eggs, sugars, vitamin A, fish, chocolate, vegetable oils, salt, caffeine and various pollens and flowers. After treatment for all the above items, her migraine headaches were completely relieved. Her blood pressure dropped from 210/120 mm. hg to 150/90 mm. hg., and stabilized there without any help of medication. She no longer suffered from varicose veins and swollen feet. Her dizzy spells and cardiac arrhythmia also subsided.

A 24-year-old woman with an eight-month-old child began to experience frequent chest pains that radiated into her left arm all the way to her ring finger. Her condition progressively worsened. A well-known cardiologist examined her and could not find anything wrong. She also began to experience rapid heartbeats occasionally. One of her friends, who was previously treated for allergies with NAET, recognized her symptoms as allergic in origin and advised her to see us. Our evaluation revealed that she was allergic to tomatoes. Her condition cleared within only eleven treatments.

Most of the time, heaviness in the chest, chest pain, and rapid heartbeat are manifestations of food allergies; although fabrics and jewelry can also cause them. A 40-year-old woman had heart palpitations whenever she wore gold, platinum and aquamarine. Her husband gave her a piece of jewelry with an aquamarine (her birthstone) set in platinum. Whenever she put the jewelry on, she experienced heart palpitations and profuse perspiration. Once, she was even taken to the emergency room for the complaints, but they found nothing wrong with her. When she was finally treated for allergies to the stone and platinum, her heart started beating normally and her perspiration lessened considerably.

HEART AND CIRCULATION

Angina pain can be caused by various allergens. Any allergen causing a blockage in the heart meridian can cause angina pains. Heaviness of the chest, pain in the chest, tightness in the chest, radiation of the pain into left arm and fingers, especially the ring and little fingers, are some of the allergy-induced angina symptoms. Plastic bags or other plastic products, coffee, chemicals in the tap water, sulfites, fats, metals and spices are some of the common items that cause angina-like symptoms.

I Don't Hurt Anymore

I had a chronic pain on the right side of my neck with the pain radiating into my right arm almost all the time ever since I can remember (maybe since I was seven or eight years old). Now I am 75 years old. I was also very obese with an enlarged liver even though I was a strict vegetarian all my life and never even touched alcohol. I had high cholesterol and my triglyceride level was 900 mgms.

I was diagnosed as diabetic for two years when Dr. Devi started treating me for various health problems. Six months after receiving treatments, I woke up one day with no pain in my neck or arm. My diabetic symptoms began to decrease gradually. Six years later, my arthritis is completely gone. I don't hurt anymore. My triglyceride level is 200 mgms now. My cholesterol is normal. My fasting sugar remains normal just by eating only non-allergenic foods. I take vitamins, and other than that, I don't take any medicines now. I weigh 120 pounds now and I am 5'5" tall. My liver is not palpable anymore.

N. Elliott
Sun Valley, CA

> *Angina Pains*
>
> *I suffered from repeated angina pain in the evenings and nights for the past ten months. My cardiologist put me on medication. Nitroglycerine and Isordil made me nauseated and bloated. I was referred by my doctor to Dr. Devi to treat for my allergy to the medications. She treated me for the medications. She also traced my chest pain to my flannel night gowns that I had bought ten months ago. I had bought three of the same kind of night gowns, in different colors, and have used them every night. After I was treated for my night gowns (flannel), I haven't had any angina pains in three years.*
>
> *Jane Brown*
> *Orange, CA*

An 11-year-old boy bought two books from the bookstore. The books were in a cute plastic bag. By the time he got to the car, he began having chest pains radiating into the left arm and fingers. His father, who was aware of allergies and their manifestations, tested him and found that the boy was allergic to the plastic bag, not the books. The allergy to the plastic bag caused a blockage in his heart meridian. The father took the books out and discarded the bag. In a few minutes, the boy's pain and discomfort was gone. He was allergic to a chemical in that particular bag.

A 39-year-old woman had some dental work done in the morning. She began having chest tightness and pains by the afternoon. She was allergic to silver in the tooth filling. Silver was causing a blockage in her heart and pericardium meridians. When she was treated for silver, her chest pains went away.

A 38-year-old woman had angina pain whenever she went to sleep. On certain nights, she had to take 4-5 nitroglycerine pills. She was allergic to the materials in her mattress and pillow, which caused blockage in the spleen and heart meridians. If the spleen meridian is blocked more than heart,

Long Standing Insomnia

When I first came to see Dr. Devi, I was only getting 2½ hours of sleep at night because my entire back, arms, neck and head were covered with an itchy rash that I was constantly scratching raw. I couldn't sleep, I was terrified of eating, and I was despondent. In just a few treatments (basic treatments) the rash started to clear up and, within a week, I was sleeping through the night. What a blessing! I will be forever grateful, and I have gotten better and better.

Margaret Lespino
Los Angeles, CA

you may have a problem falling asleep, but when you do fall asleep you may sleep through the night. If your heart meridian is blocked more than the spleen, you may not sleep through the night. You may wake up restlessly every now and then or you may have difficultly falling asleep if you wake up in the middle of the night.

Marty, 23 years old, had suffered from insomnia and chronic fatigue syndrome for four years. She suffered from severe brain fog, poor memory, sudden shooting pains in her brain, sharp pains in parts of her body, blurred vision, heart palpitation, excessive hunger, insomnia and severe constipation. She had a stainless steel implant in her right knee, which had been implanted after a football accident when she was 16 years old. After being treated for stainless steel, her brain fog decreased, and her heartbeat became regular. Her appetite regulated and the sharp shooting pains disappeared, she slept better and most of her CFS syndrome improved. The allergy to stainless steel was causing most of her unpleasant symptoms.

Peggy, age 39, suffered from severe insomnia. She was using a well-known brand of face and body cream at night. The cream, which she was highly allergic to, was the cause of her insomnia.

Fungus And Crohn's Disease

I have Crohn's disease which increases the incidence of colon cancer many times. I knew I had fungus in my body. After seeing a medical researcher demonstrate how cancer in a petrie dish would not grow in the presence of fungus, I had no interest in an NAET treatment to rid my body of fungus. A personal decision to possibly prevent colon cancer.

But the fungus was bothering me more and more. I talked to Mala about the situation. She said I could do the fungus treatment and follow that with NAET for cancer tissue. So we did the treatment for fungus. During the week following this treatment I had no usual feeling of improvement and indeed was feeling much worse. I couldn't handle stress, I came down with a virus which I couldn't successfully self treat. I had developed a new pain and soreness inside my upper thigh.

The next week I went for my treatment. I told Mala what was going on and I asked her to muscle test for cancer in my body. The muscle test showed weakness for the sample of cancer tissue. She desensitized me for that energy of cancer right away. I have never in my life experienced such immediate relief from my pain and discomfort even with prescription pain killers before. It was amazing! Not only I was relieved of my pains, the dizziness associated with the virus was no longer bothering me 20 minutes into the treatment.

I was feeling wonderful. My first clue to how much better my immune system responded to this treatment was my next trip to the grocery store. Recently, there were only one or two brands of bottled water I could drink. In testing many different bottled waters that day, just the opposite occurred. This time I couldn't find any bottled water adverse to my immune system, a complete reversal of the norm! I couldn't believe it. I could buy any brand of bottled water I wanted. I had quite a change in my immune system since the treatment for fungus. I continue to feel good after 11 months of that treatment for fungus. Dr. Devi thinks NAET for Fungus, mold and parasites are some of the essential treatments for Crohn's disease. If anyone suffers from Crohn's disease, please ask your practitioners to check these items. Then you shall enjoy freedom from your Crohn's disease too.

Thank you Mala, Dr. Devi, and Dr. Minkoff So much for helping me revive this innate ability of my body to help me live a full life!

Your's Grateful Patient,
Cathy Carlson

> ### *Blocked Arteries Caused My Chest Pains*
>
> *I was getting repeated chest pains for years. I also suffered from severe leg cramps every night. My angiogram showed that I had 80% blockage in my arteries. I am over seventy years old. I did not want any surgical procedure done on me. I was referred to Dr. Devi for pain control. She found out that I was allergic to all my food and clothes. She treated me for over two years. I got relief from my leg cramps and chest pain within 10-15 treatments. I steadily improved with each treatment. I can sleep through the night now. After two years of NAET, she sent me to my cardiologist for a check up. To my doctor's amazement and to my good fortune, the tests showed that my previously 80% blocked arteries were 90% clean now. I haven't had a chest pain in over a year and I don't get chest pains anymore.*
>
> *L. Viola, Cerritos, CA*

A 29-year-old movie producer moved into a new, expensive apartment. Soon, he began experiencing severe heart palpitations, fatigue, depression, extreme nervousness, and rashes along the heart meridian. His problem worsened day by day. Not knowing the cause of the actual problem, he had a complete physical, including cardiac and psychiatric evaluations. He even tried some counseling sessions. He had various treatments for a year but nothing helped. Throughout the year he was very sick, becoming almost disabled, and stayed at home all the time. Finally, he sought our help. Testing revealed he was allergic to all the built-in wooden structures in the apartment. Little shavings of the wood were taken from the wood structure for the NAET procedure. Soon after treatment, his health improved and he could function normally again.

Acetic acid is found in a lot of hard plastics and many other products including nail polish, food products, etc. It is a common allergen that causes cardiac arrhythmia and heart problems that mimic heart disturbances. Another common allergen is formic acid and it is found in most rubber goods. Formic acid also causes various ailments in the body such as chronic fatigue syndrome and aching feet (soles of the shoes are usually rubber). Use of rubber, pencils and liquid paper can also precipitate this syndrome.

Any allergies affecting the heart and pericardium meridians and associated muscles are capable of causing disturbances in the conduction and function of the heart and circulatory system.

A 64-year-old man, still recovering from a massive heart attack ten years ago, was told that his two major arteries were 80 - 90 percent blocked. NTT revealed he was allergic to various foods, including iron. He was also allergic to items made of iron, including the stainless steel bracelet he wore for religious reasons. His iron allergy was cleared after eighteen treatments. Before the treatments, he experienced frequent chest pains, tiredness, leg cramps, insomnia, tingling sensations in various parts of his body and frequent dizzy spells. His complaints diminished after the completion of treatments.

Buerger's disease is a condition affecting the circulatory system, causing interference with blood circulation, particularly in the hands or feet. In fact, the circulation of blood in the extremities can become completely cut off by means of a clot. Blood clots form in the blood vessels of people suffering from Buerger's disease. This condition is also known as thromboangiitis obliterans. It has been recognized that Buerger's disease occurs chiefly in heavy smokers due to allergies to tobacco. It can also be a result of an allergy to aspirin.

A 49-year-old man had such intense headaches that he resorted to taking 16-18 aspirin tablets on certain days to relieve his headaches. He also suffered from poor circulation in his hands and feet. Ironically, we discovered he was allergic to aspirin. Upon treatment for aspirin, the circulation of the distant extremities was restored to normal.

When people die form a coronary disease, the immediate cause of death is a coronary occlusion (obstruction of the blood vessels that supply the heart) by a blood clot which stops circulation in the affected artery. If one could only investigate the causes of the clots and the heart muscle spasms before they occur, many fatal incidents could be prevented. The heart is composed of muscles and contains blood vessels just like any other part of the body, which may be affected by spasms brought on by allergic reactions. Therefore, it is perfectly logical to assume that angina pectoris (spasm of the blood vessels supplying blood and oxygen to the heart) is sometimes caused by allergy.

A 44-year-old female who suffered hay fever, bronchitis, frequent pneumonia and hypoglycemia attacks since childhood, was treated by NAET, which rid her of most allergies. One night, after eating barbecued chicken, she began to experience severe chest pains that mimicked angina pectoris. She immediately tested the new barbecue sauce and discovered she was highly allergic to it. She brought the sauce to our office right away and was treated by NAET. In only a few minutes, her chest pain stopped.

The parents of a boy observed that he complained of chest pains whenever he ate mashed potatoes. He did not react to French fries. The combination of milk, butter and potatoes brought on the chest pain. His chest pain stopped after he was treated for potatoes and milk products. His mother was tested for potatoes and milk, and was also found to be allergic to them, but she never manifested chest pains. However, she did have frequent breast abscesses. Her breast abscesses have not returned since she was treated for potatoes and milk. We can conclude from this that although allergies are hereditary, they can be manifested differently.

CHAPTER 21

ALLERGY AND
THE NERVOUS SYSTEM

Commonly seen allergies of the nervous system are: epilepsy, infantile convulsions, insomnia, Meniere's disease, migraine headache, myasthenia gravis, neuralgia, pruritus, temporary paralysis of the hands, arms, or legs.

Headache can be called an allergy affecting the nervous system because it is caused by an allergy of the brain tissue. There are various types of headaches, which may be due to allergies, deficiencies, injuries and emotional disturbances. We will be discussing headaches caused by allergies.

Headaches and migraines affect millions of people all over the world. Ninety-nine percent of the migraines are due to allergies to something ingested, inhaled or contacted.

During migraine attacks, symptoms may include any one or more of the following:

■ Blurred vision, blind spots, blindness in half the field of vision in one or both eyes, blindness, flashes of light, zigzag lights, intolerance to light, pain and a feeling of protrusion in the eyes.

■ Confusion, lightheadedness, forgetfulness, excitement, tendency to scream, cry or abuse, restlessness, irritability, slowness of thought, difficulty in concentration.

■ Pallor, sweating, flushing, fever, numbness of the extremities, lips, tongue, nose, hands or feet, diminished hearing, hallucinations of hearing, taste or smell.

These symptoms are in addition to the severe headache that is present Nausea and vomiting frequently accompany migraines and may last for a few hours or continue throughout the attack. Attacks may last from a few hours to one or two days, or even a week.

There are various controversial theories prevalent about the causes of headaches, especially migraines. From our experience in treating more than 1,500 cases of migraine headaches over a three year period (with 90-95 percent recovery treating for allergies only), we conclude that the major causes of migraines are solely allergens. Like anything else, it is up to the doctor and the patient to do the detective work to locate the offending items.

None of the existing modern techniques to test for allergies work to find the culprit in migraine headaches because skin tests, scratch tests and blood tests for allergies are not able to diagnose food allergies. Elimination of foods from the diet is not efficient enough, especially when the patient is allergic to a majority of the foods he/she is ingesting. Until researchers come up with another technique, muscle response testing is the only reliable method to find the allergens in the case of migraine.

No More Migraines

I had severe migraines all my life. Whenever I got them I had to go to the emergency room to get a shot. Then I had to sleep for three to four days. Finally my migraines would go away. After Dr. Nambudripad's treatments for food allergies (about 30 treatments), I do not get migraines anymore. I haven't had one in 11 years. Thank you, Dr. Nambudripad, for discovering this revolutionary treatment!

Sara Evans
Marina Del Rey, CA

> ### *My Headaches Were From MSG*
>
> *I have suffered from headaches for years. Unbeknown to me, these headaches were caused by food allergies. I used to eat Chinese food and would get sick and get a headache. After Dr. Devi treated me for MSG, I no longer suffer when I eat Chinese food.*
>
> *Linda B.*
> *La Mirada , CA*

Many people have questions regarding the period of wellness between migraine attacks. The only hypothesis is that the brain responds to any kind of pain in the body. When a patient gets a migraine headache, he/she experiences severe pain.

The brain releases an antidote or a secretion that is a remedy for the allergen causing the existing migraine. The secretion is enough to neutralize the toxin, and the brain secretes some extra amount that stays in the body for a longer period. During this time, if the person eats or uses the same toxic product, the remaining secretion might neutralize it and prevent a further attack. Another possibility is that the very foods that cause the trouble are harmless to the patient at other times, in the presence of this neutralizing secretion. This is probably responsible for the cyclic or recurrent character of migraines. When this immunity or secretion diminishes, the body again becomes sensitive to the allergens, another attack occurs, and the brain goes through the same process again. This accounts for the periodicity of migraine headaches even when they are caused by common food items: milk, wheat, eggs, chocolate, caffeine, etc., which are constantly present in most diets.

A 44-year-old female suffered from migraine headaches, seasonal hay fever, angioneurotic edema, severe premenstrual symptoms, etc. She went to a hospital emergency room at least once a week to get an injection for pain. She slept in a dark, noise-free room for two days, until her headaches subsided. Nobody ever suspected or suggested the possibility of an allergy to this woman. When she came to our clinic, through NTT, she was found

---

No More Migraines!

I had severe migraines all my life. Whenever I got them I had to go to emergency rooms to get a shot, then I had to sleep for three to four days. Finally, my migraines would go away. After Dr. Devi's treatments for food allergies, I do not get migraines anymore. I am one of her guinea pigs from her early days of practice. NAET works! I haven't had one migraine in 14 years.

Sara Pavlov
Glendora, Azuza

---

to be allergic to almost all the foods she was eating. She was enrolled in our regular program. In two months' time, her migraines were diminished. If she got one at all, it was from milk and lasted for a few minutes to a couple of hours. It got better just by working on the pressure points, without taking any medicines. After seven additional months of treatments, she was discharged, nearly free from migraines. In the last five years, she returned only twice to our office with mild migraines.

BACKACHE

Millions of people suffer from various types of backaches. Upper backache, middle backache, lower backache and sciatic neuralgia are very common.

Upper backache

The cervical spinal segments (vertebra) and the associated spinal nerves can suffer from restricted nerve energy flow, causing pain and discomfort in the upper back. It could be the result of injuries to the upper back and the spine, (whiplash injuries in auto accidents) from sitting or sleeping in uncomfortable positions for long periods of time, or it could be from some allergens you ingested, inhaled or contacted. You may not have to suffer from the pain long if you test through NTT, and treat through NAET.

40-Year-Old Migraine

I used to have severe migraines for 40 years or so. I also developed severe arthritis. I had bad psoriasis for 20 years. When I went to Dr. Devi five years ago, I was in a mess. I was limping and walking with the help of a cane because my arthritis and bursitis were so bad. Dr. Devi treated me for food allergies. I was also treated for pollens, grasses and flowers. I do not have migraines anymore. My arthritis is almost 90 percent gone. Whenever I try a new food without testing, my ten percent of the arthritis returns. My psoriasis is almost gone, except for some pinpoint spots at the elbows. I have lots of energy. I walk four miles every morning. I am making up for the lost time in my youth due to pain. I don't have any pain now. I enjoy every precious day of my life now.

Maxine P.
Bellflower, CA

Since she was 13 years old, Mary, now 27, suffered from severe migraines. Her headaches intensified around her menstrual cycles, usually starting the first day and lasting for 4-5 days. Her doctor thought that she was having a hormone imbalance. She was placed on birth control pills when she was fifteen years old, but her headaches continued. She was evaluated through NTT, and found that an allergy to cotton was the cause of her headaches. She liked polyester and other synthetic materials and did not wear cotton fabric often. But the sanitary napkins she used were made from cotton for better absorption of the menstrual flow. The direct contact with cotton on her skin triggered the headache that continued for 4-5 days. Since she didn't use cotton much on the other days of the month she remained almost symptom-free. When she was treated successfully for cotton using NAET, the frequency, and intensity, of her migraines was reduced.

> ### My Chronic Neck And Backache Is No More!
>
> *I suffered from frequent severe stiffness of the neck and upper back-aches for the last 14 years. I was taking various prescriptions and over-the-counter pain pills for my neck and shoulder pain. I was told by many other doctors that it was from stress. When I was treated for spices by Dr. Devi, I was very sick during the first 18 hours after the treatment. When I woke up the next morning, I was free of my chronic neck and upper backache. It has not returned in three years.*
>
> *Deborah B.*
> *Artesia, CA*

Now thirty-four years old, Kim had suffered from frequent sinus congestion, headaches and upper backaches for a number of years. He often took antibiotics to keep his sinus infections under control. When he came for an evaluation we discovered, through NTT, that his sinus problems were due to tomato, garlic and onion. He ate them at every meal. After he was treated successfully for these items, his headaches diminished and his sinuses cleared. For the first time in years, he can breathe normally.

MID-BACKACHE

For two years, Michelle suffered from mid-backaches. She became health conscious two years ago, eating whole grain breads and wholesome foods. She was highly allergic to the B vitamins in the whole grain products giving rise to severe mid-backaches. When she was treated by NAET for B complex vitamins, her mid-back pain diminished.

Potatoes cause mid-backache in many people. Reggie, 39, came in with severe, constant mid-backache. She had tried various treatments for her backaches. Her back was X-rayed many times but no abnormalities were found. One of her friends, a patient at the clinic, referred her to me. I evaluated her through NTT and found that her backache was the result of her allergy to potato. She wasn't allergic to many things. Potato was her staple diet ever since she was a child. She couldn't believe that she could be allergic to potato. Since she was in acute pain I decided to treat potato immediately. In acute cases, we do not follow the basic treatment rule. Ten minutes after the treatment for potato, during the acupuncture balancing treatment, she rang the call bell from her room. I went in to check on her. She was sitting up on the table. Tears rolling down her cheeks, she asked: "Is it possible for the treatment to work this fast?" She looked anxious. "My back pain is 100% relieved now. Is it for real, doctor, or am I dreaming?" I checked her for the allergy to the potato with MRT. She was strong. "This is NAET, Reggie, and it is for real. You probably will never have another backache," I explained. Five years later, I met her in the mall one day. She ran up to me and said, "You were right, doctor, I never have had another backache ever since you treated me for potato."

LOWER BACKACHE

A recent survey reported that low backache is the second most common reason for a person to visit a primary care physician in this country.

From the time he was three years old, Ray, a 34-year-old salesman suffered from continuous nagging lower backache. He complained of severe backaches after being on the road for a day. When he didn't travel, his backaches were not as severe. He had bought a Mustang three years ago and drove it one hour to work every morning. He was found to be allergic to the acrylic seat covers in the car.

Peppers belong to the nightshade family. Nightshade family vegetables (potato, pepper, onion, eggplant, and tomato) carry a toxin like substance called *solanin*. Many people do not produce the enzyme in their body to digest solanin. This substance acts like a toxin to these people, giving rise to various health problems: asthma, heart problems, skin problems, backaches, sinus troubles, joint pains, insomnia, irritability, anxiety, headaches, etc.

Rose, 62 years old, was referred to me for her low back pain. Through NTT, I found that her low backache was related to an allergy to peppers. When I asked her if she ate peppers, she said she couldn't live without peppers. She

Lettuce and Backache

Being a former football player, I suffered occasionally from lower back pain. During one particular period, the slightest movement was causing me discomfort. I had been keeping track of what I had been eating. Dr. Devi found out that I was allergic to lettuce. After two treatments, the back pain went away and has not returned in four years. I have been a patient of Dr. Devi for over four years and I return whenever any problems occur.

Dave Almirah
Whittier, CA

picked them and ate them with every meal. After she was treated for her allergy to peppers by NAET, her low backache said good-bye to her.

Sciatic Neuralgia

John, a 52-year-old, came in with severe sciatica, with pain and numbness radiating down his left leg to the side of his foot. Through NTT, it was found that he had been using a large helping of homemade diet orange marmalade for the last few weeks. His wife had used another sugar substitute as the sweetener in the marmalade. When the problem was pinned down, he was repeatedly treated by NAET five times for the sugar substitute. After four hours of hard work, he finally responded to treatment and was free from his sciatica pain.

Joyce's husband brought her to our clinic. She was suffering from a severe sciatic neuralgia with an antalgic lean to the left that began after dinner the night before. She felt the first twinge of sciatic pain when she walked to her car that evening. When she woke up the next morning she couldn't move or get up from her bed. Evaluating through NTT, it was found that the special drink she had the night before was the cause of the sciatic neuralgia. Her husband had surprised her by taking her to dinner at a special restaurant for her birthday. To celebrate the occasion, she had red wine with

Sciatic Neuralgia

At a restaurant, chopped red onion came with the chili I ordered. So I ate it. I seldom eat onion. Within thirty minutes, my lungs reacted with wheezing and coughing. The next day my left leg was very sore. The wheezing turned into bronchitis. The leg pain kept getting worse each day with pain radiating into my left thigh, back of the knee and ankle. It continued for three weeks. I saw my internist, who pre-scribed some antibiotics and a pain killer for me. However, I contin-ued to cough and had pain in my left leg.

Dr. Devi was on vacation. After three weeks, I came to see Dr. Devi. I still had the excruciating leg pain. My cough was also still there. During her evaluation she found that I was allergic to the red on-ion I ate at that Mexican restaurant. She gave me a treatment for the onion and the leg pain disappeared in a few minutes. Two weeks later, my friend took me to the same restaurant. I ate the same chili but this time, I had no wheezing, coughing or leg pain. NAET gives me freedom to eat my favorite food in any restaurant. I have a life again!

Rosemary D.
Buena Park, CA

dinner. She was treated for the red wine by NAET and in less than half an hour she was free of her sciatic pain.

Forty-nine-year-old Betty was carried into my office by her husband and sister one afternoon. She had severe lower backache and pain radiating into her right leg. On examination, she was found to be reacting to an artichoke she ate for lunch. She was treated for artichoke immediately with NAET and, in less than 20 minutes, her pain diminished by 90 percent. After 25 hours when she came for recheck, she was 100% free of her back-ache and sciatic pain.

Cluster Headaches

I suffered from cluster headaches ever since I moved into our new house five years ago. I tried allopathic medications, Chinese herbs and homeopathic remedies without any help.

I have had allergies all my life and have just resolved to live with them. I would break out in rashes on my face; my lips and eyes would swell and itch. The doctors would give me medications and ointments and gradually it would recede temporarily for a few minutes to a few hours. No one knew the reason. But I never had cluster headaches. I was getting treatments at one of the famous hospitals in San Diego. One day (1990) I opened the San Diego Tribune newspaper and read about Dr. Devi and NAET on the cover page. I immediately made an appointment with her. In her office she discovered, by simple muscle testing, that the built-in wood work in my house was the culprit. I was asked to bring shavings from various wood fixtures, including the kitchen cabinets, from my house. After she cleared me for the wood shavings, I did not suffer from cluster headaches anymore.

Cynthia B.
Laguna Beach, CA

Marie, 67, went to dinner at her diabetic brother's house. His wife had made rice pudding with artificial sweeteners. About 10 p.m., she started having an excruciating pain on the right side of her face, which did not respond to any usual pain medications. She was treated for artificial sweeteners by NAET, and her facial neuralgia diminished 10 minutes after the treatment.

The following is a very dramatic case of a migraine headache in which the causative factor was cornstarch and corn products. The patient ate corn and corn products at least two or three times a day until he got severe headaches constantly for nine months. He had tried various treatments before he came to our clinic. After evaluation of his history and symptoms, corn was found as the main irritant. It took 28 days of consecutive treatments by NAET just to desensitize him to corn and combinations with corn. At the end of this period, not only did his headache of nine months diminish, but he had also cleared many of the other food allergies he had prior to the treatments.

Another interesting case of migraine headache is worthy of mention. Two days after his marriage, a man developed a right-sided migraine headache. Two months later, one of his friends brought him to our office. He was allergic to the bride. He was treated for her and after successfully clearing this allergy, his migraine of two months disappeared. Luckily, he was not allergic to many food items, but he was allergic to pollens and grasses. He had a history of hay fever since childhood from pollen and grasses, but never had migraine headaches before his marriage.

Any chronic or acute, unexplained headache, occurring periodically in an individual with a personal or family history of allergy, should be considered as allergic in origin unless proven otherwise.

Meniere's disease with vertigo, dizzy spells, tinnitus (ringing in the ears) is a very common complaint mainly in older or immune deficient people. Some disturbances are due to swelling in the semicircular canals that are located on each side of the head, just within the internal ear. They are composed of three

---

Will I Say Good-bye To Myasthenia Gravis?

I have suffered from Myasthenia Gravis for a few years now. My husband took me to all noted specialists in the country to find a treatment for this scary disorder. Very often, my throat closed up and my tongue felt heavy and I couldn't speak. My body felt heavy, and I couldn't move. I felt helpless during those episodes. This happened a couple of times a week in the beginning. As time went on it became more frequent. Whatever treatment I did, nothing seemed to have any affect on me. I lived in fear all the time. Then we heard about Dr. Devi and NAET through a friend. I immediately went to see her. She began treating me for allergies. After a few treatments, I can say that I am on the way to recovery from Myasthenia Gravis. I still have many more allergies to eliminate. When I restrict the use of any allergic food or products I do not have any symptoms of Myasthenia Gravis at all. If I eat an allergic item intentionally or by mistake, my symptoms return but in a milder way. But now I have hope that I am going to be free of this disorder soon with the help of NAET.

Christina S.
Laguna Beach, CA

---

connecting canals through which the perilymph circulates. These three canals are intercommunicating and lie in different positions.

On the inner mucous membrane lining of the canals are fine, very sensitive hairs or cilia, which are connected with the nerves and are constantly bathed in the circulating perilymph. This fluid moves from one part of the canal to another, depending upon the position of the body, just as a bubble moves in a carpenter's level. The semicircular canals control the balance mechanism of the body, and it is through their proper functioning that an aviator can tell whether or not he is flying upside down.

NAET Gave Me My Life Back!!

On August 18, 1999, I knew I was blessed. Earlier in the month my best friend in Atlanta Georgia called to tell me about NAET. She had been undergoing NAET treatment and had noticed a great change. After having prayed for guidance, I found Dr. Marilyn Chernoff on the net (naet.com-practitioner locator site). I had actually made an appointment with another practitioner in Santa Fe, but cancelled that appointment after speaking with Dr. Chernoff. I was diagnosed with Celiac disease at age two, and had suffered all my life with poor digestion, swelling and pain in the abdomen, depression, and fatigue. As an adult I also suffered from asthma, which I realized after many years, was "Grain" specific. Two months before meeting Dr. Chernoff I had eliminated all grains from my diet. I did however indulge on occasion and the consequences were immediate asthma.

What I did not expect was to be cleared of so many other maladies. On my first visit we discussed my chronic fatigue, forgetfullness, incontinence, hypoglycemia, swelling and pain in the abdomen. Everything was equally troubling me. I could not pinpoint one problem as being the most disabling one. I wanted to be cured from all. She did a series of NAET muscle testing on me and decided to address the issue of incontinence. With her testing skills, she determined that the incontinence had been caused by botulism. She stated that at some time in my life I had gotten very sick and had assumed it was the flu when in fact it was food poisoning. I easily remembered that my incontinence started when I was pregnant with my son 19 years ago. I had become violently ill. The incontinence started just after his birth and increased in frequency over the years. Doctors had told me that this was a consequence of birth. I had literally taken to wearing only black jeans so that I could change easily after a mishap. Girl clothes were a nightmare and on the occasions when I had to wear professional clothes for work, I walked fast and prayed, a lot...

One treatment proved the cure. I have not had an incident since that first day. After that treatment she continued with my basics then, she treated me for kidney; which turned out, were a major deterrent to my well-being. I had been wearing magnetic insoles in my shoes because I suffered from swelling in my ankles and calves.

Continued on next page)

After the second treatment, my ankles no longer swelled. My calves still swelled somewhat, but I was able to wear a short sexy dress and remain feeling sexy till after midnight. This I have to tell you first. My ankles have swelled since the late 60's. Guess who hated short dresses in those days.

All my life I had suffered from constipation. I virtually lived on laxatives. I never had a solid stool and just accepted this as a way of life. Five years ago a colonoscopy revealed that I had the colon of "an 80 year old man". (The doctor could have at least said an 80 year old woman). By the way I was 45 at the time. Needless to say this did not make me happy. Dr. Chernoff found the root cause, treated me and like magic my stool have been solid ever since. I still take a laxative, but only one herbal, and I no longer have any problem.

When she treated me for "Strep and fungus" she was able to clear my chronic bronchitis and I have not yet succumbed to any colds or flu. For about 25 hours after the treatment I felt as if someone had given me a frontal lobotomy. I walked around like a zombie. I could feel the treatment lift after the 25 hours and I had a great surge of energy.

In 1977, I was diagnosed with hypoglycemia. The doctor stated at that time that it was the worst case he had ever seen. At it's very highest my blood sugar stayed just below 100. I felt fairly good when on occasion my sugar would hit 90, but the ups and downs were difficult and I was always tired. My blood sugar controlled my vision and I never knew when my vision would turn to a blur.

My last two treatments addressed this problem and although the actual sugar treatment made me worse till I could see Dr. Chernoff one week later, the treatment for my actual hypoglycemia has given me a renewed sense of energy, joy and balance. I now eat because I am hungry, not because I am crashing.

I am sitting here working through the treatment for my salt allergy. And my next treatment is grains, (finally). You have no idea how excited I am to have reached this point.

Thank you NAET and thank you Dr. Chernoff for giving my life back for me. We still have a little ways to go but I would shout from the rooftops and sing your praises. Matter of fact, I have done that. Did I mention that I am an Insurance Adjuster handling Workers' Compensation? I have recently referred a worker to Dr. Chernoff for severe ulna neuropathy. She had a very unsuccessful surgery on her right arm due to what the physician described as pre-keloid disease.

(Continued on next page)

She had developed a very painful hypertrophic scar and was seeking something alternative to surgery for the pain in her left arm. Dr. Chernoff did two treatments and the worker is completely pain free. As a matter of fact she has since brought her mother to see Dr. Chernoff. I guess that is a testimonial to alternative health care. Workers' Compensation recognizes alternative health care. Now if only my health insurance would become aware of the health benefit and savings the NAET system of treatment provides!

I am going to tell you another story, just because it too is a miracle. My boyfriend suffered from back pain for 20 years. He too is an insurance Adjuster and Ex-Navy pilot. I tell you this so that you understand that, unlike myself, he is not into "New Age" and he saw a big difference in me, but still remained skeptical. His pain was chronic and severe, encompassing his cervical, thoracic and lumbar spine.

The first treatment addressed the heart and with that his lumbar pain disappeared. The second treatment addressed mercury and with that his thoracic and cervical pain became almost nonexistent. He never actually comprehended his level of pain before the treatment, he just knew he hurt all the time and felt he just had to live with it. It wasn't until after the treatment that he understood how much pain he had been living with. One day after having driven for 15 hours, he showed signs of being uncomfortable. Concerned, I asked if his pain was back. He stated "a little." I then asked him what it used to be. It was only then that I found out that he had lived and functioned at pain level of "nine".

Thank you Dr. Chernoff for bringing NAET into our lives and giving us back our lives. We still have work to do, but never have I found anything that has worked so well. This is not a magic. This is not faith healing, this is a matter of treat, wait and watch. This is real medicine. Any questions, please call me.

Virginia Stair
505-892-2823

Multiple Sclerosis

I was diagnosed by medical doctors in Washington State with M.S. in 1991. This condition has gotten progressively worse so that, through the years, my walking, speech, and thinking have deteriorated to the point that I had lost hope in ever believing that this condition would get any better or stop progressing.

I came down from Washington to Southern California to be treated by Dr. Devi. I have now had 12 treatments by Dr. Devi during the past three and one-half weeks and have noticed significant improvements in my walking, speech, and thinking.

N.A.E.T. treatments are pain-free, require no drugs, and have allowed me to keep true to my ethics of vegetarianism. As I stated above, the improvements in my walking have been great as I can now walk a longer distance without aid. Before these treatments my speech was weak and slurred. Now I speak more clearly, no slurring unless I am very tired, and my thinking, which had gotten impaired, has become clearer. These treatments have cleared my system of the prescription drugs and their terrible side effects, which caused hand and leg tremors. The treatments have given me something the traditional medical establishment has not; hope of a brighter future without pain and prescription drugs. My hope is that my M.S. will not get worse and I will get much better.

I must and want to return to my home in Washington this week and I will continue the N.A.E.T. treatments up there. I am doing so much better now and I do not want to stop these treatments until I have completed the full series. I feel that at last I am in control, not the M.S.

THANK YOU, Dr. Devi !!!!!

Stephanie Moon
Washington

Reflex Dystrophy

When I was nine years old I developed a sharp soreness in my little toe which was diagnosed as a bone infection. I was given antibiotics for the supposed infection, but instead of my toe getting better, it got worse and worse and soon both my feet and legs became sore and very swollen. Soon after, both my hands and arms to the elbow became sore, inflamed, and swollen. I couldn't sleep or walk. My parents were told that this was all due to a virus, which was spreading. They said they couldn't control the infection and I should immediately be hospitalized. In ten days I was seen by seven specialists and the diagnosis was the same: reflex dystrophy due to unknown virus.

My parents took me to Dr. Devi so I could get acupuncture to get some sleep before they took me to hospital. At this point I had to be carried, I could not walk.

Dr. Devi traced the problem to the ingestion of lecithin in a granola bar I had eaten 14 days before because it was the only thing that was not on my normal diet, which was watched very carefully because of my asthmatic condition. I had saved part of the granola bar in my school bag. Since I didn't like the taste, I didn't eat all. Dr. Devi treated me for the granola bar, first treating me through my mom or dad as my surrogates, and later directly on me. It took about 30 treatments every hour or so to get my advanced condition under control. Once my body no longer saw the lecithin in the granola bar as poison, the entire symptom complex vanished completely in three days. I am 24 years old now and I never had any trace of that problem again.

Preethi Puthenveetil
Cerritos, CA

Any disturbance in the passage of the fluid within the semicircular canals, any increase of fluid or swelling of the sensitive lining, will upset the balance mechanism of the body. Dizziness, staggering, or even complete loss of balance will result (falling or inability to stand erect, depending upon the severity of the disturbance). In addition to prolonged and severe dizziness, inflammation and swelling of the semicircular canals, Meniere's syndrome causes such symptoms as nausea, vomiting, temporary deafness, and sometimes convulsions. Meniere's disease is often the result of allergies that cause swelling in the semicircular canals. Food allergies are the major irritants even though inhalants, sprays, fabrics, pollens, etc., can also cause the swelling and inflammation.

A 48-year-old woman suffered from Meniere's disease and was found to be allergic to her dear pet cat. Another 58-year-old female suffering from the same disease was found to be allergic to smoke from her husband's cigarettes. A 64-year-old woman was found to be allergic to the chocolate bars she ate twice a day. All these patients were relieved of their disease after they were treated for the respective items.

But another patient, a 67-year-old female, was not as lucky. Her problem was not solved so easily. She was found to be allergic to various foods, fabrics, pollens, and inhalants. All of these items affected her balance. She cleared for all her known allergies, but she still kept having trouble with her balance. It was discovered that her hobby was tending her rose garden, and she was found to be allergic to the perfume of the rose. After treatment for the perfume, she finally got better.

Neuralgia is another disease of the nervous system often caused by allergy. It may occur in any part of the body, but is more likely to affect the head, neck, and shoulders. It occurs most frequently in patients who suffer from other allergic manifestations such as eczema, allergic migraine or GI tract allergy. As a result of allergic spasm, the pain may be due to swelling or covering of the nerves. Angioneurotic edema also may be responsible in some cases.

A middle-aged woman suffered from severe neuralgia in the right shoulder, neck, right hip, and leg, which was associated with severe headaches, drowsiness, and sleepiness due to food allergies. Many patients suffer from severe body aches and stiff neck whenever they ate string beans. Another lady, 34 years of age, suffered from neuralgia of the whole left side of the body after she ate garbanzo beans in her salad.

Many people get neuralgia from allergies to certain bacteria and viruses. Such were the cases of seven females and three males of different ages who were affected by shingles (which is caused by a virus). They were all allergic to the shingles virus. Their neuralgia got better as soon as they were treated and cleared of their respective viruses.

Epilepsy is one of the unexplainable diseases of the nervous system where allergy plays a great role. We have had many epilepsy cases, all of which were allergic in origin. When they were treated for their allergies, they all stopped having epileptic attacks. Not all seizure disorders or epileptic attacks are from allergies, but if no other etiology can be found, allergy should be considered as a possible cause.

A 67-year-old man who was subject to frequent epileptic seizures whenever he was standing in his backyard was allergic to the new acacia palm tree he had just planted there. A three-year-old female child was allergic to egg white, causing her to have seizure attacks whenever she ate an egg. A teenage boy had epileptic attacks once every two weeks, on Sunday nights. Every other Sunday, he went to the beach with his father and ate a hot dog. He was allergic to the mustard on the hot dog. A teenager was found to be allergic to apples, causing epileptic attacks. Another boy had epileptic attacks whenever he had chocolate.

Temporary paralysis is another disease affecting the nervous system. Most frequently, the allergic attacks have been so great that temporary paralysis of a certain part of the body occurs. These symptoms usually disappear after a short time. However, if the causative factor is food allergy, it might last for a long time, until the offending item is found and treated.

MULTIPLE SCLEROSIS

Multiple sclerosis could be allergy related. If so, NAET is the treatment for it.

Wanda, 36, had multiple sclerosis for the past 12 years. Her symptoms began after giving birth to her child by cesarean section. During childbirth she was injected with spinal anesthesia. She was found to be highly allergic to the spinal anesthesia that was used 12 years ago. Her symptoms improved when she was cleared for the allergy to the anesthesia.

Julia, 26, had multiple sclerosis for the last five years. When she came to our office, she was unable to walk without assistance, and she was almost blind in both eyes. Her silicone breast implant was the cause. When she was cleared for the silicone implant, her symptoms improved. She regained her sight and became steady on her feet. She was able to pass the driver's license test and drive again.

Crystal, a 24-year-old woman, was diagnosed as having multiple sclerosis. She had the typical symptoms of multiple sclerosis: numb hands, frequent headaches, bilateral lack of strength in the arms, extreme fatigue, shaking, weakness of the lower limbs, etc. She had been on a diet to lose weight for six months, when her symptoms began.

We discovered that she was highly allergic to artificial sweeteners. On her weight-loss program, she consumed a lot of artificial sweeteners. When she was treated by NAET for artificial sweeteners, these symptoms disappeared.

Pruritus or itching is a symptom that very often occurs as a result of allergy to foods, fabrics or chemicals. Pruritus is caused by an allergic response that occurs in the nerves that lie just below the surface of the skin.

A 69-year-old female came in one day complaining of generalized itching all over the body. Her history revealed that she had this itching all her life, but it had become more severe in the last 22 years. She was told by many allergists that she was allergic to all the food items, environmental items and fabrics for which she was tested. She had various size rashes and boils all over her body. She weighed 67 pounds, was 5' 6" in height, and was very malnourished. On examination in our clinic, she was found to be allergic to everything, including all foods, fabrics, and environmental substances. Her history also revealed that she had been very sick with whooping cough when she was an infant. Her parents and grandparents were quite healthy and died of old age. She could not remember any history of inherited allergies in their distant relatives.

She was tested and found to be very allergic to Bordetella pertussis bacteria and was treated by NAET for it. After successfully completing the treatment for pertussis, her itching diminished considerably and she was not reacting to most of the food items. She started eating normally and found she could assimilate the food, without any pruritus. Her allergy probably began when her body's energy pathways were blocked with the incidence of the whooping cough in her infancy.

Insomnia is another symptom of the nervous system allergy. A 26-year-old girl suffered from severe insomnia. This kept her awake the whole night, while her husband slept like a log. She was used to having a glass of milk and a banana at night, both of which she was allergic to, causing her insomnia.

Another patient, a 65-year-old woman, suffered from insomnia for 35 years. Upon questioning her, it was discovered that she was allergic to vitamin C. She ate an apple, banana, or orange every night before she went to bed. The allergy kept her awake almost the entire night.

Another woman ate fish every night for supper and had severe insomnia. When she stopped eating fish, she was able to sleep peacefully at night.

The field of nervous system allergy is still under study and it has not been explored enough as compared to other branches of allergic symptoms like migraine headaches, GI tract allergy, etc. If we do enough research and detective work in this field, no doubt we will be able to trace a lot of mental and emotional disturbances to allergy-based problems. According to Chinese medicine, if there is a blockage in the liver, stomach, and kidney meridians, nervous system and mental disorders can happen.

For many years asthma, hay fever and hives were considered to be nervous in origin. Now it is known that they are caused by allergens. An emotional upset may produce an allergic attack in an individual who is already allergic, but it is doubtful whether this ever occurs in the absence of an allergic predisposition. However, the nervous or psychic symptoms may be so pronounced, and the allergic symptom may appear so minor, that the relationship between the two is not recognized. The failure to recognize this relationship is especially the case with a number of psychiatrists who blame all such symptoms on mental disturbances and rarely consider the possibility that allergy may also be involved.

Such was the case of a 46-year-old female who was periodically very suicidal. Her friends were concerned about her behavior. They always kept her company. At a party one day, she got violently sick with an exploding type of headache, and started talking about suicide again. She refused to go to her counselor, but her friends (some of whom had had treatments for allergies by NAET) compelled her to come to our office.

Her history revealed that her headaches began after meals. She was tested for various food items. One of her friends remembered to bring a small portion of the foods she had eaten at the party. She was found to be allergic to seven out of ten items she ate, and one of them was affecting her brain. She was treated for this particular item, and in fifteen minutes her head was clear and she experienced no further headache. She had been under psychiatric care for ten years. By that time, she had been institutionalized for a while and then released with a once-a-week follow-up instruction. She could neither hold a job nor live normally. After she was treated for wheat, sugar, milk, eggs, vitamin C, and meats, she began to behave normally. Two months after her first visit to our office, she was able to work a part-time job, which eventually changed to a full-time job. She went to see the counselor once a month and continued to live normally.

Another case was that of a schoolboy who had been expelled from three schools and labeled as incorrigible. He had severe sinusitis and hay fever, but this was not taken into consideration until he came to our office and discovered that he was allergic to various food items, materials and pollens. He was treated for all of these, one by one, and after clearing them, his disposition changed completely. He got along well in school and in every way became a well-behaved youngster.

Another young boy became mentally retarded at the age of two, after he had been given various antibiotics to control a fever, which lasted for two months. At the age of nine he could not talk or respond appropriately. He was treated for various food allergies and the antibiotics that were given in childhood. At the end of the treatment for antibiotics, the boy began to ask questions, engage in conversation and respond appropriately to questions. He was found to be highly deficient in B complex. Supplements of megadoses of vitamin B complex helped to change his personality toward normalcy.

Statistics show that eight million children in the United States suffer from some form of mental disorder and 1.4 million children are hospitalized for psychiatric care every year in this country. Could their disorders be due to food allergies? Symptoms of disobedience, sulkiness, irritability, and extreme nervousness are very often found in allergic children and even in adults.

Attention deficit disorder and hyperactivity disorders are other forms of nervous system allergy. Any allergen that affects the brain and nervous system can produce hyperactivity in children and adults. Foods, fabrics, materials, environmental substances, childhood immunizations, insect bites, animals, or humans, can cause this type of allergy. An eight-year-old boy who was very intelligent could not concentrate on anything. He was allergic to various foods and was treated for almost all known food allergies. His hay fever and nasal allergies, etc., improved but his hyperactivity did not. Finally, it was discovered that he was allergic to his mother, father, grandparents and his pet dog. He was treated for each one of them. When he finished the treatments for his family members, he was not as restless and hyperactive. As he became calmer, his school work improved.

Children who are hyperactive and disobedient may be suffering from allergies to their surroundings, not foods. When left untreated, they get worse. This may be one of the reasons children turn to drugs and alcohol in search of relief from the effects of energy blockages caused by allergies.

If husbands and wives were tested and treated for allergies to each other, if mothers and children and fathers and children were tested and treated for allergies, there would be more sound, lasting marriages, fewer divorces, more stable, mentally healthy children and more productive citizens. There would be less crime, fewer people in mental asylums, fewer birth defects, less mental retardation, less disease in general and more peace in the world.

Contaminated, polluted water can also affect the nervous system. Such was the case of a 48-year-old psychologist who felt mental cloudiness, drowsiness, extreme tiredness and lacked interest in everything. She was finally placed on disability. Various medical doctors diagnosed her as having a yeast, candida infection, Epstein-Barr virus, Chronic Fatigue Syndrome, etc. No one suspected any allergy until after eight years of wandering at different medical offices and hospitals, she was found to be allergic to various food items and environmental substances. She felt better and her condition began to improve after she had allergy treatments, but she still kept having mental cloudiness and confusion. As soon as she was treated for her source of tap water and filtered drinking water, her mental cloudiness cleared and her emotional health returned.

A 46-year-old female became suicidal periodically. Her friends accompanied her wherever she went. She was also under psychiatric counseling for a year and a half, and the patient herself decided to quit counseling sessions, saying she did not feel any better. When she was evaluated in our office, it was found that she was allergic to various food items, almost all affecting her brain, resulting in her suicidal tendencies. After successfully completing treatments for all her allergies, she became very normal.

We have had hundreds of cases of allergies affecting the nervous system. In almost all cases, the patients changed from high-strung, jittery, emotionally unstable individuals into normal, calm, poised and assured people. Each day our knowledge of allergy of the nervous system is being increased, and it is hoped that the future will bring even more dramatic discoveries. However, our present knowledge has already brought great relief to patients suffering from this type of allergy.

CHAPTER 22

MISCELLANEOUS ALLERGIES

Many accidents take place as a result of brain allergies. When the allergens affect the person's mind or any part of the body, the mind and body become weak; the person can lose control and accidents can happen as a result.

A 42-year-old man went to a health food store to buy some almond oil that his nutritionist suggested to treat his dry skin. He came out to his parked car with the bottle of oil in his hands, placed the bottle on top of the car, opened the door, got in and started the car, preparing to drive away. His wife, who was in the car, reminded him to take the bottle off the top of the car. He quietly took the bottle of oil and put it near the stick shift and started driving.

Instead of turning right to get out of the shopping complex, he turned left, which led to a dead end. This was a familiar territory to him, yet he made a mistake. His wife calmly reminded him about the mistake. He obeyed silently, without any argument, unlike his normal self. Then he made a right turn into a one way street, going the wrong way, almost crashing head on into another car. His wife screamed in fear. Before he got too far, he made four more driving errors, making his wife very suspicious. Even if he had to drive blindfolded, he couldn't have made so many mistakes. She knew there had to be something terribly wrong with him. She immediately suspected the almond oil as the cause of his strange behavior. She threw the bottle into the back seat as he was driving. When they reached home, he was tested and found to be allergic to the almond oil. His liver and brain meridians were blocked from the allergy to the almond oil. That was the reason for such confused and unconscious behavior! Questioning him further, he said he felt like he was in a daze. He only vaguely remembered his wife's frequent screams as he was driving home, but did not even recall all his driving blunders. Almond oil had such an extreme effect on him.

Brain Allergy

How many accidents do you see on the road, and how many of them are caused by these kinds of brain allergies? The driver could be allergic to any material in the car, the seat, the wheel, the doors, the fabrics, the dust, fumes, pollutants, etc. They may influence the way he/she feels and, if the brain gets an allergic reaction, he/she might react unpredictably and cause accidents.

ADDICTIONS

(Sugar, Starches, Alcohol, Coffee, Chocolate, Caffeine, Smoking/Nicotine, Tobacco, Drugs and people)

Many addictions are caused by allergies. Addiction to alcohol, sugar, coffee, starches, nicotine (smoking tobacco), and drugs are caused by various nutritional deficiencies. Deficiency of the nutrients are usually caused from allergies.

B complex is the food for the nerves. Without food, nerves cannot function normally. B complex vitamins are large molecules, which require the help of sugar to travel from one area to another inside the body. Most of the enzymatic functions in the body depend on the presence of the B vitamins. Allergies to B vitamins and/or sugars can cause poor absorptions of the vital nutrients that is needed for the proper enzymatic functions in the body. In the absence of proper nutrients, incomplete enzymes are produced. These incomplete enzymes do not function properly causing to produce various allergic symptoms. This is the reason NAET treatment program stresses the importance of treating the basic treatment before treating any other allergies. NAET basics are the essential nutrients that are needed in the body for helping the body to produce normal enzymes for proper body functions. In fact, this is the secret of our successful NAET program not only in eliminating allergies permanently but in eliminating various incurable health disorders like ADD, ADHD, Autism Multiple sclerosis, ALS (Amy-

> *Sugar And Diffused Body Ache*
>
> *A grandmother in her 40's suffered from constant, diffuse body pain. She was overweight and was in the habit of eating and drinking heavily-sugared substances. Her pain vanished entirely after she cleared sugar and sugar plus organs.*
>
> *Eric Roth, M.D.*
> *New York*

olateral sclerosis), arthritis, aches and pains, etc. NAET practitioners should treat the allergy to B complex vitamins and sugars before treating addictions of any kind. This way, the patient's journey through the treatment for addictions will be a pleasant one.

Addiction to sugar

We have to admit that most of us have a "sweet tooth."

Our life-style also helps us to satisfy our sweet tooth in every possible way.

Sugar, particularly in its refined forms, has long been used in many everyday foods in all cultures. Sweetness is addictive in nature; so are foods that contain sugar, like chocolate, candy, toffee, pudding, desert, pastries and sweet drinks. The body must have sugar to maintain a supply of energy for its cells and their functions. Sugar does not have to be eaten in the form of refined sucrose. Blood can obtain glucose through digestion and enzymatic conversion from other sources. Fructose in fruits and lactose in milk are both converted to glucose. The starch in cereals, potatoes, grains, and legumes are long chains of glucose units, which are converted to glucose in the course of the digestive process.

But when you are allergic to sugar, you cannot digest or assimilate the complex carbohydrates. Refined sugar can skip a few steps of digestion so it enters the blood quickly. The brain, which is looking for some sugar for energy is momentarily satisfied and your general energy level increases. So you continue to eat the same food over and over to keep your energy level up, becoming addicted to sugar and sugar-containing foods.

Sugar and carbohydrate addiction can be tested and treated very effectively with NAET. When the allergy is eliminated, you usually lose the craving for sugar and stop overusing it.

The NAET Basic 4 treatments should be given before sugar is treated. Twenty-eight-year-old Sandra had craving for donuts, apple fritters, candies, ice creams and licorice bars. She could not satisfy her sweet tooth, no matter how much she ate. If she didn't eat sweets continuously, she became moody, agitated and irritated. She didn't care to eat other foods and wasn't overweight.

Her personality changes in the absence of sugars started interfering with her work at the sales department. When her job was threatened, she began looking for help. She took prescription drugs, hoping to cut down her addiction to sugar. When it didn't work, she tried a few natural herbal products to satisfy her cravings. She joined overeaters' anonymous, attended group therapy, was treated by a hypnotherapist, listened to the relaxation tapes given by her hypnotherapist, exercised regularly and tried to eat right. But nothing seemed to help her. She had to carry candy bars with her everywhere she went and ate them frequently to keep her in a good mood.

One of her childhood friends, now a doctor from another state, was in town to attend one of our training sessions. She visited Sandra and told her about NAET. Sandra called our office the next day and began treatment. She was found to be highly allergic to the first nine groups of allergens from the basic list (egg mix, calcium mix, vitamin C mix, B complex mix, sugar mix, iron mix, Vitamin A mix, mineral mix and salt mix). She was treated for seven of them in order. She reacted severely to the sugar group. When she completed the treatment for sugar, her sugar craving was reduced by 80%. When she completed all nine treatments, her moods and behaviors became normal .

A 39-year-old patient had a case of severe hypoglycemia. She was treated by doctors from different disciplines, a nutritionist and other holistic doctors using mega-vitamins, mineral supplements, detoxifying herbs, glandular therapy, etc. In our office, she was found to be highly allergic to sugar, carbohydrates, vitamin C, iron, protein and vitamin A. Her spleen, pancreas and heart were affected. When she was treated for all these allergens, she stopped having hypoglycemic attacks. When she started eating normal foods instead of the strict hypoglycemic diet, she regained her energy. She was no longer sleepy in the afternoons and could wake up in the morning without feeling tired. She joined an aerobic class, her favorite exercise program, something she had not been able to do for the last five years. Eventually, she became an aerobics teacher. She does not have to fight hypoglycemia anymore.

Addiction To Starches

Deficiency of B vitamins due to poor absorption and assimilation is one of the causes of addiction to eating too many starches.

A 42-year-old lady, who was 60 pounds overweight, could not keep her hands off bread and rice. She was found to be allergic to B complex and sugar, which caused blockages in her stomach and spleen meridians. After she was treated for B complex, she no longer craved breads. She was supplemented with megadoses of vitamin B complex for 3 months. Six months following the treatment, she lost all her excess weight without dieting.

Some people fall asleep an hour after they eat a big starchy meal. Starch converts into sugar, then into alcohol in the stomach in the presence of the

No More Falling Asleep after Eating!

When I first started seeing Dr. Devi in December 1988, I was falling asleep after meals and feeling weak in general. Now, several years later, I no longer fall sleep after eating, and am feeling stronger than ever before.

James F. Wiliamson
Costa Mesa, CA

stomach acids and yeast during digestion, and is released into the blood stream. If the meal contained a large amount of refined starches, a large amount of sugar and alcohol will enter the blood stream quickly. If you are not allergic to sugar or alcohol, and if you are making enough enzymes to break down the food you eat, you should feel more energetic after a big meal. On the contrary, if you are allergic to sugar or alcohol and are not producing enough enzymes to break down the food, extra energy is spent to digest the starchy food in the body. This gives the body less energy for other activities and forces it to lower the metabolism, causing you to fall asleep for a while or until the digestion is over. If you complain of falling asleep after heavy meals or take afternoon naps (activity of the yeast in the small intestine is at its peak at this time) you may be allergic to sugar, grains, refined starches, yeast and enzymes. After you are treated for all of these with NAET, you may not need to nap in the afternoon.

Addiction to Caffeine, Coffee and Chocolate

Addiction to coffee is the same as any other addiction. Normally, a caffeine-like substance is produced in the body that helps you stay alert and awake during normal waking hours. When your body does not produce this substance because of allergies, it begins to crave the substance.

Caffeinated drinks are socially accepted all over the world. But these drinks are very addictive and damaging to the central nervous system for people with allergy. Caffeine affects the cardiac function, causing heart irregularities. It also causes irritability, nervousness, constipation, twitching of the eye lids, ringing in the ears, joint pains, skin problems (psoriasis), formation of benign tumors and cysts in the ovary, uterus and/or breast. Most people with caffeine sensitivity have insomnia and other sleep disturbances. The degree of reaction is proportional to the degree of sensitivity.

People with caffeine sensitivity are usually sensitive to coffee and chocolate. Chocolate, coffee and caffeine addiction can be tested by NTT and treated very effectively with NAET. When the allergy is gone, people usually lose the craving for chocolate or coffee and stop overusing them.

Chocolate allergy treatments also trigger many past unresolved emotions, like betrayal, broken hearts, failure in love related activities, memory

> ### It Wasn't An Ovarian Cyst After All!
>
> *I was treated by Dr. Devi for a list of allergies a couple of years ago and released from her regular care. A few months later, my left lower abdomen (near ovary) began hurting. I suffered the pain for three weeks. I went in for a check-up. My gynecologist did an ultrasound on my left lower abdomen and found a lemon size cyst in my left ovary. She suggested surgery. Then I remembered to check with Dr. Devi. In her office, she tracked down my ovarian cyst to the special coffee I was drinking (5 cups/day) for the past three weeks. She immediately treated me for that coffee. She had to treat me for that particular coffee, coffee and tissue of the ovary and heat, ovary and coffee. It took four days to complete the treatment. My pain was completely gone by then. By the fifth day I saw my gynecologist and she did another ultrasound of my ovaries at my request. The cyst was not there. After five years, my ovaries still remain healthy.*
>
> *Marg Murray*
> *Eureka, California*

of impolite treatments, mental abuse, sexual abuse, rapes., etc. NAET specialists are well trained to look for emotional associations with chocolate and, if found, to eliminate them. The Basic 10 should be treated before treating for caffeine, coffee, or chocolate.

Michael, a 37-year-old school teacher, liked coffee. He drank 6-8 cups daily. Whenever he felt tired, he would make a pot of coffee and drink a couple of cups. His energy would return and he would be able to finish his work for the day. But lately, he felt tired more often, needing to increase his coffee intake even more, to 12-14 cups daily. He also developed a few dermatological problems. He started itching all over his body: on his face, the sides of his cheeks, in front of his ears, and his skin began to peel off.

Then he went to see a dermatologist. All the medicines and topical creams he received helped him temporarily. He had to take medication to get to sleep. He started to put on weight in spite of all the tennis he played. He began worrying about his health. He still kept drinking coffee. One day while he was browsing through the Internet for a solution to his itching, he read about NAET and allergies. NAET talked about addiction to coffee and immediately he saw the link between his health problems and the enormous amount of coffee he was drinking. He tried to stop drinking coffee for a day. His body trembled and his limbs turned cold and clammy. He felt extremely tired, became depressed, lost all motivation, and started getting body aches and joint pains. Finally, in the evening he drank a couple of cups of coffee and felt better. By then he realized that he had become addicted to coffee.

When he came to see me he was quite desperate. He felt embarrassed for becoming a coffee addict. He began NAET treatment right away. In five treatments (egg mix, calcium mix, vitamin C mix, B complex mix and sugar mix), his coffee cravings stopped, but he continued to have other symptoms. With every treatment his condition improved. When he finished all the basic NAET treatments, including coffee, he became normal again. Now he is satisfied with one cup of coffee per day.

ADDICTION TO SMOKING / NICOTINE / TOBACCO

Allergy to B complex is the main cause of any addiction, including smoking and nicotine addiction. After completing the treatment for B complex, it is necessary to take megadoses of B complex supplements (300-500mgs/day) for a few days to a month, as indicated by MRT testing. While going through the rest of the NAET Basic 10 treatments, you may be able to replenish your B complex deficiency before you do the treatment for smoking. (For detailed information on testing for your correct dosage, read "The NAET Guidebook," available at www.naet.com book store). After the NAET Basic 10, you will be ready to treat for the smoking and nicotine.

A 32-year-old patient was addicted to cigarette smoking, consuming three to four packs a day. His wife was suffering from asthma and frequent bronchitis. Her doctor asked him to quit smoking for his wife's sake. He tried different methods to quit. He even went through a smoking withdraw-

25 Years Of Cigarette Smoking

I smoked 3-5 packs a day for 25 years. Seven years ago, I was able to quit smoking after just one NAET treatment with Dr. Devi and didn't even miss it once.

Dee Alberts
New Jersey

al program twice. He was desperate. One of his friends who quit smoking after NAET treatments referred him to us. He was found to be allergic to B complex, sugar and nicotine, which blocked his lungs, liver and large intestine meridians. When he got treated for these items, he was able to stop smoking without any additional effort. A few years later, when he brought his daughter to the office for treatment, he said that a week after the treatment for B complex, his cravings for cigarettes diminished. He cut down his cigarette consumption, quitting completely in less than three weeks, and did not even miss it.

ADDICTION TO OVER-THE-COUNTER AND PRESCRIPTION DRUGS

Addictions to over-the-counter and prescription drugs affect people differently. They work on the nervous system to reduce pain and discomfort and induce sleep. If used in moderation, they can improve the quality of your life, but these drugs, like coffee and alcohol, can be addictive if you are not careful with their usage, whether it is for pain disorders or sleep disorders. Most people who suffer from such disorders are allergic to many things around them. When they begin taking drugs, they experience a momentary sense of well-being, which will eventually lead to overuse, then to addiction.

Allergy to drugs could be tested by NTT (Chapter 7) and treated with NAET. When the allergy is gone, the drugs can work more efficiently to give you the expected result. People usually lose the drug dependency after

NAET treatment. The Basic 10 treatments should be given before the treatments for the drug.

A deficiency of B vitamins, either due to allergies or poor intake, is one of the causes of addiction to drugs. After eliminating allergy for sugar and B complex, you need to supplement with megadoses of vitamin B complex for a couple of weeks before you can successfully treat for prescription drugs.

Many people react to lifesaving drugs: antibiotics, aspirin, penicillin, cortisone, blood pressure regulating medication, pain medication, etc. Many drug companies are sued by consumers who suffer reactions to their products. These people can be treated with NAET to remove the allergy to the drug and will then be able to use the same drug without any reactions. Sick patients may not have to go through unpleasant drug reactions and other after-effects of the drugs; frustrated doctors may not have to change drugs desperately many times a week or month on a trial and error basis to find the most suitable one; and the drug companies may be able to save millions by not paying or compensating for the law suits. If the drug companies do not have to waste large sums of money on legal expenses, they could easily reduce the price of the drugs and every drug user could benefit from paying less for their lifesaving medications.

ADDICTION TO ILLICIT DRUGS

People can also become addicted to recreational drugs. Every year we lose many lives to cocaine, marijuana and such other drugs. An addiction is due to allergy. When you treat the allergy to the drugs you lose the craving for them. After completing treatment, they will no longer have the desire to use drugs. If they ever happened to use them, they would not get any unpleasant adverse reactions.

Thirty-two-year-old Silva had a big problem with illicit drug usage. He started using drugs 7 years before under peer pressure. He tried marijuana and cocaine. He liked marijuana. Before he knew it, he found himself becoming depended on it. He couldn't sleep, relax or function without it. While he was a student, it was hard to get enough money to buy drugs, but somehow he managed to use it once a week. When he began working, the situation became easier and he began using drugs more often. Whatever he earned, he spent on drugs. Then a few months ago, he developed cardiac arrhythmia. He went through all necessary tests to check out his heart's condition. Everything seemed okay, but the cardiac arrhythmia continued. Finally, when he came to us, he was getting an irregular heartbeat at least once a day. In our office, through NTT, we discovered that he was reacting to the drugs he was taking. So, he told us his real problem. After the Basic 7 treatments, he was given megadoses of vitamin B complex. Next, he was treated for marijuana; then smoke, combinations with marijuana; smoke and serotonin. After successfully being treated for all these combinations, he quit the habit completely. Now when he gets a craving, he takes 100 milligrams of B complex. In a few minutes, he loses his craving. He hasn't touched any drug for a couple of years now.

ADDICTION TO ALCOHOL

Addiction to alcohol is an illness characterized by both intolerance and physical dependence. True alcoholism is mainly due to an allergy to B complex vitamins, especially to B-12, PABA, and also sugar, yeast and alcohol. When the nerves cannot get adequate nutrition, the starving nerves become shaky and unhappy. When the body is allergic to sugar, it cannot be absorbed through the normal digestive processes. Alcohol is able to skip the normal digestive process and part of it will be absorbed through osmosis (absorbing through the stomach lining) into the blood circulation. Momentarily, alcoholics feel better soon after they drink. This is due to the action of the sugar providing a sudden dose of energy and increasing the energy in the nervous system. When the tired brain gets a quick dose of sugar (from the alcohol), it will temporarily satisfy the partial need of the brain and it will be utilized for energy functions. Most alcoholics behave soberly when they have some alcohol in their system because the brain is getting some sugar to function. The brain gets to know this new way of acquiring sugar for its needs and issues repeated commands to bring more alcohol into the system. This will drive the person to drink more and more, leading to addiction. Only a small portion can be absorbed through the stomach lining. The rest of the alcohol will go through the digestive tract, ending up as empty calories. The "spirit" (the gaseous portion of the alcohol) will pass through the liver and get absorbed into the liver meridian, again by osmosis. The depressive action of the "spirit" overpowers the body, and the brain and nervous system become sedated and weak. The gaseous substances in the liver meridian will travel towards the brain (fig.11-12), giving rise to light-headedness, "floating in the heaven-like" sensation initially with the first few sips; later mental disturbances and strange behaviors.

The long-term effect will be on the stomach and liver. The mucous membrane lining in the stomach and the liver will be worn out by repeated filtering of alcohol if the person drinks daily for a few years, giving rise to gastric ulcers, cirrhosis of the liver, etc. After being absorbed through osmosis, alcohol finds its way into the blood stream. The corrosive action of the "spirit" will begin to eat up the blood vessel lining, causing bleeding, the appearance of prominent veins, spider veins, unhealthy looking arteries and veins, unhealthy skin, etc.

When alcoholics suppress their desire to drink, they suffer from withdrawal syndrome, which causes physical and emotional pain and physiological disturbances that are the brain's way of demanding alcohol. They go through unexplained internal fears and are unable to function properly with ease.

B complex vitamins play a great role here. If you are not allergic to B complex and you take B complex vitamin supplements, the starving nerves will be nourished. When the nerves are nourished well with the nerve food (B complex), the brain and the nervous system will not demand excess sugar from alcohol to provide energy.

Many people who go through Alcoholics Anonymous and similar groups will learn to quit drinking by practicing self-control, group therapy, support systems, etc. But most of them end up having some physical disorders or pain: migraines, backaches, neck pains, shoulder pains, insomnia, etc. When they are treated for B complex, sugar and alcohol, their physical symptoms disappear.

Before you can successfully get over a drinking problem, you need to be treated for B complex and sugar. You should receive huge amounts of B complex vitamins along with megadoses of vitamin B12 for months before you can face the real world. You need to get involved with group therapy or join AA for support while going through the treatment. I insist that my patients remain close to AA or any other support group for a long time after completion of NAET treatments. The Basic 10 should be treated first before treating for alcohol.

Alcohol treatments may bring forth trapped or troubled emotions from the past. NAET specialists are well trained to look for emotional blockages associated with alcohol and, if found, they can be eliminated through NAET.

People become alcoholics for different reasons: peer pressure, boredom, etc., or simply because alcohol is readily available. These people can drink any amount and rarely get drunk. They fall into the non-allergic category. With some will power, they can quit drinking at any time without going through physical or emotional withdrawals. Support groups and group therapy help, along with allergy elimination, to overcome addiction. Alcoholics are urged to join A A to help break the long-term habits and assure that they remain that way for the rest of their lives.

People who are allergic to alcohol have severe withdrawal symptoms when they try to quit drinking. As I stated earlier, suppressing the desire to drink may turn into physical or psychological problems. Such was the case of Susie, who tried to quit drinking by joining Alcoholics Anonymous. She ended up having severe neck pains, migraines and brachial neuralgia. Eighteen months after she quit drinking, she still suffered severe back pain. After she was treated by NAET for sugar, B complex, and alcohol, she received relief from her chronic upper backache and migraines.

Michael, 52-years old, quit drinking 15 years ago when he joined AA; however, ever since he quit drinking, he had a chronic constant lower backache. He tried different treatments, including massage therapy, physical therapy, acupuncture, etc., with no relief. When he was treated by NAET for alcohol, his 15-year-old backache diminished.

A 63-year-old woman who had suffered for two years from a severe strain on the left side of the neck, shoulder and upper arm, came to our office. She had been treated by a neurologist, an orthopedic surgeon and an internist and was in physical therapy for four months, but nothing gave her relief. Then she came to see me. During the examination, I noted some signs of long-standing addictions and liver damage by her tongue reading. In the questionnaire, she had not mentioned any addictions, only that she drank one cup of coffee, which was nothing unusual at all. This puzzled me and I asked frankly, "How much alcohol do you drink in a day?" She said, "I did not mention that I drank alcohol, did I?" I said, "I know that. I read your statement. Now I want to know, off the record, how much do you drink?" She turned pale, as if she saw a ghost. She said, "Doctor, how did you know that I was an alcoholic?" I smiled, "Your tongue gave it away."

She said she had been an alcoholic for the past 20 years. She even went to a detoxification clinic twice, but she could not stop. She worked for a telephone company but was so dependent on alcohol that she stayed home from work many times in order to drink. She hid the brandy (the only drink she used) under her bed. Her husband slept in another room, never suspecting that she was an alcoholic. Her husband worked nights and she worked days making it convenient for her to drink. She never let on that she was an alcoholic; she never drank in public. Even her family physician, who wrote excuse letters for faked migraines as her reason for not working, did not know.

She was treated for sugar and brandy. She was not allergic to B complex; this is why she could fool everyone about her drinking problem. Her large intestine meridian was blocked. After she was treated for sugar and brandy, her constant nagging pain in her neck and shoulder disappeared. Six years later, she still remains pain-free. When asked about drinking, she said that she quit drinking soon after the treatment for brandy because she did not get the "buzz" in her head anymore. Brandy tasted like tap water to her after the treatments. She drank water whenever she wanted a drink, since tap water and brandy gave her almost the same result. She concluded that she might as well drink tap water and save the money.

Fructose allergy can be a cause of sugar and alcohol addiction. Another alcoholic patient gave up drinking after she joined an AA group, but she developed very bad neck pains and bilateral elbow pain. She had taken up eating fruits and natural yogurt when she quit drinking. She was very allergic to fructose which is found in abundance in fruits. Fructose caused a blockage in the spleen meridian. After treatment for fructose, her pains went away.

We have treated many addictions to alcohol, drugs, sugar, chocolate and tobacco in the past five years. Almost all of these patients were found to be allergic to B complex and sugar. As soon as these allergies were re-moved and supplemented with megadoses of B vitamins, it was easy for most of them to break the habits. Sometimes acupuncture is needed once a week for three to four weeks to lessen the cravings and withdrawal symp-toms while they take 300-500 mgs of B complex to fill up the deficiency.

Some people do not get any unpleasant symptoms while they are drink-ing, but hangovers or migraines the morning after are quite common. They are usually allergic to the alcohol itself and not as much to the B complex or sugar. When they are treated for alcohol, they no longer have any latent symptoms.

A 36-year-old man woke up with a migraine headache every Satur-day morning for the past ten years. Most of the time, over-the-counter painkillers helped to relieve his headache. On certain days his headache was so severe that he had to go to the emergency room for medication to allevi-ate his pain. Other days nothing helped him. He had to sleep in a dark room for two days. He drank a couple of beers with his friends after work every Friday evening since he started his present job 10 years ago. Allergy to beer was responsible for the blockage in his stomach meridian, causing his Sat-urday morning headaches.

ADDICTION TO COMPANIONSHIP

Addiction can be towards anything, even toward a woman or a man. A 42-year-old woman fell in love with a married man. He spent a lot of time with her and told her that he was going to divorce his wife and marry her, but he never did it. Finally, this desperate woman told him to leave. In a few days, she became very ill. She wanted to see him so much that she called him back. When he returned, staying with her for a few hours, she felt better. This pattern was repeated. Whenever he went away for a few days, she became physically ill with joint pains, body aches, fever, etc. As soon as she saw him, she felt better. Finally, she realized that she must be allergic to him and that this allergy was turning into an addiction. She was right. She was found to be allergic to him. Her liver, spleen and gall bladder were blocked. She was able to break up with him without any repercussions after she was treated for him with NAET.

YEAST / CANDIDIASIS / MOLD / FUNGUS

Yeast infection, candidiasis, mold, fungal disease, etc., are much talked about disorders affecting men and women alike, producing anxiety and health concerns among sufferers. What is yeast? What is candidiasis? How can fungal growth and mold cause health concerns? Should we really worry about them?

In reality, they are the cleaning crew created by the universe to help keep our environment clean. They attack the unwanted organic products of the world, finding them as soon as they are produced. They do not work on the energetically sound or live products. They act only where there is no normal circulation of energy. They help to convert organic waste (the end product of any life: human, animal or plant) by immediately breaking down these substances into their original form. Carbon and hydrogen (hydrocarbon) compounds are the original life-creating form of the world.

The products of fats, proteins and carbohydrates (the organic materials from humans, animals and plants) will eventually convert into sugars during chemical reactions. Sugars will attract yeast and yeast will act upon sugars. Fermentation reaction takes place when sugar and yeast combine. Ethyl alcohol is produced by yeast fermentation of sugar. Fermentation is the production of ethanol from sugar by the action of yeast or yeast-like bacteria. The enzymes of the yeast serves as catalysts for the transformation of sugar into ethanol and carbon dioxide.

$C_6H_{12}O_6 - 2CH_3CH_2OH + 2CO_2$

Glucose (sugar) ethanol Carbon-dioxide

Ethane and carbon dioxide will evaporate and blend in with the atmosphere to begin a new life cycle.

Have you watched any organic waste dropped on the soil? If any organic waste falls on the ground and stays there, unmoved for few days, you can see these environmental cleaners going into action. First the substance will get covered with worms, molds and fungus-like growth. In a few days, it will decay by the activity of these organisms and in a few more days, the waste will not look like its original form. It will be digested completely, blending and looking like its surrounding soil by freeing the ethane and carbon dioxide.

This happens not only outside the body, but also inside the human body. Yeast and yeast-like bacteria are commonly seen in the small intestine (symbiotic relationship), where most fermentation takes place in the body. When they live just in the intestinal region, there are no unpleasant reactions in the body. For various reasons, they expand their territory and travel to other organs and into the blood circulation. Since these areas are outside of their usual habitat, they get lost, not knowing what to do. Without having a job classification in their new surroundings, they begin to work with whatever they know — to clean up the environment. They will begin their work anywhere in the body where there is dead tissue or poor energy circulation.

There are many reasons why men and women alike suffer from yeast and candida infections today. Candida overgrowth occurs in the body when food is not properly digested, resulting in poor absorption and assimilation of nutrients. Poor assimilation of nutrients leads to a weak immune system and poor circulation of energy, building up the waste products in the body, mainly in the gut. This disturbs the intestinal flora. Yeast and candida multiply by the millions to ferment the waste build-up in the gut. What a feast they have when we build up waste materials in the gut! The multiplied millions then begin to travel to other areas.

Candida Albicans

I had Candida Albicans, a severe case of yeast in my blood for over seven years. During that time I spent over $20,000 out of pocket plus insurance expenses. Two of my doctors said that I would never get over it, even by staying on a rigid yeast-free diet, taking medications and injections as well as intravenous feedings. Six months after I started seeing Dr. Devi Nambudripad, I could see the light at the end of the tunnel. Now I am at the end of the tunnel. Now I am completely free of my candida and yeast problem for the past seven years.

Charles Depoin
Laguna Beach, CA

Is This My Candida?

I have been a patient of Dr. Devi for three years. When I first started the allergy treatments, I was in pretty bad condition. My health deteriorated twelve years ago when I came down with chronic fatigue. I had constant sinus infections for years, and the antibiotics I took gave me candida. I suffered from severe systemic candida for years. I had frequent headaches, body pain, bladder infections, and a fever for over a year and a half. And my uterus was detaching and I had large cysts on my ovaries. I was exhausted all the time. I saw many doctors during the past 12 years and everyone of them diagnosed my condition as overgrowth of candida and yeast as my only problem. I went through various detox and took the mercury out of my teeth, tried to eat healthy at home, spent thousands of dollars and suffered the pain and agony everyday in spite of everything. I suffered from severe insomnia, too. Doctors could offer only drugs, surgery, and exercise. But when you have to rest to get upstairs in your house, it is pretty hard to exercise. I tried everything that I knew to get well, including a healthy diet, rest, and acupuncture with Chinese herbal teas, at great expense. This helped some, but not permanently. Little did I know I was allergic to everything I was eating and drinking, along with the environmental pollutions. Previous allergy testing only showed environmental allergies. I was 38-years old and I thought my life was over.

After I started treatment with Dr. Devi my health has steadily improved. It took about three months of basic treatments, treating the chronic fatigue and candida, after which I noticed a change. When I was treated for minerals, the cysts on my ovaries disappeared and my uterus reattached. A sonogram and examination confirmed and showed everything as normal once again.

I still receive treatments once in a while. But I have a life again. All my infections are long gone and headaches are rare. I exercise and I know I will live a long life in health and with energy.

Thank God for Dr. Devi and NAET treatment. This is a real and permanent solution for any health problems.

Janet Johnson
Riverside, CA

Poor energy circulation is caused by: an allergy to food products, leading to blockages in the energy meridians; diseases (diabetes, chronic infections, leukemia, cancer); lack of production of essential gastric juices and digestive enzymes; use of antibiotics, birth control pills, cortisone; radiation, chemotherapy, hormone imbalance, exposure to toxic chemicals; nutritional deficiencies, a high carbohydrate diet, eating refined sugar products, eating fast foods, spicy foods, poor eating habits, foods that irritate the mucous membrane of the small intestine (carbonated drinks), not drinking enough water to flush out the system, and poor personal hygiene.

When the high carbohydrate and sugars get fermented in the presence of yeast, alcohol is produced. Ethanol can become ethyl alcohol in the presence of oxygen. It will put you to sleep. Some people fall asleep after they eat a high refined carbohydrate diet, because it increases the activity of yeast. Refined sugar and starch stimulate yeast and candida growth.

Commonly seen symptoms are fatigue, poor concentration, brain fog, brain floating-like sensation, excessive sleep, sleepy in the afternoon (activity of the yeast in the small intestine at its peak time) headaches, heartburn, burning sensation around cardiac end of stomach extending to esophagus with sense of constriction, heat sensation or bloating over liver area, sweet craving, skin rashes, hives, vaginal and rectal itching, insomnia, athlete's foot, oral thrush, colic, vaginal fungal infection, vaginal discharge, pelvic inflammatory disease, arthritis and joint pains, muscle aches, dampness, bladder infection, sinusitis with purulent discharge, post nasal drip, recurrent ear infection, throat infection, depression, general body aches, abdominal bloating, constipation, diarrhea, overweight and water retention.

When you get a lot of yeast overgrowth, it is a warning sign that the body is struggling with poor energy circulation; the body is decaying.

Allergic reactions can mimic yeast-like infections. Allergy to detergents, soap, clothes, panty hose, crotches on the panty, the chemical reaction between the body and the chemicals used in fabrics, toilet paper, etc., can cause blockage in the liver and spleen meridians, causing yeast-like infections in the body.

Mary, a 38-year-old woman, went to the circus. While she was there, she used their temporary restrooms. In a few minutes she began itching and burning in her private areas, mimicking a yeast infection. She quickly re-

> ### *Perfume Causing Yeast Like Symptoms*
>
> *One of the most striking recoveries occurred with a man in his fif-ties, who experienced a liquid discharge from his ears, headache and brain fog whenever he was exposed to perfume. He was un-able to worship at Temple, and often had to leave social functions. All of his symptoms disappeared after he cleared perfume and he told me he felt as if he had his life back again!*
>
> *Eric Roth, M.D.*
> *New York*

membered the toilet paper and brought a piece to the office the next morn-ing. She was allergic to it. Her discomfort ceased soon after she was treat-ed for the toilet paper by NAET.

A woman, 28, who had yeast infections whenever she had an orange, found she was allergic to the vitamin C in the orange. A young man ate yogurt for lunch everyday. He suffered from rectal burning, anal itching, painful acne and infection around the fingernail cuticles. When he was treated for yogurt, all his symptoms cleared.

Another woman was allergic to her husband's semen, causing contin-uous yeast like infections in her. She took antibiotics everyday for years to get some relief from her discomfort. When the allergen was identified and treated with NAET, she got relief from her years-long yeast infection.

CHRONIC FATIGUE SYNDROME

This long-term illness can affect the whole body. It is characterized by debilitating fatigue and other persistent problems, such as low-grade fever, sore throat, insomnia or drowsiness, inability to concentrate, pain in the muscles and joints, enlarged or painful lymph nodes, general muscle weak-ness, headaches, forgetfulness, excessive irritability, confusion, difficulty in thinking, depression and lack of interest in life. People who suffer all or some of these symptoms fall into the CFS (Chronic Fatigue Syndrome) group. This definition of CFS was developed by researchers and published in the March 1988, "Annals of Internal Medicine." Previously, this illness was described as a chronic Epstein-Barr virus or syndrome (CEBV) or chronic mononucleosis. Researchers decided that the name Chronic Fatigue Syndrome would better reflect the major symptoms, without suggesting a cause, because no one knows the cause of CFS.

In my opinion, the major cause of CFS is allergy to: foods, (sugar, B complex, starches, alcohol, iron, fat, amino acid, minerals, copper, lead, tap water, spices, food additives, food coloring and hormones), environmental substances (chemicals, wood, formaldehyde, fabrics, carpets, detergent, newspaper, ink, pesticides and cosmetics), infectious agents (bacteria, virus, parasites and pesticides) and emotional factors (divorce, miscarriage, sudden loss of loved ones, etc.). Some people with CFS have an allergy to everything, including their own body secretions (saliva, blood, urine and mucus, etc.). We see many patients who were going to CFS clinics for years, with little result. When they are treated for allergies by NAET, they respond very well. Usually CFS patients need hundreds of NAET treatments to get back to normal life. Some of our CFS patients have been treated with two to three office visits per week for three or four years before they were able to resume a normal life.

A 35-year-old woman had been treated for CFS and EBV and was on disability for three to four years. In spite of all the treatments and the good nutrition she was receiving, her problems were getting worse. She was thoroughly evaluated in our office and was found to be allergic to almost all foods and fabrics. She was glad to know she was suffering from allergies, rather than some incurable illness. Within a few months of her initial visit, she started showing marked improvement. In her case, most of the allergens affected her spleen and heart meridians. She had four to six months of continuous treatment (three to four visits per week) to clear almost all her allergies. At the end of that period, she felt almost normal and began to work regularly.

A young woman of 28, who had been treated for EBV for seven years, was also found to be allergic to foods, external substances, fabrics and water. In her case, she was severely allergic to regular tap water. She had been on disability for seven years. Her heart, stomach, spleen, gall bladder and large intestine meridians were affected. After treatments in our office for almost a year, she was able to work full time as a teacher. Many mild to moderate cases of CFS have been treated successfully with NAET.

Genetic predisposition may play a role in chronic fatigue syndrome just as we see in cases of allergies. Most CFS patients show inherited sensitivity to allergies. We are living in an environment of electromagnetic pollution. All types of energies are bombarding our bodies from all directions, causing continuous blockages and resulting in a wide range of psychological and physiological disorders. Present day electromagnetic pollution may be causing weaknesses in the immune system. The pangs of immune deficiency diseases would not be felt so dramatically if patients had stronger immune systems. Allergies would not affect the body as much. You have to strengthen the immune system, and strengthen the function of the thymus gland, the spleen, lymph flow and bone marrow. If you suffer from CFS and other immune deficiency syndrome ailments, you may be able to fight them eventually if you make it a point to follow balancing techniques twice a day.

Electric and computer radiation can cause energy blockages in the body. We see and treat many people in our office who react to computer materials and radiation. A 48-year-old male computer programmer suffered from extreme fatigue, frequents headaches, insomnia and irritable bowel syndrome for the last 8 years. Coincidently, he worked as a computer programmer for eight years. He found that he was significantly allergic to computer radiation, which was affecting all 12 of his meridians. When he was treated with NAET for radiation and various environmental allergies, he was able to lead a normal life again. After six years, he still remains symptom-free.

Mary, 24-years-old, had been diagnosed with chronic fatigue syndrome for four years. She suffered from severe brain fog, poor memory, sudden shooting pains in her brain, sharp pains in parts of her body, blurred vision, heart palpitation, excessive hunger, insomnia and severe constipation. After a football accident when she was 16-years old, she had a stainless steel implant placed in her knee. When she was treated for the stainless steel, her brain fog decreased and her heartbeat became regular. Her appetite regulated, the sharp, shooting pains disappeared, sleep was better and her CFS syndrome improved. The allergy to stainless steel was causing most of her unpleasant symptoms.

EYE DISORDERS

Many times, eye problems are a result of allergies. Certain food items that affect the liver meridian can cause eye problems. Conjunctivitis, red eyes, watering from the eyes, cataracts, and pressure in the eyes are all probably the result of some allergy.

A 51-year-old woman complained of having blurry vision. She had to change the power of her glasses often. She was found to be allergic to various food items and environmental substances, including her contact lenses and eyeglasses. When she was treated for all her known allergies, the power of her prescription came down, and she did not suffer from blurry vision unless she ate some allergic foods.

A young boy of six had problems seeing and reading. He was taken to two different eye doctors and got exactly the same prescriptions for his glasses. He was found to be allergic to various foods. He was treated for all his known allergies; in less than two months he started reading without glasses. He said he couldn't see anything with the glasses. He was taken again to the eye doctor, and the power had changed from -3.75 to -0.25. The eye doctor did not understand how it could have happened. He concluded that the previous eye examinations were not correct.

An 18-year-old had a pea-size fatty growth on the outside of the lower left eyelid. It looked like a large pad and it bothered him a lot. He was found to be allergic to the peanut butter sandwiches he ate every day. When he was treated for peanuts, the pea-size growth disappeared. From this peanut butter reaction, a hypothesis can be formulated that benign or cancerous tumors are often the results of allergies. Finding and treating the causes of the problems can help eliminate growths and tumors.

I Can Hear Again!

I'm 47 years old, and have had a moderate to severe, bilateral, sensorineural hearing loss all my life. I've been told over and over by medical doctors and audiologists for over four decades that there is no cure...there is nothing I can do to improve my hearing. I absolutely refused to believe them, and have actively searched for the 'truth' for over 20 years. In the meantime, to help me cope, I wore hearing aids. I'm an Industrial Engineer and every day was a desperate struggle, until Friday, October 12, 2001.

I've been treated by specialists with various and sundry experimental techniques all of my adult life...with absolutely zero results. Zip, Nada, Nothing. I've been treated by chiropractors all my life, two family members are chiropractors, and my hearing never improved. Then on Thursday, October 11, 2001, I received the first treatment from Dr. Marilyn Chernoff at The Healing Center in Albuquerque, NM, using Nambrudipads Allergy Elimination Techniques (NAET). I didn't feel a thing. I must confess I was taken aback at how simple the treatment was....and just a teeny little bit disappointed.

However, on the way to work the next morning, I heard a new noise. I was wearing one hearing aid instead of two, because one was not working. I thought the engine must be knocking and fixing to go out. Then I realized I was hearing the cassette tape rewinding....I've never heard that before. At work, I went to the restroom and heard a loud electronic beeping.... I tracked it down to an electronic device on the wall that's always been there, but I've never even heard it, even with two hearing aids! All day a wonderful world of sound blossomed as I kept hearing new sounds I haven't heard before. Shoes rubbing against carpet as someone walked down the hall. The tapping of a keyboard in the next cubicle. A coffee cup being set down gently nearby. A lady chuckling several cubicles away.

(Continued on next page)

Over the weekend I could easily hear my son talking from the back seat of our noisy minivan, even when I was wearing no hearing aids. The next Monday at work, I took my hearing aid off when I realized I was hearing better out of my other ear! The next morning I wept as I listened to the richness of all the sounds of music, sounds I've never heard before from songs

I've heard all my life, on the radio as I drove in to work (again, with no hearing aids). That afternoon I actively participated in a videoconference, easily understanding conversations that was almost impossible for me to 'catch' only a week earlier. I heard the soft meow of one of our cats this morning...as he was walking away! What a beautiful sound!

Please, no matter what symptoms afflict you, help is available. Contact Dr. Marilyn Chernoff of The Healing Center at 505-292-2222 in Albuquerque, NM, or if that is not feasible, go to www.naet.com and find an NAET practitioner in your area. I profit nothing by this...except by the hope that you too can receive life-changing help.

Tim Hall
New Mexico

HEARING LOSS

Food allergies can cause hearing loss. Some children with severe food allergies begin to lose their hearing when they are very young. Ear infections, throat infections, runny noses, frequent colds and upper respiratory problems are warning signs in infants and children. When they get ear infections, their pediatricians usually explain to their parents that the canal connecting the throat and the ear is too short in children and those food particles easily escape into the ear and cause ear infections. But this explanation is not always true. When the child is allergic to the formula, the food

Weight Problem and Yeast problem Through NAET

I began gaining weight in my late teens. I continued to gain about 10 pounds every year ever since. I tried everything I could think of to get my weight down, including 10 different diet plans through the years. I barely ate to live, yet my pounds didn't go down. The more careful I got the more I just continued to pack pounds. It was awful. It was disgusting, depressing, I even tried yeastfree diets, thyroid, antidepressants and laxatives.... No one had any answer to my obesity.

Then I developed a severe nasal allergy. Burning and itching inside and outside my nostrils. I also developed vaginal candidiasis. Again none of the treatments I tried was working on me. It seemed that I was resistant to all types of treatments. I met a lady in a healthfood store. She suggested NAET. I had no hope with NAET either. As a last resort, I decided to start NAET treatments. What is there to lose?

To my surprise my practitioner found the cause of my problem on the very first visit. I was allergic to everything I ate. By the time I finished the basic NAET treatments, I was seeing results. My nasal allergy stopped and my weight began dropping, slowly but surely. I was happy because finally something was working on me. I continued NAET regularly, three times a week for the last three years. After about 150 NAET treatments in my practitioner's office and many many self-treatments at home, I can say that I am fairly healthy now and weigh 50 pounds less than three years ago.

Every morning I weigh myself and if I see a weight gain even if it is one pound, I muscle test (O-ring test) myself and find the food or drink I ate previous day that caused a weight gain and I self-treat every 15 minutes for 6 times before I eat anything. Thank God this is working well and keeping my weight normal and yeast infection problem completely under control for the first time in years.

Thanks again to NAET.

Jane Jones,
Los Angeles, CA

or formula may get into the ear canal and cause an allergic reaction that mimics an infection. If the parent or the pediatrician decides to change the child's food menu to non-allergic items, the child will not have to suffer ear infections or most of the other unwanted childhood diseases.

A two-month old infant who had a history of vomiting after each meal, along with chronic constipation, caught a common cold accompanied by a mild fever, a runny nose and an ear infection. The baby was fed with the formula prescribed by the pediatrician and was given antibiotics for 14 days without any results. The child's grandmother visited them during that time and she thought the formula he was drinking could be the cause of his health problems. She advised the mother to stop the formula and all the medicines, and feed him with 50 percent low fat, regular, homogenized milk. The child's ear, throat and upper-respiratory tract infection, and the low-grade fever cleared up in two days. He began to have regular bowel movements. This child was not allergic to regular cow's milk, but to all other formulas. Every child may not be as lucky as this one, but it would help if parents and doctors could find a non-allergic formula.

A 4-month-old infant was exhibiting mild cold symptoms. His pediatrician gave him antibiotics for ten days. He said that the child had an ear infection, but from the time of the second dose of medicine the infant began crying continuously day and night, without stopping. He cried for three days and two nights, without any sleep or food. He was found to be allergic to the antibiotic. When he was successfully treated for the antibiotic, he stopped crying and began sleeping for the first time in three days. He was also found to be allergic to the milk he was drinking, which had caused the ear infection in the first place.

If the child's food allergy had been allowed to continue untreated or ignored, in time he would have built up more and more allergic reactions and self-damaging toxins affecting the energy pathways, neural pathways, organs and related structures. If the target of the toxin were the ear, hearing loss would be the result.

Most people begin to lose hearing in their old age. These are the people who probably fall in the mild to moderate allergy group. They may not have too many allergic manifestations in their youth. But toxins accumulated from minor allergies may affect their hearing in old age. If you did not have allergies, hearing loss need not occur just because you are old. Hearing loss due to old age is not a proper diagnosis. Many people with hearing loss who begin to eat the right (non-allergenic) foods experience improved hearing. If the problem is caught in the initial stages, complete recovery is possible. If the damage is less than 20 percent, regeneration of the damaged tissue is possible, and you can expect a complete cure after successful treatment for all allergies. It might take months or years before you can get satisfactory results. If the damage to the tissue is more than 20 percent, then further damage can be prevented with the treatment. Complete reversal may not be possible unless you are under 16, in which case complete reversal is possible if the problem is allergy-related.

Ever since Valentine's Day, a 32-year-old woman was suffering from a severe earache and headache on one side of the body. She visited her internist and an ear specialist and had taken 20 days of antibiotics and painkillers, all without any relief. When she came to our office, escorted by one of her friends, she was wearing a tiny, single-stone, diamond ear ornament that had been given to her by her husband on Valentine's Day as a token of his love. She was found to be allergic to the earring top. She removed it and put it away, and in a few minutes her pain and discomfort disappeared. Eventually, she was treated for the earring top, so that she could wear it and please her husband.

Another interesting case of hearing loss was a young man who was eighteen-years old. After Christmas, he complained of congestion and fullness in his left ear for about a month. He also suffered from frequent ringing in the ears, lightheadedness, and mild to moderate deafness in the left ear. He thought he was getting the flu for a few days and did not do anything about it. When the symptoms persisted, he saw a medical internist, who diagnosed a mild ear infection and prescribed a decongestant and an antibiotic. He tried them but they did not do much good.

Finally, he came to our office. When he was evaluated, he was found to be highly allergic to metals. He was wearing a brand new, yellow metal wristwatch, and he informed us that it was his girl friend's Christmas gift to him and he had worn it ever since, even to bed. This watch was touching "San Jiao 5," one of the main points of the San Jiao acupuncture meridian, which is responsible for the well-being of hearing and other related functions. The watch was irritating this point constantly and created a continuous blockage in that meridian, causing all his symptoms. Unless treated, the blockages would have become larger and the related tissues would have been damaged. The end result would have been complete deafness.

TINNITUS

Food additives and preservatives can cause ringing in the ears. Hanan suffered from ringing in the ears (tinnitus) for seven months. He saw an ear, nose and throat specialist and took many laboratory tests, but the ringing in his ears persisted. When he was evaluated in our office through NTT, it was revealed that his problem was related to a grain he was eating everyday. He was found to be allergic to a particular cereal he was eating daily for breakfast. His wife, who had accompanied him, remembered that he had started to eat that brand of cereal seven months ago. He liked it so much that on certain days he craved it and even ate it for supper. After he was

---

Ringing In The Ear

I suffered from severe ringing in the ears for many years. It wasn't severe in the beginning and it happened only when I was resting. Gradually it got worse and it began bothering me all day long. I tried different treatments, nothing worked. Finally I heard about NAET. In her office, Dr. Devi evaluated me and asked me if I used feather pillows. I had used feather pillows and comforters since childhood. I loved my pillows. I carried them with me wherever I went, even on vacation. She said that they were causing my problem. She treated me for feathers and asked me to stay in a hotel until the 35 hours were over since I had so many feather pillows and feather particles flying all over the house. That night I slept very well. The next morning when I woke up, I was free of the ringing in my ears. After 35 hours, I returned home. I am still free from the ringing in the ears.

Casey N.
Costa Mesa

---

treated for that brand of cereal, the ringing in his ears stopped, and he did not crave it anymore.

VERTIGO

Mary, a 48-year-old, had vertigo for one week when she came to the office. Questioning her, it was discovered that for the past week she had been substituting a particular artificial sweetener for the sugar in her coffee. Upon clearing her allergy for that particular sugar substitute, the vertigo left her.

Yeast, virus, bacteria, food colors, food additives, etc., can cause vertigo in many people. Energy blockages in the kidney or liver meridians are affected in people with vertigo. Using city water on certain days (rains, extreme heat, etc.) has been found to cause inner ear imbalance and vertigo in many patients in the greater L.A. area. After NAET, they get relief from their vertigo.

PAIN DISORDERS / FIBROMYALGIA

Fibromyalgia syndrome is very frequently allergy-related. Fibromyalgia means pain in the muscles, ligaments and tendons. In many cases, the cause of FMS is allergies to foods (egg mix, calcium, vitamin C, sugar, B complex, whole grains, yogurt, yeast, starches, alcohol, iron, fat, amino acid, minerals, vegetables, tomato, potato, bell pepper, onion, garlic, egg plant, cigarette, nicotine, phosphorus, copper, lead, tap water, spices, food additives, food coloring and hormones), environmental substances (chemicals, wood, formaldehyde, fabrics, carpets, detergent, newspaper, ink, pesticides and cosmetics), and emotional factors (divorce, miscarriage, sudden loss of loved ones, etc.). Some people with FMS have an allergy to everything, including their own body secretions such as saliva, blood, urine and mucus, etc.We see many patients who were going to FMS clinics for years with little or no result. When they are treated for allergies by NAET, they respond very well. Usually FMS patients need many NAET treatments to get back to normal life. Some of our FMS patients have received treatments two to three times per week for three or four years before they were able to resume a normal life.

Most patients with fibromyalgia say that they ache all over. Their muscles may feel like they have been pulled. Sometimes the muscles twitch and other times they burn. More women than men get this disorder, but it shows up in all ages and both sexes.

Symptoms associated with this disorder are deep muscular aching, burning, throbbing, shooting and stabbing pain. The pain and stiffness are worse in the morning. Fatigue, brain fog, sleep disorders, irritable bowel syndrome, migraine headaches, severe premenstrual syndromes, irritable bladder, lightheadedness, dry mouth, skin, and eyes are some of the commonly seen problems with fibromyalgia patients.

Fibromyalgia patients react to most foods and chemicals. Since whole grains are harder to digest, it is advisable for people to eat partially processed foods until they eliminate the allergy to the wholesome products.

Amy, 32, suffered from FMS since she was 18 years old. She was allergic to everything around her. She reacted to all kinds of foods, body secretions (blood, saliva, urine, etc.), detergents, chemicals, fabrics, tiles, floor coverings, carpets, bed sheets, plastics, her pets (cat, dog), newspapers, grasses, molds, trees, food additives, thyroid supplements and her pain medications. She was one of many who had to take hundreds of NAET treatments to get some relief from her pains. After 5 years of regular treatments (at least once a week), she is 80 percent pain-free now. She tried various types of treatments for her FMS in the past. Since this is the only treatment that has given her some relief from her pain syndrome and hope for a pain-free future, she continues, without losing her enthusiasm, to explore all avenues of NAET to get completely well.

Mike, 27, suffered from fibromyalgia for 9 years. On the first visit, he was treated for eggs and chicken. He reported on his next visit that he was 90% better. His major allergy was proteins. After receiving the Basic 10 treatments, he is 99 percent pain-free.

For 4 months, Susan, a 51-year-old, suffered from constant, intense sciatic pain radiating from the right hip to the ankle. She saw various specialists dealing in pain management: chiropractors, acupuncturists, herbalists and a physical therapist, but her pain continued. She had given up hope of getting better. Then one day her daughter saw us on television, called our office, and brought her in for evaluation.

Through NTT, we discovered that one of her supplements was the culprit. She had stopped taking all vitamin-mineral supplements, but contin-

> ## My Neck Pains And Osteoporosis?
>
> *For decades, I suffered from severe neck pain which was attributed to disc degeneration that was first diagnosed by X-ray in my late 20's. By my late 40's, the pain was severe and a neuro-radiologist told me that, based on a recent M.R.I., if I didn't have my neck fused, I was at risk to become a quadriplegic. After treating my calcium allergy, including many combinations, the pain left. I plan to retake X-rays in one year to monitor the remineralization of the cervical vertebrae.*
>
> *Elena Oumano, Ph.D.*
> *New York*

ued to take the hormone pill her doctor had prescribed four months ago. She was immediately treated for the pill. After 30 minutes, she left the office free of pain in her leg. Her pain hasn't returned in 2 years.

Tina ate potato for lunch in her salad. She immediately began having mid-backache. She brought a sample of her lunch to the office. When she was treated for potato, her mid-backache cleared.

Margie, a 24-year-old female, complained that her hands fell asleep whenever she slept. She had suffered from this unique problem that mimicked carpal tunnel syndrome for the past nine weeks. With the kinesiological diagnostic technique, it was discovered that she was eating cream-filled arrowroot cookies every night before she went to bed. When she was treated for the cookies, her hands did not fall asleep when she went to bed.

Newspaper and newspaper ink can cause carpal tunnel syndrome among its readers. NAET has given great relief to people suffering carpal tunnel syndrome.

INFECTIONS

When the immune system gets low, infectious agents can attack it, causing various infectious diseases. When the immune system is strong, bacteria or virus may not bother us.

If you suspect that you are getting a cold or flu, immediately take a sample of your saliva or urine and balance your body, using the points described in Chapter 11. It may prevent you from getting a flu or cold.

Jill, 55-years-old, suffered from the Epstein-Barr virus and various allergies. After treatment for the virus, her response was very encouraging. Questioning her, it was found that her Japanese parents, uncles and aunts died of tuberculosis. She was immediately tested and treated for tuberculosis and became allergy-free and healthy once again.

Patient Regains Use of Hand Through NAET

A man in his 30's, who worked as a manual laborer, sustained a crush injury to his dominant right hand while working. I saw him about three years after the accident. During that time he was unable to work or use his right hand, which was frozen in a clenched position, and he was in constant pain. The clinic where I work was unable to do physical therapy because his hand was very sensitive to touch. So, I asked him to try NAET. Muscle testing revealed that he was allergic to all of the Basic 10. As he cleared each item, he improved steadily. By the time he was clear for the final item, he had full use of the hand, no pain, and he was able to return to work.

Eric Roth, M.D.
(Board Certified Physiatrist, Certified Acupuncturist, Osteopath)

No Radiation Burns!

I am a cancer survivor. My treatments for cancer included severe chemotherapy over a seven month period, followed by 33 days of radiation therapy. Prior to beginning radiation therapy my sister-in-law told me of her positive experience of NAET. At her request, and despite my skepticism, I went for treatments to Dr. Eric Thompson. I received the NAET treatment for Radiation therapy. Doctor (my oncologist) and nurses that had warned me of radiation burns (and the need for a break after the 2nd or 3rd week) were shocked that after 31 days of radiation I had only red "sun-burn" like skin, and only minor burns following the last of the 33 cycles. They had never seen anyone go through this type of therapy with such minor side effects. I honestly believe that the NAET treatments given to me by Dr. Eric Thompson and Tess are what made the difference.

A short time later I developed Lymphoedema due to the removal of eleven lymph-nodes in a cancer related surgery. My leg would frequently swell and cause me enough pain that I could not sleep some nights. I wore a special compression-stocking to reduce the swelling but it was not always effective and was very uncomfortable. Then he treated me for "Lymph system" treatment using NAET and it helped dramatically. My leg will still swell on occasion but it does so rarely and does not get nearly as bad as used to be. I no longer need the compression stocking either.

I had many food allergies as well as environmental and chemical sensitivities. I have been treated for "Trees" and am now able to walk through a park or go camping and enjoy the smell of pine trees free from the worrying about any allergic reaction. I don't get sick on foods anymore. I have been able to enjoy my life more than ever now since I don't react adversely to most foods, chemicals or environmental substances around me anymore.

Dr. Eric and Tess have helped me so much that I aked them if there was some way for me to help or support them in return. They said a testimony of my experiences would be nice.

Well, this letter is a testimony, but most of all it is a chance for me to say "THANK YOU" for the many ways in which they have helped me to improve the quality of my life through NAET treatments.

C.S., WA
NAET Practitioners: Drs. Eric and Tess Thompson, Richland, WA

My Child Doesn't Have Lupus Athritis Anymore!

I would like to express my sincere gratefullness and happiness to Dr. Devi Nambudripad for taking care of our daughter Nithya Menon age 3 with ANA level 7.4H on 8/15/2001.

My daughter was in pain and unable to climb staircase at home and walk. Her pediatrician wanted to refer her to a specialist of pediatric rheumatoid arthrology and a pediatric ophthalmology for treatment of Lupus.

When the pediatrician informed me that my 3 year old child may be a victim of Lupus, I couldn't think for a few seconds. Finally when I pulled together, I refused to believe it. I didn't say anything to our considerate pediatrician. She was only trying to help my child with what she knew. She had no concept of alternative medical approach. She had no idea that treatments like NAET existed outside the medical regimen. Last year when my mother-in-law suffered from a bleeding gastric ulcer for three months, when the gastroenterologist couldn't help her with all the medication she was taking, we saw Dr. Devi and she detected an allergy to the rice she was eating everyday was the cause of her gastic bleeding. Soon after she completed the treatment for rice, she stopped bleeding. She hasn't had the problem ever since.

I immediately called Dr. Devi's office and made an appointment for my daughter (8/31/2001). She took a sample of her venous blood treated her for vitamin C first, then with a combination of vitamin C and blood. By the same evening she began walking again without pain. She did a few more basic treatments with combinations and told us to wait a month to repeat the lab work. We did blood work through the pediatrician's office on October 2, 2001 and the the doctor called to notify us that the ANA level has dropped to 1.6 H and Rheumatoid factor negative.

Copies of the laboratory reports dated 2/11/2000 showing her ANA as 2.3H, 6/27/2000 ANA as 3.4H, 8/15/2001 ANA as 7.4H, 10/5/2001 ANA showing 1.6H (after NAET treatments) are attached with this testimony as a proof of what we have stated above. With our utmost thanks.

Ravi & Sathi Menon, Irvine, CA

ALLERGY TO DENTAL ANESTHESIA

For three weeks, a 28-year-old woman had complained of excruciating pains in her right jaw, along with swelling of the right side of the face. She had some dental work done exactly three weeks before. She returned to her dentist many times with the same complaint following the initial work. Following her dentist's advice, she applied cold and hot compresses, took antibiotics and pain pills. Nothing gave her any relief. When she came to our office, testing through NTT revealed that she was allergic to the dental anesthetics used in the procedure. She was treated for the exact anesthetic with NAET. The result was amazing: halfway through the acupuncture balancing treatment, the final step of NAET, a period of less than 20 minutes, her facial swelling was absolutely gone. By the end of the treatment, she had no pain at all and it has never returned.

Charles, 40, had some dental work done five months ago. Ever since, he suffered from a funny "burned charcoal-like taste" in his mouth. He brushed and gargled many times a day to remove the funny taste, but his mouth felt the same. He also felt the sensation of electrical current in his mouth every now and then, which made him very uncomfortable. He told his dentist about these unusual sensations many times. The dentist checked his mouth thoroughly and sent him home, saying everything looks just right; but it just didn't feel right.

When he came to me, he appeared very miserable. I evaluated him through NTT and traced the problem to the crown in his mouth. He had one gold crown with a silver filling. These two metals were interacting and he felt the energy of their interaction as electrical current. The burnt smell was the result of the interaction of the energy with the enamel of the teeth. After he was treated for gold, silver, enamel and all in combination, his bad taste and sensitivity diminished.

Twenty-eight-year-old Tina had sensitive teeth for five months. She felt uncomfortable whenever she drank hot or cold drinks. Her dentist gave her a special toothpaste. He examined her and found that her gums were receding. Surgery was the only way to correct the problem. But the dentist, who was also a trained NAET practitioner, found some allergy involvement in her dental condition. He referred her to me. Through NTT, it was discovered that she was allergic to her toothbrush, which she had been using for

Periodontal Disease

I know I wrote a letter already about the wonderful effects of NAET, but I have to send you another about the most recent discovery. On 4/15/96 I went for a regular check-up with my dentist. The hygienist took a "sample" from my gums and put it under a slide. To my horror, I had stuff I did not want to look at. I was advised that I had the beginnings of gum periodontal disease. Yuk! Here's the data:

Initial Exam 4/15/96

Selenomonas spp	*too many to count*
Amoeba	*13-24 on a screen*
Actinobacillus	
Actinomycetemeomitans	*07-12 on a screen*

*Note: underlined numbers indicate my count is on the high end.

I came in to your office for a treatment on 4/17/96. My hygienist agreed to do another slide exam to determine if the treatment had been effective. She was amazed!! She said no one improves that quickly when the counts are as high as mine were. Here's the data:

As of 4/25/96

Selenomonas spp	*none*
Amoeba	*1-6 on a screen*
Actinobacillus	
Actinomucetemeomitans	*1-6 on a screen*

I think the data says it all. The dentist's office staff were amazed. They are not typically open to alternative methods of treatment. They called me and asked for Dr. Trott's number. My hygienist even suggested that I get another treatment from Dr. Trott and come back for another test to see if there was even further improvement.

Phyllis Stewart, LMSW, ACP

(Pt of Dr. Gary Trott, TX)

the past five months. After she was treated for that brand of toothbrush, in less than four months, her receding gums were naturally repaired.

PEDIATRIC PROBLEMS:
AUTISM, ADD, ADHD, ASTHMA, INFECTIONS & FEVER

According to the Autism Society of America, more than 500,000 Americans have some form of autism. The developmental disability typically appears during the first three years of life and is characterized by problems interacting and communicating with others. Many individuals exhibit repeated body movements such as hand-flapping, rocking, and may resist changes in routine. In some cases, they may display aggressive or self-injurious behaviors.

Milk and dairy products cause attention deficit and hyperactivity disorders. Milk is also one of the culprits in autism. These people cannot break down the milk protein and undigested protein might get into the circulation to the brain, causing irritability and abnormality in behaviors. After successful NAET treatments, the body will learn to make the appropriate digestive enzymes to break down the proteins.

Many infants are allergic to various things in their surroundings: crib material, the finish on the crib, fabric covering on the mattress, plastic and metal ornaments and toys, baby carriages, clothes, bottles, nipples, lotions, diapers, formulas and other foods, etc., can cause various health conditions in an infant. Infants and children can also react to their immunizations and vaccinations. When your infant is normal during infancy and suddenly develops developmental delays or any other unusual health conditions, please check all the new items you have introduced the infant to: foods, drinks, toys, clothes, coloring books, crayons, vitamins, immunizations, antibiotics, new baby seat, training panty, training chair, a new friend, visiting a new place, etc.

Many children become autistic due to an allergy to childhood immunizations. One of the major causes of ADD, ADHD, and/or AUTISM is allergy to something the child was eating, drinking, breathing and/or injecting (immunizations).

Diaper Rash

My daughter was five-days old when Doctor Devi began to treat her for cotton so she could wear her diapers. When my baby returned for the next treatment, it was for a terrible diaper rash because she had a reaction to my breast milk. Dr. Devi traced this to cauliflower I had eaten. Caitlin, my baby girl, had thrown up and had diarrhea all night long. Her bottom, as a result was "raw" by morning. After Dr. Devi treated the baby and me for the allergy to cauliflower, the rash and rawness disappeared completely and exactly in 24 hours.

Cindy Burch

Orange, CA

A 6-year-old boy had a low grade fever, about 100 to 101 degrees, throughout the day for three to four weeks. His parents tried many different treatments, including antibiotics, but nothing they gave him lowered his fever. Finally, his mother recalled that four weeks earlier, he drank a glass of eggnog and vomited almost all of it a few minutes after he drank it. His mother remembered that was also the beginning of his fever. One of the ingredients of the eggnog was nutmeg. MRT showed that he was highly allergic to nutmeg. After treatment for nutmeg with NAET, his fever broke and his temperature became normal a few hours later.

Many children suffer from chronic ear infections. The major cause of ear infections in children is due to food and environmental allergies. At the first sign of onset, if the cause is traced through NTT and eliminated through NAET, your child may not have to suffer unnecessary pain and discomfort due to ear infection.

VOMITING

Another 4-year-old girl started vomiting and ran a fever of 103 degrees. Her parents took her to the family doctor, who prescribed antibiotics. After three days of oral medication she was not any better. Her vomiting and fever continued. Finally, she was brought to our clinic. We discovered that she had been given cactus pickle by her sitter. She was highly allergic to cactus. After treatment for cactus, she stopped vomiting and, within a few minutes, her temperature became normal.

TEMPORARY PARALYSIS

A 3-year-old girl was at a friend's birthday party. After the party, as all the guests were about to depart, her mother noticed that she was crawling on the floor. Her mother thought that she was tired and sleepy from running and playing the entire evening. She fell asleep in the car. Her parents carried her to the house and to her bed. The next morning, when she refused to wake up, her parents got worried and called the paramedics. The child was still breathing, but unresponsive. She was taken to the hospital in a coma. After 72 hours, she woke up to find her legs paralyzed below the waist. She was kept in the hospital nine days, until her general condition stabilized, and was sent home with instructions to follow up with physical therapy. When she was out of the hospital, her parents, who were already familiar with NAET, brought her straight to our clinic. We found that she had eaten a large piece of pineapple cake with chunks of pineapple in it. It was the first time she had ever eaten pineapple. She was found to be allergic to pineapple. She had several treatment sessions by NAET for pineapple, and upon finishing the treatments, she started walking on her own. She did not go back for physical therapy. Her temporary paralysis was due to her allergy to pineapple.

STREP-THROAT

An 11-year-old girl got a sore throat and was very sick. Her pediatrician took a throat swab and found that she had strep throat. She took antibiotics for seven days. Instead of getting better, her sore throat got worse. Then she was brought to our clinic. Through a kinesiological examination, we were able to trace the allergy cause of her strep-like symptoms. She had eaten a particular candy bar nine days earlier that was the cause of her sore throat. When she was treated for the particular candy bar, her strep-like symptoms cleared in minutes.

ABDOMINAL CRAMPS

A 12-year-old girl suffered from frequent abdominal cramps. She stayed home from school so often that she was given home schooling. Her doctor put her on some medication that made her sleepy. Her stomach discomfort continued. One day her mother brought her to the clinic. Examining her through NTT, it was found that she was allergic to cauliflower. Because her mother had become vegetarian a few months earlier, they ate a lot of cauliflower daily. When she was treated for the allergy to cauliflower by NAET, she no longer had stomach cramps.

CANKER SORES

Allergy to milk, magnesium, vitamin D, sugar, spices, braces in the mouth, and dentures can cause canker sores in many people. Canker sores are very painful and irritating. As in any pain disorder, people with canker sores are unable to eat normal foods and function normally.

A 13-year-old girl suffered from painful multiple canker sores, making it difficult to eat any normal food. She drank a few glasses of milk every day. She tried various prescription and over-the-counter medications for her canker sores but nothing seemed to give her any relief. Finally, she found out about NAET and came to see me. Through NTT, it was discovered that she was allergic to milk, which was causing her canker sores. She was treated for milk and had to stay away from it for 72 hours after the treatment. When she returned, her canker sores had healed and have never returned.

SIDS (SUDDEN INFANT DEATH SYNDROME)

John, an infant, was one week old when his mother found him in his crib one day without any signs of life. He wasn't breathing. She grabbed him and shook him. Her husband called the paramedics. Within three minutes, the paramedics arrived and found his heart had stopped. They used a defibrillator and revived him. John was alive once again, his breathing and heartbeat restored.

He was taken to the hospital and monitored for 48 hours, after which he was sent home with a beeping monitor. Whenever he stopped breathing, the beeper went off. Back home his beeper was going off frequently, at least

An Allergy To My Asthma Medicine

I have been asthmatic for approximately 13 years. I first went on medication in small doses. I didn't realize it at the time, but I wasn't getting as much help as I should have been. After my doctor told me we needed other means of help (ten years of medication, hospitalization and breathing treatments) because I was on maximum medication, I was told about Dr. Devi. After I started treatment with her, I found I was allergic to the very thing that was supposed to be helping me. Since then, I have been treated for asthma medication and now I am experiencing good health and working full-time.

Miriam B.
Fullerton, CA

five to eight times a day. His mother, grandmother and father watched closely for 24 hours. Although he was doing fine at the hospital, he was having breathing stoppages frequently at home. Later on, it was found that he was allergic to the attractive, plastic covering and other plastic accessories on his crib. After he was treated for these items by NAET, he did not have any breathing problems.

PHARMACY

According to the April 15, 1998, issue of *The Journal of the American Medical Association*, side effects from common prescription and over-the-counter medications are the fifth leading cause of death in the United States.

It is estimated that over 40,000 Americans each year have to be hospitalized due to the side effects of these nonsteroidal, anti-inflammatory drugs (NSAIDS): aspirin, acetaminophen (Tylenol, Anacin 3, Excedrin) and Ibuprofen (Advil, Nuprin). Over 6,000 Americans actually die every year from NSAIDS related complications. Side effects happen due to an allergy to the particular drug. In many of these cases, the suggested dose of the pain reliever has caused severe intestinal bleeding. If you take some of these NSAIDS along with alcohol, your chance of internal bleeding increases dramatically. Long term use of NSAIDS can also cause ringing in the ears, digestive problems and loss of motor skills, liver and kidney damage. If you take them before going to bed, you will likely cut your body's production of melatonin, a hormone that helps you sleep.

Many people have allergic reactions to various drugs like antibiotics, analgesics, hormone pills, decongestants, antidepressants, anti-asthmatics, etc. When one drug does not work or gives an allergic reaction, the doctor will prescribe another one until all the drugs are exhausted.

Finally, the patient who hoped to get a magical recovery with the drug will lose patience and trust in the efficacy of the pharmaceuticals and even the doctors. The patient's reaction can be so severe, survival from the episode may be doubtful. If the drug was tested for allergy and effectiveness before it was administered, patients, doctors and pharmacists would not have to go through such trying times. Kinesiological testing for allergies and effectiveness should be taught in the schools of pharmacy, nutrition, western med-

---

Aspirin, Does It Cause Arthritis?

I was asked to take one aspirin a day to keep my blood thin. A week after I started this treatment, I noticed that I was developing joint pains and stomach upsets, which I never had. Dr. Devi traced these new symptoms to the allergy to the aspirin. After the successful treatments for aspirin, my indigestion of 11 months is gone, thanks to Dr. Devi.

Edward Degrass
Costa Mesa, CA

---

icine, chiropractic medicine, dentistry and all other medical schools. Operating room assistants and surgeons should be taught to test for allergies to the surgical materials, transplant materials, organs for transplants, etc., with the patients to make sure they are not allergic to them. When the non-allergic materials are used in a procedure, chances of reactions and rejection of the transplants are minimal, giving more satisfaction not only to the patients and family, but also to the treating doctor.

Many people take an aspirin every day to keep their blood thin in order to prevent heart attacks. If you are allergic to aspirin, it does just the opposite of what it is supposed to do. So, it is very important to test the aspirin and, if you are allergic, treat it with NAET before you take it daily.

Allergy to asthma medication has been found to worsen the condition. Usually doctors try to change medications, to find which one works better, by trial and error. It is not necessary to play that game anymore. Doctors and pharmacists should learn NAET muscle testing to detect allergies before they prescribe or supply the medication. If an allergy to the prescribed medication is found, it can be changed to a non-allergic one before it is supplied to the patient.

Mariah, a schoolteacher in her mid-30's, had frequent severe itching and hives for many years. She said her problems started after taking some penicillin injections a few years ago. She was found to be allergic to penicillin and treated by NAET. Her skin problem diminished dramatically after the penicillin treatment.

Mike 42, developed severe asthma. NTT revealed that he was reacting to a drug that he was taking. The daily aspirin he was taking to keep his circulation healthy was found to be the cause of his asthma. He was treated for aspirin. It took seven treatments to free his allergy to aspirin. When he finished the treatment successfully, his asthma stopped.

RESTLESS LEG SYNDROME

Many people suffer from restless leg syndrome, which is caused by blockages in the spleen and kidney meridians from allergens. Legs feel tingly and uncomfortable in any position. The sufferer keeps moving back and forth or rolls from side to side. Sometimes, legs feel heavy. Cereals, hot dogs, fruit juices with additives, colors, food additives, chemicals, detergents, fabrics, pillows, bed sheets, etc., can cause restless leg syndrome.

Elena, 67, suffered from restless leg syndrome for many years. She heard about NAET and decided to check it out. She was found to be allergic to the furniture in her bedroom: her chest of drawers, side tables, the bed frame and headboard. After she was treated for her furniture, she stopped having restless leg syndrome.

Patty, 38, was allergic to her bed sheets and pillows. Her restless leg syndrome diminished when she was treated for her bed sheets and pillows.

URINARY DISORDERS

Jose, 49-years-old, had urinary problems for seven years. He urinated frequently, especially at night. He couldn't sleep, having to get up at least 10 to 12 times a night. An elementary school teacher, he felt very tired most of the time due to lack of sleep. Urologists examined him many times, prescribing various antibiotics for a possible urinary tract infection and prostatitis. None of the medicines worked for him and his problem persisted. He was desperate and gave up teaching for a while.

When he came to our office, he was absolutely miserable. His history revealed that every morning he had two to three cups of coffee with an artificial sweetener. He always had a couple of tuna sandwiches at night, between 8 and 10 p.m. Further testing confirmed that he was highly allergic to artificial sweeteners. The sweet relish in the tuna sandwiches contained artificial sweeteners, which caused him to urinate frequently throughout the night. After he was treated by NAET for artificial sweeteners, his long-standing problem was solved.

Marianne, 72-years-old, complained of frequent urination for ten years. She was forced to get up at least five to six times each night. She could not get continuous sleep, which made her very tired. She was examined by urologists and given a few antibiotics for possible bladder infections. Nothing worked in her case. She also started waking up with severe headaches in the mornings. She was in an extreme neurotic condition when she was evaluated in our office. The woman was found to be highly allergic to cotton. Using cotton under garments gave her constant bladder irritation and frequent urination, which mimicked a bladder infection. Her nephew had given her a cotton nightdress a year earlier for her birthday. Whenever she slept in that nightshirt, she experienced fainting spells or woke up with migraine headaches. After she was treated for cotton by NAET, she was able to overcome her problems permanently.

SJOGREN'S SYNDROME

Sjogren's syndrome is a chronic autoimmune disorder in which immune cells attack and destroy the glands that produce tears and saliva. The major symptom is dry mouth and dry eyes. It is named after the Swedish ophthalmologist who first described it, Dr. Henrik Sjogren.

Sjogren's syndrome can also cause problems in other parts of the body, including the joints, lungs, muscles, kidneys, nerves, thyroid gland, liver, pancreas, stomach, and brain (see Figure 1). In addition, Sjogren's syndrome may cause skin, nose, and vaginal dryness, and may affect other organs of the body, including the kidneys, blood vessels, and lungs. Blindness is a rare complication of Sjogren's.

The causes of Sjogren's syndrome are not known. But we have been seeing good response just by treating basic allergies, virus, and bacteria in combination with vitamin F and mucous membrane.

VULVODYNIA

A variety of symptoms are associated with what is known as "vulvodynia." Translated from its Greek roots, vulvodynia means "vulvar pain." It has come to refer to a specific type of vulvar pain.

Women with this condition often have generalized vulvar skin pain and discomfort, including pain and/or itching, stinging, parchedness, drying, swelling, and drawing sensations all over the vulvar skin, or only certain parts of it, as well as in the rectal or anal skin.

Hypersensitivity along the edge of the small labia, which makes it difficult to walk, is common. Also, pain or discomfort on touching or pulling pubic hair is common. Some women cannot even wear underwear for these reasons. Often there is itching and stinging in the grooves between the large and small labia. Sometimes the clitoris is painful or hypersensitive, and sometimes pain shoots up the abdomen from the clitoris.

The pain of vulvodynia is characteristically a burning pain that usually occurs primarily in response to pressure or stretching. However, there can also be residual pain, and sometimes the pain is experienced constantly.

Twenty-three-year-old Shana suffered from vulvodynia since she was ten years old. Her parents took her to different doctors, including western medical doctors, a naturopath, and even a shaman, hoping to get some relief of the constant, nagging pain their little girl suffered. Her uncle, a medical practitioner, heard about treating vulvodynia while attending an NAET seminar. The next day, she was flown into our office from another state. She started with the basic treatment. When treated for the NAET sample vitamin C group, she needed repeated treatment to desensitize the vitamin C group. The oxalic acid in the vitamin C group was the culprit in her case. After two years, her vulvodynia is still in emission.

We have treated a few other cases with the same pain syndrome. Another woman was allergic to all her fabrics and suffered from the same type of pain. A few women suffered from childhood emotional traumas that caused vulvodynia. Each individual case should be evaluated separately and their individual needs determined in order to receive satisfactory results.

Vestibulitis is one particular type of vulvar pain. The term refers to pain in the "vestibule," or entrance to the vagina.

Some, but not all, women with vestibulitis experience painful sex (dyspareunia). The pain may be felt only with sexual intercourse, on inserting or tolerating tampons, and/or on sitting. Many women with vulvar pain also have urological symptoms to some degree. They may be as minor as having to get up more frequently during the night. However, frequent cystitis attacks, constant urgency and frequency, and even interstitial cystitis, are common.

Toxic Shock Syndrome

Some Women often react severely to tampons and sanitary napkins, often known as "Toxic Shock Syndrome." Women with this complaint should treat each batch of tampons and sanitary napkins to avoid unexpected health hazards. All these disorders have been traced to various allergies and can be treated successfully with NAET.

HEALTH DISORDERS OF YOUR PETS

Animals can suffer from similar types of disorders as humans. They are part of the family to many. Their health is equally important.

Getting Pregnant through NAET Treatments!

NAET is one treatment that not only eliminates the illness but also determines what really causes it. For me, Dr. Devi Nambudripad definitely opened a whole new world of the real allergy elimination, thereby giving much hope for all generations to come.

I'm Carol Sy. My first encounter with NAET was in 1995 here in the Philippines. After consulting Millet Ting, a trained NAET practitioner here in Manila, I never thought that I would be facing a battle with my problem. All I was concerned about NAET was to determine what was causing my cold allergy and further eradicate it from my system. I also had frequent backaches and dysmenorrhea. It took quite some time for me to understand and take the treatment seriously until the time I realized that I was setting myself free from all my allergies.

(Continued on next page)

In 1997, after 6 years of marriage and failing to get pregnant, my husband and I decided to seek medical help. In this course, we found out that I had endometriosis, that was the reason I failed to get pregnant according to my doctor.

Millet told me she can treat my endometriosis with NAET. We decided that I was to treat my endometriosis with NAET and would undergo laparoscopy to remove the cysts. I had laparoscopy in March of 1998 to speed up the process. Then I continued NAET with combinations of uterus and hormones.

At the same time, I was still consulting my ob-gyne. She performed artificial insemination but it failed. This time, she told me that it was the low sperm count of my husband that became the problem. Frustrated, I decided to stop seeking medical help.

In June 1999, I went to the U.S. and had the chance to meet Dr. Devi Nambudripad in her clinic. She repeated my treatment of hormones and gave me herbs to strengthen my uterus. Confidently, she told me that I could get pregnant after 6 months. I went back to Manila and set aside what Dr. Devi had told me. Determined to get pregnant, we went back to my ob-gyne in November and we already considered I.V.F. (in-vitro fertilization) to be performed in Belgium. I have given up hope to get pregnant the natural way. December came, we started preparing the requirements for the process. All this time I was praying hard that I still wanted to get pregnant the natural way. I thought it would be just another year.

January 2000, my menstruation was delayed. It was the moment I have been waiting for. I was already pregnant! Counting back the months, I realized it was exactly six months after my consultation with Dr. Devi.

I am now a mother to a healthy baby boy. I could say that my life would never have been this happy and fulfilled without NAET. Forever will I be grateful to Dr. Devi for having found the solution and the cure to most unanswered health questions.

My Practitioner: Mila Ting, Pharmacist, MT,
Manila, Philippines

Animals can also have allergic symptoms and diseases: allergy to food, water, chemicals, formaldehyde, carpet, and emotions. They should be treated for the Basic 10 groups, dry foods, wet foods, garlic, insects, drinking water, leash and collar, toys, sleeping mattress, grass, pesticides, other allergens from the environment, fungus, viruses, and emotions to their owners. After eliminating allergy, all animals, like dogs and cats, should be given a clove of garlic daily to keep the pests and fleas away.

Susan and her family were looking for a watch dog and, finding Bat, her children fell in love with him. When they bought him from his previous owners, two-year-old Bat appeared scared all the time. He was startled by any minute sound. His family loved him dearly. Since he was so scared, his owners had to take him with them everywhere they went. He refused to come out of the car and would hide under the car seat. He could not function as a watch dog. One morning he began vomiting. Through MRT, Emily found out that the dog was allergic to water. She brought him in for NAET treatment. She said that Bat vomited a couple of times a week without fail. During the examination through NTT, I discovered that he was reacting to water emotionally. When he was a baby he had been abandoned and rejected. These emotional blockages were affecting him when he drank water. He was treated for those emotional issues using NAET and was sent home.

A week later, Emily brought him for a recheck. "The treatment worked!" She exclaimed. "He is not afraid anymore. He comes out of the car and inspects the environment. He has become a real watch dog.."

So far, NAET is the preferred treatment for allergies and the elimination of most health problems that arise from allergies. This is absolutely a new revolutionary approach.

Until these disorders are fully understood and treatment is made widely available, professionals are encouraged to begin to view their patients in terms of environmental illnesses. They need to recognize the potential for cure that the holistic techniques of kinesiology, chiropractic and acupuncture have to offer.

GLOSSARY OF TERMS

Acetaldehyde: An aldehyde found in cigarette smoke, vehicle exhaust, and smog. It is a metabolic product of Candida albicans and is synthesized from alcohol in the Liver.

Acetylcholine: A neurotransmitter manufactured in the brain, used for memory and control of sensory input and muscular output signals.

Acid: Any compound capable of releasing a hydrogen ion; it will have a pH of less than 7.

Acute: Extremely sharp or severe, as in pain. Can also refer to an illness or reaction that is sudden and intense.

Adaptation: Ability of an organism to integrate new elements into its environment.

Addiction: A dependent state characterized by cravings for a particular substance if that substance is withdrawn.

Additive: A substance added in small amounts to foods to alter the food in some way.

Adrenaline: Trademark for preparations of epinephrine, which is a hormone secreted by the adrenal gland. It is used sublingually and by injection to stop allergic reactions.

Aldehyde: A class of organic compounds obtained by oxidation of alcohol. Formaldehyde and acetaldehyde are members of this class of compounds.

Alkaline: Basic, or any substance that accepts a hydrogen ion; its pH will be greater than 7.

Allergenic: Causing or producing an allergic reaction.

Allergen: Any organic or inorganic substance from one's surroundings or from within the body itself that causes an allergic response in an individual is called an allergen. An allergen can cause an IgE antibody mediated or non-IgE mediated response in a person. Some of the commonly known allergens are: pollens, molds, animal dander, food and drinks, chemicals of a different kind like the ones found in food, water, air, fabrics, cleaning agents, environmental materials, detergent, make-up products etc., body secretions, bacteria, virus, synthetic materials, fumes, and air pollution. Emotional unpleasant thoughts like anger, frustration, etc., can also become allergens and cause allergic reactions in people.

Allergic reaction: Adverse, varied symptoms, unique to each person, resulting from the body's response to exposure to allergens.

Allergic shiners: Dark circles under the eyes, usually indicative of allergies.

Allergy: Attacks by the immune system on harmless or even useful things entering the body. Abnormal responses to substances usually well tolerated by most people.

Amino acid: An organic acid that contains an amino (ammonia-like NH3) chemical group; the building blocks that make up all proteins.

Anaphylactic shock: Also known as anaphylaxis. Usually it happens suddenly when exposed to a highly allergic item; but sometimes, it can also happen as a cumulative reaction. (The first two doses of penicillin may not trigger a severe reaction, but the third or fourth one could produce an anaphylaxis in some people). An anaphylaxis (a life-threatening allergic reaction) is characterized by: an immediate allergic reaction that can cause difficulty in breathing, lightheadedness, fainting, sensation of chills, internal cold, severe heart palpitation or irregular heart beat, pallor, eyes rolling, poor mental clarity, tremors, internal shaking, extreme fear, angio-neurotic edema, throat swelling, drop in blood pressure, nausea, vomiting, diarrhea, swelling anywhere in the body, redness and hives, fever, delirium, unresponsiveness, or sometimes even death.

Antibody: A protein molecule produced in the body by lymphocytes in response to a perceived harmful foreign or abnormal substance (another protein) as a defense mechanism to protect the body.

Antigen: Any substance recognized by the immune system that causes the body to produce antibodies; also refers to a concentrated solution of an allergen.

Antihistamine: A chemical that blocks the reaction of histamine that is released by the mast cells and basophils during an allergic reaction. Any substance that slows oxidation, prevents damage from free radicals and results in oxygen sparing.

Assimilate: To incorporate into a system of the body; to transform nutrients into living tissue.

Autoimmune: A condition resulting when the body makes antibodies against its own tissues or fluid. The immune system attacks the body it inhabits, which causes damage or alteration of cell function.

Basophils: A type of white blood cell that mediates inflammatory reactions. They are functionally similar to mast cells and are found in mucous membranes, skin, and bronchial tubes.

B-cell: A white blood cell. It produces antibodies as directed by the T-cells.

Binder: A substance added to tablets to help hold them together.

Blood brain barrier: A cellular barrier that prevents certain chemicals from passing from the blood to the brain.

Buffer: A substance that minimizes changes in pH (acidity or alkalinity).

Candida albicans: A genus of yeast-like fungi normally found in the body. It can multiply and often cause severe infections, allergic reactions or toxicity.

Candidiasis: An overgrowth of Candida organisms, which are part of the normal flora of the mouth, skin, intestines and vagina.

Carbohydrate, complex: A molecule of sugar linked together, found in whole grains, vegetables, and fruits. This metabolizes into glucose slower than refined carbohydrate.

Carbohydrate, refined: A molecule of sugar that metabolizes quickly into glucose, e.g., white flour, white sugar, and white rice.

Catalyst: A chemical that speeds up a chemical reaction without being consumed or permanently affected in the process.

Cerebral allergy: Mental dysfunction caused by sensitivity to foods, chemicals, environmental substances, or other substances like work materials etc.

Chronic: Of long duration.

Chronic fatigue syndrome: A syndrome of multiple symptoms most commonly associated with fatigue and reduced energy or no energy.

Crohn's disease: An intestinal disorder associated with irritable bowel syndrome, inflammation of the bowels and colitis.

Cumulative reaction: A type of reaction caused by an accumulation of allergens in the body.

Cyclic allergy: A type of allergy which, with abstinence and/or non-exposure, will disappear and will not reappear unless there is overexposure to the substance.

Cytokine: A chemical produced by the T-cells during an infection as our immune system's second line of defense. Examples of cytokines are interleukin 2 and gamma interferon.

Desensitization: The process of building up body tolerance to allergens by the use of extracts of the allergenic substance.

Detoxification: A variety of methods used to reduce toxic materials accumulated in body tissues.

Digestive tract: Includes the salivary glands, mouth, esophagus, stomach, small intestine, portions of the liver, pancreas, and large intestine.

Disorder: A disturbance of regular or normal functions.

Dust: Dust particles from various sources irritate sensitive individuals, causing different respiratory problems like asthma, bronchitis, hay fever-like symptoms, sinusitis, and cough.

Dust mites: Microscopic insects that live in dusty areas, pillows, blankets, bedding, carpets, upholstered furniture, drapes, corners of the houses where people neglect to clean regularly.

Eczema: An inflammatory process of the skin resulting from skin allergies causing dry, itchy, crusty, scaly, weepy, blisters or eruptions on the skin. Skin rash frequently caused by allergy.

Edema: Excess fluid accumulation in tissue spaces. It could be localized or generalized.

Electromagnetic: Refers to emissions and interactions of both electric and magnetic components. Magnetism arising from electric charge in motion. This has a definite amount of energy.

Elimination diet: A diet in which common allergenic foods and those suspected of causing allergic symptoms have been temporarily eliminated.

Endocrine: Refers to ductless glands that manufacture and secrete hormones into the blood stream or extracellular fluids.

Endocrine system: Thyroid, parathyroid, pituitary, hypothalamus, adrenal glands, pineal gland, gonads, the intestinal tract, kidneys, liver, and placenta.

Endogenous: Originating from or due to internal causes.

Environment: A total of circumstances and/or surroundings in which an organism exists. May be a combination of internal or external influences that can affect an individual.

Environmental illness: A complex set of symptoms caused by adverse reactions of the body to external and internal environments.

Enzyme: A substance, usually protein in nature and formed in living cells, which starts or stops biochemical reactions.

Eosinophil: A type of white blood cell. Eosinophil levels may be high in some cases of allergy or parasitic infestation.

Erythrocyte: Red blood cell.

Exocrine: Refers to substance released through ducts that lead to a body compartment or surface.

Exogenous: Originating from or due to external causes.

Extracellular: Situated outside a cell or cells.

Extract: Treatment dilution of an antigen used in immunotherapy, such as food, chemical, or pollen extract.

Fibromyalgia: An immune complex disorder causing general body aches, muscle aches, and general fatigue.

Fight or flight: The activation of the sympathetic branch of the autonomic nervous system, preparing the body to meet a threat or challenge.

Food addiction: A person becomes dependent on a particular allergenic food and must keep eating it regularly in order to prevent withdrawal symptoms.

Food grouping: A grouping of foods according to their botanical or biological characteristics.

Free radical: A substance with unpaired electrons, which is attracted to cell membranes and enzymes where it binds and causes damage.

Gastrointestinal: Relating both to stomach and intestines.

Heparin: A substance released during allergic reaction. Heparin has anti-inflammatory action in the body.

Histamine: A body substance released by mast cells and basophils during allergic reactions, which precipitates allergic symptoms.

Holistic: Refers to the idea that health and wellness depend on a balance between physical (structural) aspects, physiological (chemical, nutritional, functional) aspects, emotional and spiritual aspects of a person.

Homeopathic: Refers to giving minute amounts of remedies that in massive doses would produce effects similar to the condition being treated.

Homeostasis: A state of perfect balance in the organism also called as Yin-Yang balance. The balance of functions and chemical composition within an organism that results from the actions of regulatory systems.

Hormone: A chemical substance that is produced in the body, secreted into body fluids, and is transported to other organs, where it produces a specific effect on metabolism.

Hydrocarbon: A chemical compound that contains only hydrogen and carbon.

Hypersensitivity: An acquired reactivity to an antigen that can result in bodily damage upon subsequent exposure to that particular antigen.

Hyperthyroidism: A condition resulting from over-function of the thyroid gland.

Hypoallergenic: Refers to products formulated to contain the minimum possible allergens: some people with few allergies can tolerate them well. Severely allergic people can still react to these items.

Hypothyroidism: A condition resulting from under-function of the thyroid gland.

IgA: Immunoglobulin A, an antibody found in secretions associated with mucous membranes.

IgD: Immunoglobulin D, an antibody found on the surface of B-cells.

IgE: Immunoglobulin E, an antibody responsible for immediate hypersensitivity and skin reactions.

IgG: Immunoglobulin G, also known as gammaglobulin, the major antibody in the blood that protects against bacteria and viruses.

IgM: Immunoglobulin M, the first antibody to appear during an immune response.

Immune system: The body's defense system, composed of specialized cells, organs, and body fluids. It has the ability to locate, neutralize, metabolize and eliminate unwanted or foreign substances.

Immunocompromised: A person whose immune system has been damaged or stressed and is not functioning properly.

Immunity: Inherited, acquired, or induced state of being, able to resist a particular antigen by producing antibodies to counteract it. A unique mechanism of the organism to protect and maintain its body against adversity of its surroundings.

Inflammation: The reaction of tissues to injury from trauma, infection, or irritating substances. Affected tissue can be hot, reddened, swollen, and tender.

Inhalant: Any airborne substance small enough to be inhaled into the lungs; eg., pollen, dust, mold, animal danders, perfume, smoke, and smell from chemical compounds.

Intolerance: Inability of an organism to utilize a substance.

Intracellular: Situated within a cell or cells.

Intradermal: Method of testing in which a measured amount of antigen is injected between the top layers of the skin.

Ion: An atom that has lost or gained an electron and thus carries an electric charge.

Kinesiology: Science of movement of the muscle.

Latent: Concealed or inactive.

Leukocytes: White blood cells.

Lipids: Fats and oils that are insoluble in water. Oils are liquids in room temperature and fats are solid.

Lymph: A clear, watery, alkaline body fluid found in the lymph vessels and tissue spaces. Contains mostly white blood cells.

Lymphocyte: A type of white blood cell, usually classified as T-or B-cells.

Macrophage: A white blood cell that kills and ingests microorganisms and other body cells.

Masking: Suppression of symptoms due to frequent exposure to a substance to which a person is sensitive.

Mast cells: Large cells containing histamine, found in mucous membranes and skin cells. The histamine in these cells are released during certain allergic reactions.

Mediated: Serving as the vehicle to bring about a phenomenon. For example, an IgE-mediated reaction is one in which IgE changes cause the symptoms and the reaction to proceed.

Membrane: A thin sheet or layer of pliable tissue that lines a cavity, connects two structures, selective barrier.

Metabolism: Complex chemical and electrical processes in living cells by which energy is produced and life is maintained. New material is assimilated for growth, repair, and replacement of tissues. Waste products are excreted.

Migraine: A condition marked by recurrent severe headaches, often on one side of the head, often accompanied by nausea, vomiting, and light aura. These headaches are frequently attributed to food allergy.

Mineral: An inorganic substance. The major minerals in the body are calcium, phosphorus, potassium, sulfur, sodium, chloride, and magnesium.

Monocyte: A type of white blood cell.

Mucous membranes: Moist tissues forming the lining of body cavities that have an external opening, such as the respiratory, digestive, and urinary tracts.

Muscle Response Testing: A testing technique based on kinesiology to test allergies by comparing the strength of a muscle or a group of muscles in the presence and absence of the allergen.

NAET: (Nambudripad's Allergy Elimination Techniques): A technique to eliminate allergies permanently from the body towards the treated allergen. Developed by Dr. Devi S. Nambudripad in 1983 and practiced by over 4,500 medical practitioners worldwide. This technique is completely natural, non-invasive, and drug-free. It has been effectively used in treating all types of allergies and problems arising from allergies. It is taught by Dr. Nambudripad in Buena Park, CA to currently licensed medical practitioners. If you are interested and want to learn more about NAET or attend a seminar, please visit the website: www.naet.com.

Nervous system: A network made up of nerve cells, the brain, and the spinal cord, which regulates and coordinates body activities.

Neurotransmitter: A molecule that transmits electrical and/or chemical messages from nerve cell (neuron) to nerve cell or from nerve cell to muscle, secretory, or organ cells.

Nutrients: Vitamins, minerals, amino acids, fatty acids, and sugar (glucose), which are the raw materials needed by the body to provide energy, effect repairs, and maintain functions.

Organic foods: Foods grown in soil free of chemical fertilizers, and without pesticides, fungicides and herbicides.

Outgasing: The releasing of volatile chemicals that evaporate slowly and constantly from seemingly stable materials such as plastics, synthetic fibers, or building materials.

Overload: The overpowering of the immune system due to massive concurrent exposure or to low level continuous exposure caused by many stresses, including allergens.

Parasite: An organism that depends on another organism (host) for food and shelter, contributing nothing to the survival of the host.

Pathogenic: Capable of causing disease.

Pathology: The scientific study of disease; its cause, processes, structural or functional changes, developments and consequences.

Pathway: The metabolic route used by body systems to facilitate biochemical functions.

Peak flow meter: An inexpensive, valuable tool used in measuring the speed of the air forced out of the lungs and helps to monitor breathing disorders like asthma.

Petrochemical: A chemical derived from petroleum or natural gas.

pH: A scale from 1 to 14 used to measure acidity and alkalinity of solutions. A pH of 1-6 is acidic; a pH of 7 is neutral; a pH of 8-14 is alkaline or basic.

Phenolics: (also known as terpenes). They are seen naturally in plants to give color and fragrance to the leaves, bark, flowers, fruits and saps. They are derivatives of benzene that are made synthetically, also to give flavor and color to foods and to help preserve them.

Postnasal drip: The leakage of nasal fluids and mucus down into the back of the throat.

Precursor: Anything that proceeds another thing or event, such as physiologically inactive substance that is converted into an active substance that is converted into an active enzyme, vitamin, or hormone.

Prostaglandin: A group of unsaturated, modified fatty acids with regulatory functions.

Radiation: The process of emission, transmission, and absorption of any type of waves or particles of energy, such as light, radio, ultraviolet or X-rays.

Receptor: Special protein structures on cells where hormones, neurotransmitters, and enzymes attach to the cell surface.

Respiratory system: The system that begins with the nostrils and extends through the nose to the back of the throat and into the larynx and lungs.

Rotation diet: A diet in which a particular food and other foods in the same "family" are eaten only once every four to seven days.

Sensitivity: An adaptive state in which a person develops a group of adverse symptoms to the environment, either internal or external. Generally refers to non-IgE reactions.

Serotonin: A constituent of blood platelets and other organs that is released during allergic reactions. It also functions as a neurotransmitter in the body.

Sick building syndrome: (Also known as building materials related illness). This term is used when one or more occupants of a building develops similar symptoms related to some indoor pollutants. Many of these symptoms involve reactions to carpets, formaldehyde, pressed woods, paints, fiber glass, tile work, chemical cleansers, leaking gas from plastic and other synthetic materials.

Steroid: A substance of naturally occurring lipid molecules such as hormones, bile acids, precursors for vitamins, and certain natural drugs; in pharmacology, a synthetic compound used to suppress the action of the immune system.

Stress: Anything that places undue strain upon normal body functions. Stress may be internal in origin (disease, malnutrition, allergic reaction), or external (environmental factors).

Sublingual: Under the tongue, method of testing or treatment in which a measured amount of an antigen or extract is administered under the tongue, behind the teeth. Absorption of the substance is rapid in this way.

Supplement: Nutrient material taken in addition to food in order to satisfy extra demands, effect repair, and prevent degeneration of body systems.

Susceptibility: An alternative term used to describe sensitivity.

Symptoms: A recognizable change in a person's physical or mental state, that is different from normal function, sensation, or appearance and may indicate a disorder or disease.

Syndrome: A group of symptoms or signs that, occurring together, produce a pattern typical of a particular disorder.

Synthesis: Combining of separate elements and substances to make a new, coherent whole.

Synthetic: Made in a laboratory; not normally produced in nature, or may be a copy of a substance made in nature.

Systemic: Affecting the entire body.

Target organ: The particular organ or system in an individual that will be affected most often by allergic reactions to varying substances.

T-cell: A white blood cell that instructs B-cells to produce antibodies in an allergic reaction, or immune reaction.

Tolerance: The capacity of the body to withstand repeated exposure without symptoms.

Tolerance threshold: The maximum amount of allergens, stress, and exposures that an individual can tolerate without having symptoms.

Toxicity: A poisonous, irritating, or injurious effect resulting when a person ingests or produces a substance in excess of his or her tolerance threshold.

Toxin: Poisonous, irritating, or injurious substance.

RESOURCES

**Nambudripad Allergy
Research Foundation**
6714 Beach Blvd
Buena Park, CA 90621
(714)523-0800

NAET Seminars
6714 Beach Blvd
Buena Park, CA 90621
(714)523-8900

Delta Publishing Co.
6714 Beach Blvd.
Buena Park, CA 90621
(714)523-0800
E-mail: naet@earthlink.net

Environmentally Safe products

Quantum Wellness Center
Drs. Dave & Steeven Popkin
1261 South Pine Island Rd.
Plantation, FL 33324
954-370-1900
Fax: 954-476-6281
E-mail: buddha327@aol.com

**Cotton Gloves and other Envi-
ronmentally Safe Health Products**

Janice Corporation
198 US Highway 46
Budd Lake, NJ 07828-3001
(800) 526-4237

Herbal Supplements
Kenshin Trading Corporation
1815 West 213th Street, Ste. 180
Torrance, CA 90501
(310) 212 3199

Phenolics
Frances Taylor/Dr. Jacque Krohn
Los Alamos Medical Center,
Ste.136
3917 West Road
Los Alamos, NM 87544
(505) 662 9620

Enzyme Formulations, Inc
6421 Enterprise Lane
Madison, WI 53719

Allergies Life Style & Health
5520 Lake Otis Parkway, Ste.101
Anchorage, AK 99507
(907) 562 2672

Lotus Herbs
1124 N. Hacienda Blvd.
La Puente, CA 91744
(818) 916-1070

American Environmental
Health Foundation
8345 Walnut Hill Circle, Ste. 200
Dallas, TX 75231
(800) 428-2343
(760) 944 1030

Apex Energetics Inc.
1701 E. Edinger Ave, Ste.A-4
Santa Ana, CA 92705

Chiro-Tech, Inc.
628 Calle Plano
Camarillo, CA 93010
(805) 388-7127

BIBLIOGRAPHY

Abehsera, Michel, Ed., *Healing Ourselves,* 1973

Ali, Majid M.D., *The Canary and Chronic Fatigue,* Life Span Press, 1995

American Medical Association Committee on Rating of Mental and Physical Impairments, *Guides to the Evaluation of Permanent Impairment,* N.P., 1971

American Psychiatric Association, *Diagnostic and Statistical Manual of Mental Disorders,* 4th. ed., 2000

Austin, Mary, *Acupuncture Therapy,* 1972

Beeson, Paul B., M.D. and McDermott, Walsh, M.D., Eds., *Textbook of Medicine,* 12th edition, 1967

Bender, David, and Bruno Leone, *The Environment, Opposing Viewpoints,* Greenhaven Press, 1996

Blum, Jeanne Elizabeth, *Woman Heal Thyself,* Charles E. Tuttle Co., 1995

Brodal, A., M.D., *Neurological Anatomy in Relation to Clinical Medicine,* 2nd ed.

Cecil Textbook Of Medicine, 21st ed., 2000

Cerrat, Paul L., *"Does Diet Affect the Immune System?"* RN, Vol. 53, pp. 67-70 (June 1990)

Chaitow, Leon, *The Acupuncture Treatment of Pain,* Thomsons Publishers, 1984

Collins, Douglas, R. M.D., *Illustrated Diagnosis of Systematic Diseases,* 1972

Cousins, Norman, *Head First, The Biology of Hope and the Healing Power of the Human Spirit,* Penguin Books, 1990

Daniels, Lucille, M.A, and Catherine Wothingham, Ph.D., *Muscle Testing Techniques of Manual Examination,* 3rd ed., 1972

Davis, Rowland H., and Weller, Stephen G., *The Gist of Genetics,* Jones and Bartlett Publishers, 1996

East Asian Medical Studies Society, *Fundamentals of Chinese Medicine,* Paraadigm Publications, 1985

Elliot, Frank, A., F.R.C.P., *Clinical Laboratory,* 1959

Fazir, Claude A., M.D., *Parents Guide to Allergy in Children,* Doubleday & Co., 1973

Fratkin, Jake, *Chinese Herbal Pattent Formulas,* Institute of Traditional Medicine, 1986

Fujihara, Ken and Hays, Nancy, *Common Health Complaints,* Oriental Healing Arts Institute, 1982

Fulton, Shaton, *The Allergy Self Help Book,* Rodale Books, 1983

Gabriel, Ingrid, *Herb Identifier and Handbook,* Sterling Publishing Co., 1980

Gach, Michael Reed, *Acuppressure's Potent Points,* Bantam Books, 1990

Goldberg, Burton and Eds. of Alternative Medicine Digest, *Chronic Fatigue and Fibromyalgia & Environmental Illness*, Future Medicine Publishing, 1998

Goldberg, Burton and Eds. of Alternative Medicine Digest, *Definitive Guide to Headaches,* Future Medicine Publishing, 1997

Golos, Natalie, and Frances, *Coping With Your Allergies,* Simon and Schuster

Goodheart, George, J., *Applied Kinesiology,* N.P., 1964

---. *Applied Kinesiology,* 1970 Research Manual, 8th ed. N.P., 1971

---. *Applied Kinesiology,* 1973 Research Manual, 9th ed. N.P., 1973

---. *Applied Kinesiology,* 1974 Research Manual, N.P., 1974

---.*Applied Kinesiology,* Workshop Manual, N.P., 1972

Gray, Henry, F.R.S., *Anatomy of the Human Body,* 27th, 34th, and 38th eds., 1961

Graziano, Joseph, *Footsteps to Better Health,* N.P., 1973

Guyton, Arthur C., *Textbook of Medical Physiology,* 2nd ed., 1961

Haldeman, Scott, *Modern Developments in the Principles and Practice of Chiropractic,* Appleton-Century-Crofts, 1980

Hansel, Tim, *When I Relax I Feel Guilty,* Chariot Victor Publishing, 1979

Harris H. M.D., and Debra Fulghum Bruce, *The Fibromyalglia Handbook,* Holt and Co., 1996

Hepler, Opal, E., Ph.D., M.D., *Manual of Clinical Laboratory Methods,* 4th ed., 1962

Heuns, Him-Che., *Handbook of Chinese Herbs and Formulae,* Vol V., 1985

Hsu, Hong-Yen, Ph.D., *Chinese Herb Medicine and Therapy,* Oriental Healing Arts Institute, 1982

---. *Commonly Used Chinese Herb Formulas with Illustrations,* Oriental Healing Arts Institute, 1982

---. *Natural Healing With Chinese Herbs,* Oriental Healing Arts Institute, 1982

Janeway, Charles A., and Travers, Paul, and Walport, Mark, and Shlomchik, Mark, *Immunobiology,* Garland Publishing, 2001

Kandel, Schwartz, Jessell, *Principles of Neural Science,* McGraw Hill, 4th ed., 2000

Kennington & Church, *Food Values of Portions Commonly Used,* J.B. Lippincott Company, 1998

Kirschmann J.D. with Dunne, L.J., *Nutrition Almanac,* 2nd ed., McGraw Hill Book Co., 1984

Krohn, Jacqueline, M.D., and Taylor, Frances A., M.A. and Larson, Erla Mae, R.N., *Allergy Relief and Prevention*, 2nd. ed, Hartley & Marks, 1996

Krohn, Jacqueline, M.D., and Taylor, Frances A., M.A., *Natural Detoxification,* 2nd. ed, Hartley & Marks, 2000

Lawson-Wood, Denis, F.A.C.A. and Lawson-Wood, Joyce, *The Five Elements of Acupuncture and Chinese Massage,* 2nd ed., 1973

Lyght, Charles E., M.D., and John M. Trapnell, M.D., Eds., *The Merck Manual,* 11th ed., Merck Research Laboratories, 1966

MacKarness, Richard, *The Hazards of Hidden Allergies,* Mc Ilwain

Merkel, Edward K., and John, David T., and Krotoski, Wojciech A., Eds., *Medical Parasitology*, 8th. ed., W.B.Saunders Company, 1999

Milne, Robert, M.D., and More, Blake, and Goldberg, Burton, *An Alternative Medicine Definitive Guide to Headaches,* 1997

Mindell, Earl, *Vitamin Bible,* Warner Books, 1985

Moss, Louis, M.D., *Acupuncture and You,* 1964

Moyers, Bill, *Healing and the Mind,* Doubleday, 1976

Nambudripad, Devi, *Living Pain Free,* Delta Publishing Company, 1997

Nambudripad, Devi, *Say Good-bye to ADD and ADHD,* Delta Publishing Company, 1999

Nambudripad, Devi, *Say Good-bye to Allergy-related Autism,* Delta Publishing Company, 1999

Nambudripad, Devi, *Say Good-bye to Children's Allergies,* Delta Publishing Company, 2000

Nambudripad, Devi, *Say Good-bye to Environmental Allergies,* Delta Publishing Company, 2002

Nambudripad, Devi, *Say Good-bye to Chemical Sensitivities,* Delta Publishing Company, 2002

Nambudripad, Devi, *Survivimg Biohazard Agents,* Delta Publishing Company, 2002

Nambudripad, Devi, *The NAET Guidebook,* Delta Publishing Company, 2001

Northrup, Christiane M.D., *Women's Bodies, Women's Wisdom,* Bantam Books, 1998

Palos, Stephan, *The Chinese Art of Healing,* 1972

Pearson, Durk, and Shaw, Sandy, *The Life Extension Companion,* Warner Books, 1984

Pert, Candace B., Ph.D., *Molecules of Emotion,* Scribner, 1997

Pitchford, Paul, *Healing with Whole Foods,* North Atlantic Books, 1993

Radetsky, Peter, *Allergic to the Twentieth Century,* Boston, Little, Brown and Co., 1997

Randolph, Theron, G., M.D., and Ralph W. Moss, Ph.D., *An Alternative Approach to Allergies,* Lippincott and Conwell, 1980

Rapp, Doris, *Allergy and Your Family,* Sterling Publishing Co., 1980

Rapp, Doris, *Is This Your Child?* Quill, William Morrow, 1991

Shanghai College of Traditional Chinese, *Acupuncture, a Comprehensive Text*

Shealy, C. Norman, M.D., Ph. D. and Caroline Myss, Ph. D., *The Creation of Health,* Stillpoint Publishing, 1993

Shima, Mike, *The Medical I Ching,* Blue Poppy Press, 1992

Sierra, Ralph, U., *Chiropractic Handbook of Applied Neurology,* Mexico, 1956

Somekh, Emile, M.D. *The Complete Guide To Children's Allergies,* Pinnacle Books, Inc. 1979

Smith, CW, Electromagnetic Man: *Health and Hazard in the Electrical Environment*, Martin's Press, 1989, 90, 97

Smith CW, Environmental Medicine: *Electromagnetic Aspects of Biological Cycles,* 1995:9(3):113-118

Smith CW., *Electrical Environmental Influences on the Autonomic Nervous System,* 11th. Intl. Symp. on *"Man and His Environ ment in Health and Disease"*, Dallas, Texas, February 25-28, 1993

Smith CW., *Electromagnetic Fields and the Endocrine System,* 10th. Intl. Symp. on *"Man and His Environment in Health and Disease"*, Dallas Texas, February 27- March 1, 1992

Smith CW., *Basic Bioelectricity: Bioelectricity and Environmental Medicine,* 15th. Intl. Symp., on *"Man and His Environment in Health and Disease"*, Dallas, Texas, February 20-23, 1997. (Audio Tapes from: Professional Audio Recording, 2300 Foothill Blvd. #409, La Verne, CA

Smith, John, H., D.C., *Applied Kinesiology and the Specific Muscle Balancing Technique.*

Sui, Choa Kok, *Pranic Healing*, Samuel Wiser, 1990

Weiss, Jordan, M.D., *Psychoenergetics,* 2nd. ed., Oceanview Publishing, 1995

Zong, Linda, *"Chinese Internal Medicine,"* lectures at SAMRA University, Los Angeles, 1985

Case Histories from the Author's private practice,1984-present

Index